D0950072

The Plant Paradox

THE

Plant
Paradox

THE HIDDEN DANGERS IN "HEALTHY" FOODS THAT CAUSE DISEASE AND WEIGHT GAIN

Steven R. Gundry, MD

with Olivia Bell Buehl

HARPER WAVE
An Imprint of HarperCollinsPublishers

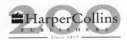

THE PLANT PARADOX. Copyright © 2017 by Steven R. Gundry. All rights reserved. Printed in the United States of America. No part of this book may be used or reproduced in any manner whatsoever without written permission except in the case of brief quotations embodied in critical articles and reviews. For information, address HarperCollins Publishers, 195 Broadway, New York, NY 10007.

HarperCollins books may be purchased for educational, business, or sales promotional use. For information, please email the Special Markets Department at SPsales@harpercollins.com.

FIRST EDITION

Designed by Bonni Leon-Berman

Library of Congress Cataloging-in-Publication Data

Names: Gundry, Steven R., author.
Title: The plant paradox : the hidden dangers in "healthy" foods that cause
    disease and weight gain / Steven R. Gundry, MD, FACS, FACC,
    FCCP, FASA with Olivia Bell Buehl.
Description: First edition. | New York, NY : Harper Wave, 2017. | Includes
    bibliographical references and index.
Identifiers: LCCN 2016052864 (print) | LCCN 2017001993 (ebook) |
    ISBN 9780062427137 (hardcover) | ISBN 9780062427144 (eBook)
Subjects: LCSH: Plant lectins. | Plant toxins. | Plants—Nutrition. | BISAC:
    HEALTH & FITNESS / Nutrition. | HEALTH & FITNESS / Weight Loss. |
    HEALTH & FITNESS / Diseases / Immune System.
Classification: LCC QK898.L42 G86 2017 (print) | LCC QK898.L42 (ebook) |
    DDC 582.13—dc23
LC record available at https://lccn.loc.gov/2016052864

18 19 20 21   LSC   20

To all my patients:
Everything contained in this book I either learned from you or
discovered because of your willingness to join me in this journey.
If people see me, it is because I stand on your very tall shoulders!

Contents

Introduction
It's Not Your Fault

Suppose that in the next few pages I told you that everything you thought you knew about your diet, your health, and your weight is wrong. For decades, I believed those lies as well. I was eating a "healthy" diet (after all, I'm a heart surgeon). I rarely ate fast food; I consumed low-fat dairy and whole grains. (Okay, I will admit to having a penchant for Diet Coke, but that was better than drinking the original sugar-filled brew, right?) Nor was I a slouch in the fitness department. I ran thirty miles a week and worked out at the gym daily. Despite the fact that I was hauling around excess weight, had high blood pressure, migraine headaches, arthritis, high cholesterol, and insulin resistance, I continued to believe that I was doing everything right. (Spoiler: I'm now seventy pounds lighter and no longer have any of these health issues.) But a nagging voice inside my head kept asking the same question: "If I'm doing everything right, why is this happening to me?"

Does this sound eerily familiar?

If you're reading this book, you, too, probably know that something isn't right, but you don't know what. Maybe you simply can't take control of your raging appetite or cravings for certain foods. Low-carb, low-fat, Paleo, low-glycemic, and other diets haven't helped and were unsustainable—or after initial success, the lost weight quickly crept back. Nor has running, speed walking, weight training, aerobics, CrossFit, yoga, core training, spinning, high-intensity interval training, or whichever exercise program(s) you've embarked upon banished those stubborn extra pounds.

Excess weight (or being significantly underweight) is a serious problem, but perhaps your primary concern is food intolerances and cravings, digestive issues, headaches, brain fog, lack of energy, aching joints, morning stiffness, adult acne, or a host of other conditions you just can't shake. Possibly, you suffer from one or more autoimmune diseases or a disorder such as type 1 or type 2 diabetes, metabolic syndrome, or a thyroid or other hormonal condition. Perhaps you have asthma or allergies. You may feel that somehow you're at fault for your poor health or your excess pounds, adding guilt to your heavy load. If it is any comfort, you are not alone.

All that is about to change for you. Welcome to *The Plant Paradox.*

First, repeat after me: "I am not to blame." That's right: your health problems are not your fault.

I have the solution to what ails you, but please prepare to have all your assumptions about what you thought you knew about living a healthy life challenged. This information will dispel myths that are embedded in our culture, and introduce concepts that may initially blow your mind. But here's the really good news. The secrets I'll share with you will reveal what is keeping you sick, tired, depleted of energy, overweight (or underweight), fuzzy headed, or in pain. And once you discover and remove the roadblocks standing in the way of vibrant health and a slim body, your life will change.

You see, with all modesty, I've found there is a common cause for most health problems. It is based on ample research, including my own papers, published in peer-reviewed medical journals, but no one has put it all together before. While health "experts" have pointed to our laziness, our addiction to fast food, our consumption of beverages full of high-fructose corn syrup, and the host of toxins in the environment as causes for our current ailments (among many others), sadly, they are wrong. (Not that these things don't *contribute* to poor health!) The real cause is so well hidden that you would never have noticed it. But I am getting ahead of myself.

Starting in the mid-1960s, we have seen a rampant rise in obesity, type 1 and type 2 diabetes, autoimmune diseases, asthma, allergies and sinus conditions, arthritis, cancer, heart disease, osteoporosis, Parkinson's disease, and dementia. Not coincidentally, in the same period, there have been many seemingly imperceptible changes in our diet and in the personal care products we use. I've discovered a significant part of the answer to the mystery of why our collective health has declined and our collective weight has risen so drastically in just a few decades—and it starts with plant proteins called lectins.

You've probably never heard of lectins, but you are definitely familiar with gluten, which is just one lectin among thousands. Lectins are found in almost all plants, as well as some other foods. In fact, lectins are present in the vast majority of foods in the current American diet, including meat, poultry, and fish. Among their other functions, lectins level the playing field in the war between plants and animals. How so? Long before humans walked the earth, plants protected themselves and their offspring from hungry insects by producing toxins, including lectins, in the plants' seeds and other parts.

It turns out the same plant toxins that can kill or immobilize an insect can also silently destroy your health and insidiously impact your weight. I titled this book *The Plant Paradox* because while many plant foods are good for you—and form the bedrock of my eating plan—others that have been regarded as "health foods" are actually to blame for making you sick and overweight. That's right, most plants actually want to make you ill. Another paradox: small portions of some plants are good for you but large amounts are bad for you.

We'll delve into more detail on all of this shortly.

Have you ever been told, "You're just not yourself today"? As you'll learn, thanks to subtle changes in the foods we eat most often, the way food is prepared, the use of certain personal care products, and the drugs that you assume will improve your health, you really aren't "yourself" anymore. To borrow a term from the computer world, you've been hacked. The entire collection of cells, the inputs and outputs within you, and the way your cells communicate with one another have been altered.

Not to worry. This alteration can be reversed, allowing your body to heal and achieve a healthy weight. To begin the restoration of our collective health, we need to take a step back—actually several steps—in order to move forward. We chose the first wrong fork in the road thousands of years ago and have continued to take additional wrong paths at almost every opportunity. (Just to be clear, the so-called Paleo diet is the furthest thing from what I am talking about.) This book will provide the road map to get back on track, starting with eliminating our overreliance on certain foods as our primary form of sustenance.

What you have just read might seem so unbelievable that you may be wondering about the experience I've had that could have led to such claims, or if I'm even really a doctor. I assure you I am. As a bit of background, after graduating from Yale University with honors, I got my MD from the Medical College of Georgia and then entered the cardiothoracic surgery program at the University of Michigan. I later won a prestigious fellowship in research at the National Institutes of Health. I spent sixteen years as a professor of surgery and pediatrics in cardiothoracic surgery and head of cardiothoracic surgery at Loma Linda University School of Medicine, where I saw tens of thousands of patients with a spectrum of health issues, including cardiovascular disease, cancer, autoimmune conditions, diabetes, and obesity. Then, in a move that stunned my colleagues, I left Loma Linda.

Why would a successful practitioner of conventional medicine leave such an important position at a prestigious medical center? When I turned my own health around and went from obese to slim, something in me had shifted: I realized that I could reverse heart disease with diet instead of surgery. To this end, I established the International Heart and Lung Institute—and within it the Center for Restorative Medicine—in Palm Springs and Santa Barbara, California. I published my first book, *Dr. Gundry's Diet Evolution: Turn Off the Genes That Are Killing You and Your Waistline*, which described the changes my heart, diabetic, obese, and other patients experienced on my diet plan—and which revolutionized my medical practice and changed the lives of hundreds of thousands of readers. It also helped propel me on the path that ultimately led to *this* book.

In addition to being a physician, I'm a medical researcher and inventor of many of the devices used to protect the heart during heart surgery. With my former partner, Leonard Bailey, I performed more infant and pediatric heart transplants than anyone in the world. I hold multiple patents on medical devices and have written extensively on transplant immunology and xenotransplantation. That mouthful of a word refers to fooling the immune system of one species to accept the organ of another species. Thanks to my work with xenotransplantation, I happen to hold the record for the longest-surviving pig-to-baboon heart transplant. So, yes, I know how to fool the immune system—and I know when the immune system is being fooled. I also know how to fix it.

Unlike so many authors and so-called health experts, this isn't my first rodeo. I wrote my senior thesis at Yale University about how food availability at different times of year prompted the evolution of great apes into modern humans. As a heart surgeon, cardiologist, and immunologist, my entire career has been about how the immune system makes decisions about what is its friend and what is its foe. The wealth of these experiences made me uniquely qualified to discover the solution to your health and weight problems introduced in this book.

In my evolving role as a health sleuth, I came to find that many patients who had used my diet to reverse coronary artery disease, hypertension, or diabetes (or a combination of two or three) related that their arthritis also quickly began to subside and their heartburn disappeared. My patients also noted improved mood and resolution of fairly chronic bowel issues. Excess pounds disappeared effortlessly, along with food cravings. As I studied the results of the elaborate lab tests I devised for each patient and experimented with the allowed foods, certain striking patterns emerged, which made me start tinkering with the original dietary program.

Rewarding as these results were, it wasn't enough for me just to see these dramatic improvements in my patients. I needed to know the whats and whys. (Remember, I'm a researcher as well as a physician.) What altered that had made them ill and overweight? Which items on the lists of "good" and "bad" foods that I gave all my patients restored their health? Or, more important, which eliminated foods had been part of the problem? And were factors other than dietary changes also playing a role?

A meticulous review of my patients' histories, physical conditions, specialized lab tests, and tests on the flexibility of blood vessels convinced me that most of them (and most likely you, as well) are literally at war with themselves, thanks to common "disruptors" that interfere with the body's natural ability to heal itself. These

disruptors encompass changes in how food animals are themselves fed, as well as in some foods that are regarded as healthful—
whole grains, lentils, and other beans, for example—plus a host
of chemicals, including herbicides like Roundup, and the use of
broad-spectrum antibiotics. On top of that, I've found that antacids,
aspirin, and other nonsteroidal anti-inflammatory drugs (NSAIDs)
have drastically changed the environment in your gut.

Over the past fifteen years, I have presented my findings at prestigious academic medical conferences such as the American Heart
Association and published them in peer-reviewed medical journals, all the while refining my program.[1] As a result of this work, I
have become an acknowledged expert on the human microbiome,
the bacterial and other organisms that live in you and on you.

As it stands, the Plant Paradox Program consists of a cornucopia
of vegetables, limited amounts of high-quality protein sources, as
well as certain fruits (but only in season), tree nuts, and certain
dairy products and oils. Equally important are the foods I omit,
at least initially—namely, grains and the flours made from them,
pseudo-grains, lentils and other legumes (including all soy products), fruits that we call vegetables (tomatoes, peppers, and their
kin), and refined oils.

You may be in a rush to get started on the Plant Paradox Program
ASAP, but I've found that my patients are far more likely to succeed in healing themselves when they understand the root causes
behind their poor health. So, before we get to the "solution," I'll
spend Part I explaining the often shocking and frequently amazing story of those root causes and how they have affected most of us
over the last several decades. When you get to Part II, you'll learn
how to start the program with a three-day cleanse. Then you'll find
out how to repair your damaged gut and feed your gut microbes the
food they need to thrive, including a group of foods called resistant

starches, which conveniently also help you feel satiated and shed unwanted pounds and inches. Once you've stabilized your health, you'll move on to Phase 3 of the Plant Paradox Program, which becomes your blueprint for longevity. The program includes regular modified fasts to give your gut a mini-vacation from the hard work of digestion. At the same time, it allows the energy-producing mitochondria in your brain and cells a chance to enjoy a well-deserved rest. For those of you with acute health needs, I've provided a chapter on the Plant Paradox Intensive Care Program. In Part III, I'll provide meal plans and simple but delectable recipes for all three phases of the Plant Paradox Program. They'll make you forget those problematic foods that once kept you plump, sick, and in pain.

While modifying your eating habits is a significant component of the program, I'll also recommend other changes, such as eliminating certain over-the-counter drugs and personal care products. Follow the complete program and I promise you will banish most, if not all, of your health problems, achieve a healthy weight, reboot your energy level, and elevate your mood. Once you start experiencing the effects of this new approach to eating and living—my patients start to feel better and lose weight within days—you'll understand the remarkable changes that occur when you feed your body (and your microbiome) foods on which it thrives. As an added reward, you will simultaneously eliminate the disruptive ingredients and other agents that stand in the way of enjoying a long, healthy life.

Turn the page so I can begin to share this life-changing experience with you.

PART I

The Dietary Dilemma

The War Between Plants and Animals

Don't let the title of this chapter worry you. You haven't mistakenly dipped into a botany textbook or parachuted into the set of *Avatar*. You have my assurance that this book will help you learn how to be slim and energized and lay the foundation for vibrant health and longevity. If you wonder why knowing how plants operate could possibly affect you—to say nothing of whether plants possess intention—fasten your seat belt and prepare to be amazed as we take a brief tour through the last 400 million years. Along the way, you'll come to understand that leaves, fruits, grains, and other vegetable foods aren't just sitting there accepting their fate as part of your dinner. They have their own sophisticated ways of defending themselves from plant predators like you, including the use of toxic chemicals.

But first, let me make one thing crystal clear. There is no question that consuming certain plants is essential for good health—and therein lies the paradox. They power your body and provide most of the hundreds of vitamins, minerals, antioxidants, and other nutrients that you need not just to live, but also to thrive. Over the last fifteen years, more than ten thousand of my patients have found that following my Plant Paradox Program results in both weight loss and remarkable reversals of numerous health problems. Meanwhile, people whose digestive issues had made them unable to keep pounds on were finally able to achieve and maintain a healthy weight. Unlike the Paleo diet and other low-carb or even ketogenic diets, all of which stress heavy meat consumption, you'll be dining mostly on certain plant foods, as well as a small amount of wild fish and shellfish and the occasional serving of pastured meat. I also provide vegan and vegetarian variations.

Now here's a shocker to start off your reeducation: the more fruit I removed from an individual's diet, the healthier he or she became and the more his or her cholesterol numbers and markers for kidney function improved. The more I removed vegetables that have lots of seeds, such as cucumbers and squash, the better my patients felt, the more weight they lost, and the more their cholesterol levels improved! (By the way, any so-called vegetable that has seeds, such as a tomato, cucumber, or squash, and even string beans, is botanically a fruit.) Plus, the more shellfish and egg yolks the patients ate, the lower their cholesterol numbers. Yes, that's correct. Eating shellfish and egg yolks dramatically reduces total cholesterol.[1] As I said in the Introduction, forget everything you thought you knew was true.

It's All About Survival

EVERY LIVING THING possesses the drive to survive and pass on its genes to future generations. We consider plants our friends because they feed us, but plants regard all plant predators, including us, as enemies. However, even enemies have their uses. Therein lies the dilemma we plant eaters face: the very foods we need to eat have their own ways of discouraging us from consuming them and their offspring. The result is an ongoing battle between the animal kingdom and the plant kingdom.

But not all plants are created equal. Some of the very vegetables and fruits that sustain us simultaneously contain substances that can harm us. We've been glossing over this paradox for literally ten thousand years. Gluten, of course, is one example of a plant component that is problematic for some people, as the recent gluten-free craze has spotlighted. But glutens are just one example of the kind of protein known as a lectin and one factor in the Plant Paradox, and they may well have sent us off on a wild goose chase, as you'll soon learn. I'll introduce you to the larger world of lectins later in this chapter.

The Plant Paradox Program introduced in this book offers a broader, more nuanced, and more comprehensive look at how plants can sometimes hurt us and also reveals the link among lectins (and other defensive plant chemicals), weight gain, and disease. Humans and other plant eaters are not the only ones with an agenda. Quite simply, plants don't want to be eaten—and who can blame them? Like any living thing, their instinct is to propagate the next generation of their species. To this end, plants have come up with devilishly clever ways to protect themselves and their offspring from predators. Again, let me make it crystal clear that I am not anti-plant. If you have ever had lunch with me, you'll know that I am a devoted plant predator! That said, I will guide you through the confusing garden of plant options to teach you which are your friends, which are your foes, and which can be tamed in one way or another, perhaps with certain preparation methods or by eating them only in season.

In the deadly game of predator versus prey, an adult gazelle can often outrun a hungry lioness, an alert sparrow can take flight when stalked by a domestic cat, and a skunk can let loose a spray of noxious liquid to temporarily blind a fox. The stakes aren't always rigged against the prey. But when the prey is a plant, the poor thing is helpless, right? No way!

Plants appeared on land about 450 million years ago,[2] long before the first insects arrived 90 million years later. Until those plant predators turned up, it must have truly been a Garden of Eden for plants. There was no need to run, hide, or fight. They could grow and thrive in peace, unfettered in their production of the seeds that would become the next generation of their species. But when insects and other animals (and eventually our primate ancestors) arrived, it was game on. These species saw those tasty greens and seeds as dinner. And although plants don't want to be eaten any more than you would, animals would seem to have the advantage, with wings and/or legs to propel them over to that grove of immobile greens to gobble them up.

Not so fast. Plants have actually evolved an awesome array of defensive strategies to protect themselves, or at least their seeds, from animals of all shapes and sizes, including humans. Plants may use a variety of physical deterrents, such as color to blend into their surroundings; an unpleasant texture; sticky stuff such as resins and saps that entangle insects, provide protective cover by making sand or soil clump,[3] or attract grit that makes them unpleasant to eat; or a simple reliance on a hard outer coating, such as a coconut, or spine-tipped leaves, such as an artichoke.

Other defensive strategies are far subtler. Plants are great chemists—and alchemists, for that matter: they can turn sunbeams into matter! They have evolved to use biological warfare to repel predators—poisoning, paralyzing, or disorienting them—or to reduce their own digestibility to stay alive and protect their seeds, enhancing the chances that their species will endure. Both these physical and chemical defensive strategies are remarkably effective at keeping predators at bay, and even sometimes at getting animals to do their bidding.

Because their initial predators were insects, plants developed some lectins that would paralyze any unfortunate bug that tried to dine on them. Obviously, there is a quantum size difference between insects and mammals, but both are subject to the same effects. (If you are suffering from neuropathy, take notice!) Clearly, most of you won't be paralyzed by a plant compound within minutes of eating it, although a single peanut (a lectin) certainly has the potential to kill certain people. But we are not immune to the long-term effects of eating certain plant compounds. Because of the huge number of cells we mammals have, we may not see the damaging results of consuming such compounds for years. And even if this is happening to you, you don't know it yet.

I learned of this connection via hundreds of my patients who respond almost instantly, often in fascinating ways, to these mischievous plant compounds. For this reason, I call these patients my "canaries." Coal miners used to take caged canaries into the mines with them because the birds are especially subject to the lethal effects of carbon monoxide and methane. As long as the canaries sang, the miners felt safe, but if the chirping stopped, it was a clear signal to evacuate the mine posthaste. My "canaries" are more sensitive to certain lectins than the average person, which is actually an advantage in terms of seeking help sooner rather than later. You learn about some of them in the Success Stories throughout the book. (Note that all but a few names are pseudonyms to protect people's privacy.)

SUCCESS STORY

An Unhappy "Canary" Sings Again

Paul G. is thirty-two years old, a computer programmer, and formerly an active outdoorsman. He suffered from POTS syndrome (sudden low blood pressure) and was allergic to almost everything, breaking out regularly in severe hives. He couldn't leave his own house or go to his parents' house without experiencing a powerful reaction. Paul also had dangerously high cortisol and inflammation levels. Because he was allergic to most foods, he was emaciated. After ten months of following the Plant Paradox Program, Paul's POTS syndrome was gone and his cortisol level was normal, as were his markers for inflammation. He now takes no medications and is enjoying camping and other outdoor activities. He is gaining weight and can now visit his parents' home and other places without any allergic reactions.

Plants Are Master Manipulators

A LITTLE BOTANY lesson here: Seeds are actually the plant's "babies," which become the next generation of a plant species. (No, I'm not being sentimental or anthropomorphic. Botanists and other scientists regularly refer to plant seeds as babies.) It's a tough world out there for those potential plants, so a lot more are produced than will ever actually take root. Plant seeds can be divided into two basic types. Some are babies that plants actually want predators to eat. These seeds are encased in a hard coating designed to survive a trip all the way through the predator's GI tract, although a large baby, such as a peach seed, might not be swallowed, and instead simply be left behind. Then there are "naked babies," which lack such a protective coating; the plant does *not* want these to be eaten (more on them shortly).

Fruit trees, which bear seeds enclosed in a hull, are one example of the first type of plant seeds. The mother plant relies on animals to eat the seeds before they fall to the ground. The objective is to have their babies wind up some distance away from the mother plant, so that they don't have to compete with it for sun, moisture, and nutrients. This increases the species' chances of survival while also broadening its range. If the swallowed seed remains intact, it emerges from the animal along with a nice dollop of poop, to boost its chance of sprouting.

Thanks to the protective hull, there is no need for such plants to resort to a chemical defense strategy in the seeds. In fact, quite the opposite! The plant uses several devices to attract the predator's attention, thereby encouraging the predator to eat its offspring. One is color. (For this reason, all animals that eat fruit have color vision.[4]) But the plant doesn't want its babies to be eaten before the protective coating is completely hardened, so it uses the color of unripe fruit (usually green) to convey the message "not yet" to the predator. Just in case the predator can't interpret this signal, the plant often increases the toxin levels in the unripe fruit itself to make it absolutely clear that the time is not right. Before such things as the Granny Smith apple were introduced to this country, youngsters of my generation who ate green apples learned the hard way, via the green apple two-step (diarrhea), not to eat fruit before it was ripe.

So, when is the *right* time for the predator to consume the fruit? Again, the plant uses the color of the fruit to signal to predators that it is ripe, which means that the seed's hull has hardened—and therefore the sugar content is at its height. Incredibly, the plant has chosen to manufacture fructose, instead of glucose, as the sugar in the fruit. Glucose raises insulin levels in primates and humans, which initially raises levels of leptin, a hunger-blocking hormone—but fructose does not. As a result, the predator never receives the normal message that it is full, which would signal it to stop eating. (Would it surprise you that great apes gain weight only during the time of year when fruit is ripe?) That makes for a win-win for predator and prey. The animal obtains more calories, and because it keeps eating more and more fruit and therefore more seeds, the plant has a better chance of distributing more of its babies. Of course, this is no longer a win-win for most modern humans, who don't need the additional calories in *ripe* fruit that were so essential for hunter-gatherers and our ape relatives. And even if we still needed those calories, until the last few decades, most fruit was available only once a year, in the summer. As will soon become clear, year-round availability is making you sick—and overweight!

Timing Is Everything . . . but Looks Can Be Deceiving

So as we've learned, plants use color to communicate the message that their fruit is ready to harvest, meaning the mature seed hull is hard and has the best chance of making it through the predator's digestive tract unscathed. In this case, green means "stop" and red (and orange and yellow) means "go." Red, orange, and yellow signal sweetness and desirability to your brain, a concept that food marketers have long known about and employed. Next time you are in the snack food aisle in the supermarket, check out the packaging and signage and you'll see that both forms of marketing are dominated by these warm colors.

Plants have long taught us to associate red, yellow, and orange colors with ripeness; however, now when you buy fruit in North America in December, it was likely grown in Chile or another country in the Southern Hemisphere, picked slightly unripe, and then given a blast of ethylene oxide when it arrived at its destination. The ethylene oxide exposure changes the color to make the fruit *appear* ripe and ready to eat, but the lectin content remains high because the protective coating of the seed never fully matured and the fruit never got the message from the parent plant to reduce the lectin content. Again, when fruit is allowed to ripen naturally, the parent plant reduces the amount of lectins surrounding the seeds in the fruit and skin and then communicates this information by changing color.

In contrast, gassing artificially changes the color of the fruit, but the lectin protection system remains in effect. Thanks to the high lectin count, eating fruit picked too early is detrimental to your health. That's one reason, in Part II, I recommend that you eat only locally grown produce and only during key times during the year. In Europe, most out-of-season fruit is grown in Israel or North Africa. Because it does not have to travel a long distance over several days, it may be picked ripe and not have to be gassed. It's possible that eating naturally ripened fruit with lower lectin content helps explain why Europeans are generally healthier and slimmer than those of us on the other side of the "pond."

Biological Warfare

IN THE CASE of naked seeds, plants use a divergent strategy. These grasses, vines, and other plants that grow out in the open fields have already chosen a fertile spot in which to grow. They want their babies to fall in place and take root there. That way, after the parent plants die off in the winter, the babies will sprout the following season, replacing the earlier generation. There is no advantage to being carried off, so the plant must discourage insects or other animals from consuming its babies and transporting them elsewhere. Instead of a hard casing, the naked seed contains one or more chemicals that weaken predators, paralyze them, or make them ill, so they won't make the mistake of eating the plant again. These substances include phytates, often referred to as anti-nutrients, which prevent absorption of minerals in the diet; trypsin inhibitors, which keep digestive enzymes from doing their job, interfering with the predator's growth; and lectins, which are designed to disrupt cellular communication by, among other things, causing gaps in the intestinal wall barrier, a condition known as leaky gut. Whole grains actually contain all three of these defensive chemicals in the fibrous hull, husk, and bran. (Teaser alert: This is just one reason that the idea of "whole-grain goodness" is a huge misconception, as you'll learn in chapter 2.)

Still other plant-predator dissuaders include tannins, which impart a bitter taste, and the alkaloids found in the stems and leaves of the nightshade family. You may already know that nightshades, which include such culinary favorites as tomatoes, potatoes, eggplants, and peppers, are highly inflammatory. We'll come back to the nightshade family, which also includes goji berries, as well as to grains and to beans and other legumes, later.

Do Plants Think?

PLOTTING TO HARM us? Concocting chemicals to deter predators? Convincing animals to transport their seeds to other locales to expand their territory? Such strategies suggest that plants are capable of intention, perhaps even of learning. Now you're thinking, come on, surely they can't do that. To be sure, plants don't think in the way you and I conceive of thinking. But any living thing wants to survive and reproduce. In terms of evolutionary strategy, whether you are a "simple" plant or a complex "super" organism like a human being, any compound that can be produced, even if by accident, and ensures more copies of your genes will survive and be propagated gives you an advantage. If you're a plant, any compound that makes your predator think twice about eating your offspring is a good thing from your viewpoint. Think about that the next time you encounter a jalapeño pepper.

Did you know that a plant knows when it is being eaten? Well, as recent research reveals, it does, but it doesn't just sit there and accept its fate. It deploys troops to defend itself, in an effort to stop the predator.[5] In this case, the research subject was a plant called thale cress (*Arabidopsis thaliana*), a member of the cabbage family. Thale cress was the first plant to have its genome sequenced, so researchers have a better understanding of its inner workings than of most other plants. To find out if the plant was aware of being eaten, the scientists re-created the vibrations that a caterpillar makes as it eats the leaves. They also recorded other vibrations that the plant might experience, such as that of wind blowing. Sure enough, the cress responded to the vibrations that mimic a munching caterpillar by upping its production of mildly toxic mustard oils and delivering them to the leaves to deter predators. The plant showed no response to wind or other vibrations.

Another example is the sensitive plant (*Mimosa pudica*), which is deserving of its name. It has learned to protect itself from being disturbed, which includes being eaten, by defensively folding its leaves in response to touch. In fact, the leaf-folding behavior is more pronounced and persistent when it grows in an area where it has been particularly subject to interference than when it grows in an undisturbed area.[6] Whoa! Thinking, reasoning plants! This isn't their first rodeo either.

Plants also respond to circadian rhythms, just as humans and other animals do.[7] In one study, researchers found that the so-called clock gene in plants determines the time of day a plant will produce an insecticide to coincide with the time a predator is likely to be on the prowl. When the researcher removed the clock gene from the plant, it lost its ability to produce the toxin.[8]

Finally, let's focus on the plant chemical you had probably never heard of until you picked up this book: lectins. Yes, you are reading that word correctly. It is lectin, not lecithin (a fatty substance in a plant or animal) or leptin (the appetite-regulating hormone mentioned above). When bugs start eating leaves on one side of a plant, the lectin content doubles almost immediately on the other side,[9] as the plant valiantly struggles to dissuade further consumption. As you'll come to learn, lectins play a key role in the defensive strategies that plants use to protect themselves, and they also play a key role in harming us.

Edible Enemies

SO, WHAT ARE lectins anyway? For the most part, with one important exception, they are large proteins found in plants and animals, and they are a crucial weapon in the arsenal of strategies that plants use to defend themselves in their ongoing battle with animals. Scientists discovered lectins in 1884 as part of their investigation into different blood types. Until now, you have probably been familiar with only one famous—or, rather, infamous—lectin: gluten. There are many more, and soon I'll introduce you to the most important of these—and believe me, you'll want to know them. (Just as a teaser, 94 percent of humans are born with antibodies to the lectin in peanuts.)

How exactly do lectins help plants defend themselves? Well, lectins in the seeds, grains, skins, rinds, and leaves of most plants bind to carbohydrates (sugars), and particularly to complex sugars called polysaccharides, in the predator's body after it consumes the plant. Like smart bombs, lectins target and attach themselves to sugar molecules, primarily on the surface of the cells of other organisms—particularly fungi, insects, and other animals. They also bind to sialic acid, a sugar molecule found in the gut, in the brain, between nerve endings, in joints, and in all bodily fluids, including the blood vessel lining of all creatures. Lectins are sometimes referred to as "sticky proteins" because of this binding process, which means they can interrupt messaging between cells or otherwise cause toxic or inflammatory reactions,[10] as we'll discuss later. For example, when lectins bind to sialic acid, one nerve is unable to communicate its information to another nerve. If you have ever experienced brain fog, thank lectins. Lectins also facilitate the attachment and binding of viruses and bacteria to their intended targets. Believe it or not, some people—those who are more sensitive to lectins—are therefore more subject to viruses and bacterial infections than others. Think about that if you seem to get sick more often than your friends do.

In addition to the potential to cause health problems, lectins can also stimulate weight gain. The reason that wheat became the grain of choice in northern climates is thanks to a uniquely small lectin in wheat, known as wheat germ agglutinin (WGA), which is responsible for wheat's weight-gaining propensity. You read that correctly. Wheat helped your ancestors gain or maintain weight in ancient times when food was often scarce; back then, a "wheat belly" was a great thing to possess! And guess what? That WGA in the "ancient" forms of wheat is just as present in modern wheat— hence the weight gain. We will explore these implications further in the following chapters.

A plant will do just about anything to keep your mouth off its

seeds and save its babies, including sacrificing its leaves. By design, lectins either kill any animal that dares to eat it outright or at
the very least make that animal feel unwell. After all, a weakened
enemy is more vulnerable. Assuming they survive their initial encounter with such a plant, insects and other animals quickly learn
not to eat any plant (or its seeds) that makes them feel bad or fail to
thrive. The animal decides that that plant is not worth eating and
moves on to greener fields and other species, while the plant and
its babies survive. Again, it's a win-win situation and the détente
prevails.

Ancient humans developed a host of ways to deal with lectins.
Unfortunately, modern humans aren't so savvy. Instead, if we eat
something that doesn't agree with us or makes us sick, we find or
invent something—think Nexium, a stomach-acid reducer, or a drug
such as ibuprofen that lessens pain—so we can continue to eat a substance designed to destroy, cause pain in, or at least weaken us.

Speaking of stomach acid, get this: Not only do we keep eating foods that are designed to hurt us, but we also feed them to
animals in the food chain, which suffer similarly from their
diet. Left to their own devices, cows would never consume corn
and soybeans—their natural diet is grasses and other forage—but
that is exactly what they are fed on industrial farms. The lectins
in corn and soy are far more effective than grass in making the
cow heavier and giving them a better ratio of fat. (That same corn
and grain in processed foods bulk you up as well, as you will learn
in chapter 5.) Both soy and corn are laden with lectins foreign to
cows, causing them to develop such severe heartburn and pain
in swallowing that they actually stop eating. Yes, cows develop
heartburn from these lectins, just as you do. To keep their beasts
eating more of this fattening food, farmers dose them with calcium carbonate, the active ingredient in Tums.[11] In fact, half of

the world's production of this compound is added to cattle feed to stop the heartburn, ensuring that cows continue to eat their unnatural diet of corn and soybeans.

You Really Are What You Eat

THE LECTINS IN beans and other legumes, wheat and other grains, and certain other plants are especially problematic for humans. First, not enough time has elapsed to allow our species to develop immunological tolerance to these substances; nor has sufficient time elapsed for the human gut microbiome to become fully capable of breaking down these proteins. Numerous health problems are the result, with gastric distress as just the tip of the iceberg. (If you are impatient to know the range of the resultant potential health problems, turn to pages 68–70, and prepare to be shocked.) Such plants are not the only place in which you'll encounter lectins; they also turn up in animal products. When cows and other animals eat grain- or soy-based feed, both of which are full of lectins, these proteins wind up in the animals' milk or meat. The same thing happens with the meat and eggs of chickens raised on feed full of lectins. Ditto for farm-raised seafood, which dine on soy and corn as well. Until I saw firsthand in many of my "canaries" how removing such foods from their diet was the final key to restored health, I would not have believed this.

In the mid-1980s, a personal experience effectively drove this point home. I had moved my wife and two young daughters to London, where I was a heart surgery fellow at Great Ormond Street, the renowned children's hospital. At that time, chickens in England were fed primarily ground-up fish meal. My girls missed their favorite American food of fried chicken, so as a special treat I took them to the only KFC in town for dinner. No sooner had they bitten into a piece of chicken than they turned up their noses, claiming it was fish, not chicken. I tried to persuade them it was indeed chicken, but in a way, they were right. Because it had been fed fish, the chicken was actually a fish. At that time, I didn't give any thought to the fact that a chicken fed corn or soybeans isn't actually a chicken, but instead a clucking, walking grain or bean.

As the old saying goes, "You are what you eat." But you are also what the thing you ate, ate. When you consume organically raised produce and pastured animal products—and I do *not* mean free-range—the nutrients in the plants and the nutrients the plants got from the soil (as well as the plants the animals ate) pass into your body and are incorporated into every one of your cells. Knowing how the food you eat was grown and raised is not just a lifestyle choice; it also directly affects your health.

There is now conclusive evidence that organically grown vegetables and fruits do contain more vitamins and minerals than conventionally grown produce,[12] but, more important, they contain more polyphenols. (Without getting too technical, these beneficial plant chemicals are found in tea, coffee, fruits and berries, and some vegetables.) The same applies to eating pastured animal foods. But the implications of being what you eat (or what the thing you ate, ate) don't stop there. The lectins in the grain and soy fed to conventionally raised animals end up in the flesh, milk, or eggs of these animals, and ultimately in your gut, where they can still work their damage.

Even organic and so-called free-range animals contain these lectins because they, too, are fed soy and corn, albeit organic versions. (And by the way, it is perfectly legal to keep an animal inside a warehouse its entire life and call it free-range, as long as a door to the outside is open for a mere five minutes a day. Never mind that it is unlikely that any single bird packed cheek by jowl with thousands of other chickens ever manages to work its way to this door.) There is a vast difference in a burger (or milk or cheese) made from a cow that grazed on grass in the summer and ate hay in the winter and a burger made from an animal raised in a stockyard on lectin-rich corn and soy.[13] To start, there's the difference in the ratio of omega-3 to omega-6 fats. With certain exceptions, omega-6 fats are inflammatory and omega-3 fats are anti-inflammatory. Corn and soy contain primarily omega-6 fats, while grass is high in omega-3 fats. But there's more to it than that. Remarkably, those same soybeans and grains make cows much fatter than do the equivalent number of calories in grass.[14] This means that the *source* of calories plays an important role in how you metabolize them. Keep that in mind when we discuss weight gain. And compounding the issue, of course, is that in the United States, almost all soy and corn is also produced from genetically modified seed. We'll delve further into the effects of consuming GMO foods in chapter 4.

SUCCESS STORY

Life After Chicken

Yvonne K., a fifty-year-old Los Angeles woman, had severe lupus with joint pain, fatigue, and rashes, despite taking immune-suppressing drugs and practicing meditation. After a friend suggested she see me, I put her on the Plant Paradox Program. Within a month, the joint pain, fatigue, and most of the rashes had resolved. She stopped her immunosuppressant medications and continued to do well. When I saw Yvonne about four months later, she was ecstatic about what had happened, except for some persistent eczema on her eyelids. She told me she was vigilant about avoiding all bad foods, and we went over the lists of good foods and bad foods with a fine-tooth comb. When we got to the good food list, I asked if she was eating any chicken. She replied that she ate only organic free-range chicken. And that's when we figured it out: she was effectively eating what the chickens had eaten—namely, corn and soybeans. She was an indirect grain and legume eater! We immediately removed chicken from her diet, and sure enough, within two weeks Yvonne's eczema vanished. Three years later, it is still gone, and so is the free-range chicken.

The Balance of Power

SO, WHERE DO humans stand in the war between the plant and animal worlds? Are we just pushovers for the damage that plant lectins and other chemicals can inflict on our poor bodies? Not at all. It's important to understand that although lectins can be toxic or inflammatory and have the ability to mess with your body's internal messaging system, all animals, including humans, have developed their own defensive systems to render lectins harmless or at least mitigate their effects. A four-pronged defense mechanism protects us from the toxic effects of plants, and specifically of lectins.

1. **THE FIRST LINE OF DEFENSE** is the mucus in your nose and saliva in your mouth, collectively called mucopolysaccharides (meaning many sugars). Guess what those sugars are there for? To trap lectins. Remember, lectins like to bind to sugars. The next time your nose runs after eating spicy foods, you'll know

that you've just eaten some lectins. That extra dose of mucus not only traps the lectins you just ate but also adds an additional coating to your esophagus as your meal works its way down.

2.   **THE SECOND LINE OF DEFENSE** is stomach acid, which in many cases does the job of digesting certain lectin proteins, although not all of them.

3.   **THE THIRD LINE OF DEFENSE** is the bacteria in your mouth and gut (part of your microbiome), which have evolved to efficiently consume lectins before they have the opportunity to interact with the wall of your gut. The longer you have been eating particular plant lectins, the longer you have been producing gut bacteria specifically designed to defuse them.[15] That's why if you eliminate all gluten from your diet, the gluten-eating bugs die off; then when you do revert to eating gluten or eat something you don't realize contains gluten, you cannot digest them, causing discomfort.

4.   **THE FOURTH AND FINAL LINE OF DEFENSE** is a layer of mucus produced by certain cells throughout your intestines. Like the mucus in your nose, mouth, throat, and extending all the way to your anus, this layer of gut mucus acts as a barrier. It keeps the plant compounds you have eaten in the gut where they belong, using the sugars in the mucus to trap and absorb lectins. If you're a *Star Wars* or *Star Trek* fan, think of this mucosal layer as an activated force shield!

Taken all together, it's an effective system. Nevertheless, the more troops in the form of lectins thrown at these defenses, the more the sugar molecules in the mucous layer are used up, and the more likely lectins are to get where they really want to go: the living cells that line your gut. This is where the rubber meets the road.

Of course, you do have another powerful weapon to employ in

your battle with lectins—your brain. Once you know that certain foods are problematic, you should avoid them, eat them rarely, or mitigate their effects with the sorts of preparation methods our forebears long knew about, which we'll discuss in good time. You'll also soon learn why the use of drugs that eliminate stomach acid and the adoption of a completely gluten-free diet are ill advised except in that small portion of the population diagnosed with celiac disease. Once you understand more about your gut and the microbes that call it home, you can use your brain to better correct these missteps.

So there you have the human defense strategy—and I'll share with you the specifics of how to fortify your defenses in Part II—but like the setup for an NFL football game, let's now look at the lectin offensive lineup. Plants attack your formidable defense system with their own three-pronged approach, making you feel sick on several fronts.

LECTIN ATTACK STRATEGY #1: Get Through the Gut Wall

The first mission of lectins is to pry apart what are called tight junctions between the cells in the mucosal wall lining your intestine. Believe it or not, the lining of your intestine is only one cell thick, while its surface area is equivalent to the size of a tennis court.[16] Imagine that a wall just a single cell thick is responsible for manning this huge border. Your intestinal cells absorb vitamins, minerals, fats, sugars, and simple proteins, but not large proteins—and lectins are relatively large proteins. If all is well with your gut health and its mucous layers, lectins should not be able to squeeze past the mucosal cells. But if you ever engaged in the old playground game of red rover, think of how the big kids tried to pry your arms apart to break through the line. That's exactly what happens when lectins attack your mucosal wall.[17]

If one or more of the four lines of defense detailed above are breached, lectins can pry apart the tight junctions in the intestinal wall by binding with receptors on certain cells to produce a chemical compound called zonulin. Zonulin opens up the spaces between the cells of the intestinal lining, which enables lectins to access the surrounding tissues, lymph nodes and glands, or bloodstream, where they have no business being. Once there, they act like any foreign protein, prompting your body's immune system to attack them. Think of when you get a splinter under your skin, and how your body's response is to attack the splinter with white blood cells, creating swelling and redness. While you can't see that response to lectins gaining access to off-limits territory in your body, I assure you that invading lectins prompt your immune system to respond in a similar fashion. I routinely see this when I measure inflammatory cytokines, which act like air raid sirens to alert the immune system to an incoming threat.

LECTIN ATTACK STRATEGY #2: Confuse the Immune System with Molecular Mimicry

There are many examples in the animal kingdom of creatures that mimic other species to their own advantage. Some moths mimic spiders to get their spider predators to leave them alone. The harmless scarlet king snake looks remarkably like the deadly coral snake, creating a powerful deterrent to predators. Likewise, plants may mimic birds or insects to keep from being eaten by them. One insect, the well-named walking stick, looks just like a dried twig, helping protect it from predators. Therefore, we shouldn't be surprised to discover that plants purposely make lectins that are virtually indistinguishable from other proteins in your body, a tactic called molecular mimicry.

Lectins are nearly indistinguishable from certain other proteins in your body. By mimicking such proteins, lectins fool the host's immune system, causing it to attack the body's own proteins. Or the lectins bind to cell receptors, acting like a hormone or blocking a hormone, thus disrupting communications within the body and wreaking havoc (see below). I'm sure that on more than one occasion, you have had a passerby hail you down, using someone else's name, only to apologize when he or she realizes it is a case of mistaken identity. Molecular mimicry is similarly a case of inappropriate pattern matching.

Our immune system cells and other cells use "bar-code" scanners called TLRs (toll-like receptors) to identify proteins as friend or foe. These pattern receptors, built over hundreds of millions of years, have been subjected to new patterns in certain foods that unfortunately mimic a whole different set of compounds that instruct cells—particularly, immune and fat cells—what to do. For instance, these compounds instruct fat cells to store fat when they shouldn't be storing fat, or they tell our white blood cells to attack our own bodies in a case of mistaken identity. Some of these compounds are so new that most of our ancestors never encountered them until five hundred years ago. And some, the really bad ones, we've encountered for only the last fifty years! We'll go into greater detail on the insidious effects of molecular mimicry in chapter 2.

LECTIN ATTACK STRATEGY #3: Disrupt Cellular Communication

Some lectins also disrupt transmissions between your cells by mimicking or blocking hormonal signals.[18] Hormones are proteins that fit into actual docking ports on the walls of all cells and release information about what the hormone wants a cell to do. For example, the hormone insulin enables cells to allow glucose to enter and provide fuel. If there is excess glucose, insulin attaches to fat cells and directs them to store the glucose as fat for use when there's less food. Once the hormone releases information, the cell informs the hormone that the message has been received and the hormone backs out of the dock, so the dock is ready for the next hormone. In order to do any of these things, the docking port for insulin has to be open and available. However, lectins can bind to important docking ports on cell walls, either giving wrong information or blocking release of the correct information. For example, the lectin WGA bears a striking resemblance to insulin.[19] It can attach to the insulin docking port as if it were the actual insulin molecule, but unlike the real hormone, it never lets go—with devastating results, including reduced muscle mass, starved brain and nerve cells, and plenty of fat. Ouch!

A Plant-Based Diet

JUST TO REITERATE, I am not anti-vegetable. Far from it! And therein lies the paradox. We may be at war with plants, but they (or at least most of them) contain the vitamins, minerals, and a long list of flavonoids, antioxidants, polyphenols, and other micronutrients essential for our microbiome's health—and, consequently, our health.

The Plant Paradox Program is actually a microbiome- and mitochondria-centric program that recommends a diverse array of the right plant foods at the right time, prepared the right way, in the right amounts. By the time you have finished reading this book, you'll know exactly which plant foods to eat, which to avoid, and how to prepare certain foods to mitigate the impact of lectins.

But you won't subsist on plants alone. The source of most of the animal protein you'll be eating is wild seafood, so I call this program a "vegaquarian" diet. Naturally, as a longtime professor at Loma Linda University School of Medicine, a Seventh-day Adventist vegetarian institution, I also provide an empowering approach for vegetarians and vegans to achieve optimal health.

Half of my patients seek me out because they have failed to show improvement on other famous gut-healing regimens, such as the GAPS diet, the SCD, and the Low FODMAP diet. What my colleagues in gut health don't recognize is that while numerous factors are important in healing leaky gut, you must remove the offending proteins that are forcing the wall of the gut open in the first place. Until you do this, you are merely doing the equivalent of bailing water out of a leaky boat. Unless you fill the holes and stop making new ones, the boat (and you) will continue to sink.

Fortunately, there are ways to outwit the damaging effects of lectins, which I will reveal in the following chapters. Following the three phases of the Plant Paradox Program, you will initially remove the most problematic lectins so that you can heal your gut. Most people can later reintroduce some lectins, properly pretreated, in moderation. Nor is everyone equally sensitive to individual lectins. The longer your ancestors had been eating a certain leaf or other plant part that contains a lectin, the more opportunity your immune system and microbiome had to evolve to tolerate that lectin. At some point, they both evolve to merely shrug their shoulders when confronted with this particular protein.

In the next chapter, we'll delve deeper into the world of lectins to understand how they are leading the charge in the war within your body. We'll also explode the myth of many so-called healthy foods, which, as you'll learn, are actually the hidden cause of heart disease, diabetes, arthritis, obesity, and all autoimmune diseases.

Lectins on the Loose

Now that you've been introduced to the mischievous proteins known as lectins, let's address the obvious questions: If our fore-bears have been eating most of these lectin-containing foods for thousands of years, why are they only now undermining our health? And what, if anything, has changed in recent years to make that the case?

This is where it gets really interesting. Lectins have actually been making trouble for humans for thousands of years. Through trial and error, any animal, including our own species, learned which plants to avoid. But about one hundred thousand years ago, humans made a discovery that catapulted us past all other crea-tures in our war with plants: fire! Cooking partially breaks down many lectins. Plus, it is an easy way to break apart the cell wall of a plant. Previously, only gut bacteria were capable of both feats. This allowed our early ancestors to evolve in a way that dramatically lessened the amount of energy (and surface area of the intestines) required for digestion—a change that made calories more accessi-ble to our energy-demanding brain. While not a perfect solution, cooking also allowed us to utilize the underground starch storage system of plants called tubers—think of sweet potatoes—by break-ing down these previously indigestible plant compounds.

After cooking came about, things were looking pretty good for

Homo sapiens for about ninety thousand years. Plentiful animals and tubers produced tall, robust humans. In fact, up until ten thousand years ago, the average human stood about six feet tall. But when the last Ice Age ended, trouble began. The huge beasts that thrived in the cold rapidly died off, requiring a new resource for calories for mankind. Enter agriculture and the domestication of grains and beans (legumes) in the fertile triangle of the Middle East. Both could be stored and used later, unlike fruit, which needs to be consumed when ripe. The cultivation of grains and legumes was the ultimate double-edged sword of the plant paradox. Entirely new lectins entered our guts for the first time in millions of years, and we were, and still are—excuse the pun—ill prepared. But as you'll soon understand, grains and beans were both the best and worst things that could have happened to our species.

Two Types of Lectins

IN THE LAST chapter, you learned about two kinds of seeds, those with and without hard casings. You also learned about the two divergent defensive strategies plants use—either to deter predators from eating their seeds or conversely to encourage predators to eat and transport them. Not surprisingly, plant predators also fall into two categories. Grazers evolved to consume single-leaf plants (monocotyledons, or monocots, for short), which we tend to think of mostly as grasses or grains. Meanwhile, tree dwellers evolved to consume tree leaves and other two-leaf plants (bicotyledons) and their fruits. The lectins in one-leaf plants are totally different from the lectins in two-leaf plants, so the sets of gut microbes in grazers and tree dwellers also evolved in two distinct paths. Gut microbes in grazers digest the lectins in single-leaf plants, while the tree dwellers have a different set of microbes capable of processing the lectins in two-leaf plants.

We know that the longer you are exposed to a compound, the more you become tolerant of it and don't vigorously react to it. Think of how allergy shots give you a little dose of an allergen until eventually you can handle that food or other substance. But in this case, the time frame necessary for us to come to tolerate certain lectins isn't weeks or months; rather, it is millennia.

The predecessors of cows, sheep, antelope, and other grazers have had millions and millions of years to develop and pass on microbes capable of handling lectins in single-leaf plants. By handling, of course, I mean digesting and eliminating those lectins; and if not eliminating these lectins, then "educating" the immune system not to be overly bothered, since it has been encountering them for millions of years. Mice and rats evolved as grain eaters at least 40 million years ago and have had far longer to become tolerant of these lectins: on the order of four thousand times longer than we humans. Rodents also have hundreds of times more enzymes called proteases in their gut to break down lectins in seeds, which means a rodent's intestinal wall is not under the constant threat that lectins pose to your gut.

We humans certainly aren't grazers, at least in the original use of the term. (We do love to graze on snack foods all day! But I can assure you that the Plant Paradox Program will cure you of that tendency.) Therefore, we are categorized as tree dwellers, or at least the descendants of a long line of tree dwellers that initially were tree shrews. I know. That may seem hard to believe, but it was at least 40 million years ago. And over that time, the microbes that now call your body home and can handle the lectins of two-leaf plants were passed down from generation to generation.[1]

✴

Four Cataclysmic Changes in the Human Diet

OUR GUT BACTERIA play an important role in "educating" our immune system as to which compounds should be accepted as relatively harmless and allowed in, and which are cause for concern and should be barred from entry.[2] This "border patrol" known as our immune system has been built over 80 million years, beginning long before *Homo sapiens* emerged. But only relatively recently have we (and our microbes) been subjected to new patterns in certain foods. Unfortunately, compounds in these foods mimic a whole different set of compounds that tell our cells, particularly immune and fat cells, what to do.

The four major disruptions in human eating patterns outlined below have upset the sophisticated balance of power between plants and humans, which allowed both of us to coexist and thrive for millennia. Each of these disruptions has forced us to accommodate (or not) a changing diet. And it's only recently that we have uncovered the role that lectins play in this disruption. The epidemics of obesity, type 2 diabetes, and other health problems provide proof positive that we are now losing this war. To understand why this is happening now and what we can do about it, let's take a short trip back to mankind's ancient origins.

CHANGE #1: The Agricultural Revolution

The advent of the agricultural revolution about ten thousand years ago meant that a totally new source of food—grain and beans—became the dietary staple of most cultures relatively quickly. At that point, the human diet shifted from primarily leaves, tubers, and some animal fat and protein to primarily grains and beans. Until then, the human microbiome had never encountered lectins in grasses (grains) or legumes, and therefore the human gut bacteria, microbes, and immune system had zero experience handling them.

Fast-forward five thousand years or so. Thanks to its granaries full of wheat, ancient Egypt was able to feed its people, including the slaves who built its pyramids, enabling its rise to a great kingdom. However, analysis of thousands of Egyptian mummified remains has revealed the health status of those wheat eaters, and it wasn't good. They died overweight, with clogged arteries. Their teeth were also decayed from a diet high in grains, which are full of simple sugars, and worn down to the gums from grinding the grains.[3] The mummified remains of Queen Nefertiti suggest that she most likely had diabetes. The legendary queen was not the only one with problems related to her grain-heavy diet. In fact, oatmeal has been associated with dental problems even in modern times. In 1932, researchers found that putting young children with dental cavities and malformed teeth on a diet free of oatmeal but fortified with vitamin D and cod liver oil for a period of six months resulted in almost complete elimination of both new cavities and regression in the growth of existing ones.[4] These results were dramatically better than previous efforts using only vitamin D supplementation but that allowed the children to continue to consume oatmeal.

To varying degrees, we can see that the lectins in oats and other grains, legumes, and certain other plants have always been toxic—but given the choice between starvation and some serious health trade-offs, humans will always opt for survival. Our ancestors did come up with ways to minimize the effects of lectins once the agricultural revolution brought them to our plates, using fermentation and various other ingenious preparation techniques. And clearly, without grains and beans, civilization as we know it would not have occurred.

CHANGE #2: A Mutation in Cows

About two thousand years ago, a spontaneous mutation in Northern European cows caused them to make the protein casein A-1 in their milk instead of the normal casein A-2. During digestion, casein A-1 is turned into a lectinlike protein called beta-casomorphin. This protein attaches to the pancreas's insulin-producing cells, known as beta cells, which prompts an immune attack on the pancreas of people who consume milk from these cows or cheeses made from it.[5] This is likely a primary cause of type 1 diabetes.[6] Southern European cows, goats, and sheep continue to produce casein A-2 milk, but because casein A-1 cows are hardier and produce more milk, farmers prefer them. The most common breed of cows worldwide is the Holstein, whose milk contains this problematic lectinlike protein. If you think that drinking milk gives you a problem, it's almost certainly the cow's breed that is at fault, not milk per se. The black and white Holstein is the classic example of the A-1 cow, while the Guernsey, Brown Swiss, and Belgian Blues are all casein A-2. That's why I recommend that if you consume dairy, you opt for only casein A-2 dairy products, which grocery stores have recently started selling, particularly on the West Coast. Alternatively, use goat or sheep milk products to be safe.

SUCCESS STORY

It's the Breed of Cow!

Allison M., a longtime sufferer of rheumatoid arthritis, came to me for help. In her fifties, she had decided that spending the rest of her life on immune-suppressing drugs, which might promote cancer, was too much to deal with. Instead, she stopped the drugs and started the Plant Paradox Program. She began to thrive, and her pain disappeared—and with it the inflammatory markers. But it was the call I got from the Napa Valley that makes this success story so poignant. It seems that Allison was visiting a girlfriend who offered her some yogurt from grass-fed cows on a nearby farm, knowing that she was on this "crazy Gundry diet." My patient declined, saying that it wasn't the right breed of cow, which made her friend belittle the diet, saying that was ridiculous. As if the breed of cow made a difference! Allison laughed and agreed that it *was* silly, and that surely a little bit couldn't hurt. So to be polite, she ate a couple of tablespoons of yogurt. That night she awoke with three finger joints in her left hand swollen and bright red. She called me, not in panic, but in delight! It *was* the breed of cow, after all. She told me that never had anything that hurt so badly felt so good, because now she knew that she had the secret formula for lifelong good health.

CHANGE #3: Plants from the New World

It would seem that we should have become pretty tolerant of these new lectins over the past ten thousand years, but let's take one more trip back in time. Five centuries ago, the last of the major changes in lectin exposure—and perhaps the biggest disruption of all—occurred when Europeans reached the Americas. The explorers brought New World foods back to their native countries, and the Columbian Exchange, named after Christopher Columbus, exposed the rest of the world to a whole array of new lectins. They include the nightshade family, most of the bean family (legumes, including peanuts and cashews), grains, pseudo-grains such as amaranth and quinoa, the squash family (pumpkins, acorn squash, zucchini), and chia and certain other seeds. All are foods that until then no European, Asian, or African had ever seen, much less eaten. Half of the foods you have been told to eat for good health are actually New World plants that most of mankind had no prior exposure to, meaning your body, your gut bacteria, and your immune system are ill prepared to tolerate them. Getting to know a new lectin in five hundred years is equivalent to speed dating in evolution!

CHANGE #4: Contemporary Innovations

In the last five decades we have faced yet another unleashing of lectins in processed foods and most recently in genetically modified organisms (GMOs), including soybeans, corn, tomatoes, and rapeseed (canola). Our bodies have never before encountered any of these lectins. Moreover, with the introduction of broad-spectrum antibiotics, other drugs, and a vast array of chemicals, we have totally destroyed the gut bacteria that would have normally given us a chance to process these lectins and educate our immune system about them. We'll discuss these deadly disruptors further in chapter 4.

All four of these factors have profoundly disrupted normal messaging within our bodies. There is no way we (and our microbiome) can adapt to deal with these onslaughts of lectins in such a short time span. (Just think about those poor cows that had never encountered corn and soy lectins until about sixty years ago and are treated with Tums in order to get them to eat their weight-promoting new food.) This is particularly true if we make a practice of killing most of our microbiome daily by ingesting certain medications, including antibiotics, and other substances such as artificial sweeteners. It's akin to expecting one of the first personal computers developed in the 1970s, with perhaps 250 bytes of memory, to allow you to stream videos, check your Facebook page, pay bills, reserve airline tickets, order groceries, and perform countless other functions now possible on even the most basic modern-day computers.

Why Now?

IF ONLY ONE of these four factors is based on modern-day changes, why are we suddenly so much more sensitive to lectins today? The answer to that question is nuanced. As we discussed in the contemporary innovations section above, several recent changes have impacted how we respond to lectins. The pace of these shifts is approaching warp speed, outpacing our ability—and that of our microbiome—to adapt in a comparable time frame.

In the last half century, we have abandoned many of the tried-and-true ways of eating and preparing foods, opting instead for fast food, processed food, ultraprocessed food, microwave meals, and on and on. The makeup of our diet has also changed significantly. Corn, soy, and wheat, all packed with lectins, are in most processed foods. The lectin load on humans is higher than ever before, but there's much more to the story. In this same five-decade time span, an onslaught of herbicides, biocides, drugs, fertilizers, food additives, skin-care products, and a host of other chemicals has also disrupted your internal messaging system, your gut, and the microbes in your gut. That chemical overload has compromised your ability to deal with grains, legumes, and other lectin-bearing plants.

As I alerted you in the Introduction, much of what I will be telling you can initially be difficult to accept. It may make you question the very concept of who you are. It will challenge your notions of what causes health and disease. It will upend your concepts of what constitutes healthy foods, good foods, bad foods, and even organic foods—and it will certainly make you question the U.S. Dietary Guidelines. At the most basic level, I want you to understand why you cannot ignore the past in order to enjoy a long, healthy future.

Our present-day food supply looks very different from the one that sustained people for generations.

Consider this: In just the last fifty years, the following significant changes have taken place:

- We now eat far more wheat, corn, and other grains, as well as soybeans, in the form of processed foods, which have displaced unprocessed carbohydrates, including leafy greens and other vegetables.[7]
- More than 43 percent of the average household food budget is spent outside the home, up from just under 26 percent in 1970.[8]
- Instead of home-cooked meals, we increasingly rely on prepared foods to pop in the microwave, ultraprocessed foods full of questionable ingredients, and take-out meals.
- We have forgotten (or ignored) tried-and-true ways to neutralize the negative effects of consuming certain lectin-containing foods.
- Many once-familiar plants are now grown using petrochemical fertilizers and modified to be more pest resistant, ripen sooner, minimize or eliminate bruising or denting, and to make other changes that increase production and facilitate moving produce long distances.
- Even our healthy vegetables are not being raised with the eons-old help of soil bacteria, which have been wiped out by modern farming techniques and biocides. Levels of zinc and magne-

sium, key elements that prevent diabetes and metabolic syndrome, in the soil have also dropped significantly.[9]
- Although we don't necessarily connect them to obesity and other
health problems, nonfood products such as over-the-counter
and prescribed drugs, room fresheners, hand sanitizers, and
countless other disruptors are not just a problem in their own
right but also compound the negative effects of eating lectins.

What Is Healthy Food?

AS YOUR HEALTH is so dependent on your diet, it all depends upon
your choice of foods and their relative amounts, as well as the
preparation techniques you use. But ironically, most of my patients
with disease conditions were already eating "healthy"! Or at least
so they thought.

In my original diet plan for my patients, I banished white foods
such as flour, sugar, potatoes, and milk, and limited brown foods
such as certain whole grains and legumes. But when I subsequently
removed *all* grains and all pseudo-grains (quinoa, buckwheat,
and the like) along with all legumes, including tofu, edamame,
and other soy products, my patients experienced even greater improvements. It seemed that the more supposedly healthy foods
that I eliminated, the more their health improved. Their cancers
regressed or disappeared—yes, you read that right—as did their
type 2 diabetes, coronary artery disease, fibromyalgia, and autoimmune diseases. How could that be? After all, we've been eating
these healthy foods for thousands of years. Or have we?

Many foods, including those that contain lectins, have both
good and bad properties. Additionally, individuals have different
tolerances for lectins, depending upon the state of their health. But

to a large extent, your individual health depends on the health of your gut lining, your microbiome, and its instructions to your immune system. And it's become clear to me that lectins are leading the charge in the war within your body.

Even when organically raised, certain lectin-heavy foods are the cause of so-called autoimmune diseases, while lectin avoidance in my patients and as reported in scientific literature has been found to cure autoimmune diseases.[10] These claims may seem outrageous, but the evidence walks in and out of my waiting room every day. In one study, twenty women with rheumatoid arthritis (RA) were put on a water fast, during which the RA disappeared in all twenty—and when they were put on a vegan diet following that, half remained in remission, meaning that their gut had healed. But the RA recurred in the other 50 percent of the patients on the vegan diet.[11] In fact, my studies have shown that eating "healthy" lectin-rich foods causes RA. We need to reframe our definition of what defines healthy, which should include limiting the intake of lectin-rich foods.

SUCCESS STORY

Hoping for a Second Child

Beautiful and full of life, twenty-seven-year-old Suzanna K. and her husband were seeking my help. Shortly after delivering her first child, Suzanna had developed devastating rheumatoid arthritis. She was placed on steroids and an immunosuppressant drug, but she still had extremely swollen joints. Any movement was painful, making it impossible to hold her child. Moreover, she and her husband desperately wanted another baby, but they knew that being on these drugs made it too dangerous for Suzanna to contemplate another pregnancy.

Suzanna was ready to try anything. Her blood work showed that even on these powerful drugs, her immune system was nonetheless in full attack mode. Her tests also showed the marker for lectin sensitivity. So we instituted the Plant Paradox Program and stopped her medications. It was tough going at first. We used natural anti-inflammatory compounds such as boswellia extract and high-dose fish oil and vitamin D_3. With each passing week, her pain began to subside and her inflammation markers slowly descended, approaching normal. She could now play with her son without pain, and lift or hold him without wincing. About a year into her program, I met with her again, along with her husband and mother, who had both joined the program to help her stick with it. I told her that her markers had improved to the point where I thought she could try to get pregnant. Her face lit up mischievously. "I knew you would say that," she declared, "so I jumped the gun. I just got the test back, and I'm four weeks pregnant!"

Suzanna recently gave birth to a normal baby girl, and unlike the first go-round, her rheumatoid arthritis hasn't flared seven months postpartum.

And how about her husband and mother? Despite being a fitness nut, her husband had been plagued by chronic sinus issues, which have disappeared since he started the program. Why might that be? Lectins are the cause of sinus issues, because excessive mucous production is the first line of defense to entrap the lectins we consume. Next time your nose runs after you eat spicy salsa, remember this. And Mom? Her diabetes, high cholesterol, and arthritis are gone, she's off all of her medications, and she's thirty pounds lighter—just by helping her daughter change her diet. The issues faced by these three people might seem disparate, but they were all united by lectin sensitivity—and they all found success upon removing lectins from their diet.

Getting to the Bottom of Gluten Sensitivity

AS YOU NOW know, gluten, the protein found in wheat, barley, rye, and often in oats, is just one form of lectin, and the one that has received the lion's share of attention in recent years. Consumption of any or all four of these "healthy foods" can trigger celiac disease, a life-threatening gut condition. Other people display sensitivity to gluten in an array of symptoms, including brain fog, joint pain, and inflammation.

All gluten foods contain lectins, although not all lectin foods contain the particular plant proteins known as glutens. What's perhaps worse is that almost all grains and pseudo-grains contain glutenlike lectins. And there are thousands of other lectins—unfortunately, the standard American diet, aptly abbreviated to SAD, is bursting with them. Moreover, many other lectins are more detrimental than gluten. So-called gluten-free products are actually full of lectins in the form of flours made from corn, oats, buckwheat, quinoa, and other grains and pseudo-grains, as well as soybeans and other legumes. That explains why so many people whom I see in my practice who have eliminated barley, rye, oats, and wheat (BROW) continue to have digestive and other health problems, including being overweight or underweight, particularly if they eat "'gluten-free" (but not lectin-free) products.[12] In fact, weight gain is a frequent result of going (supposedly) gluten-free. Another issue can arise from going gluten-free as well: we all typically have bacteria that eat gluten, but if you omit all gluten from your diet, the food supply disappears, and the gluten-digesting bugs depart. Then if you are exposed to gluten at a later date, as you almost certainly will be, gluten will create problems for you.[13]

The Gluten-Free Myth

Clarence V. cured himself of type 2 diabetes with my dietary changes. However, when I later diagnosed him with celiac disease, he began eating gluten-free breads and cookies, which are sugar bombs. Not surprisingly, he once again became a rip-roaring diabetic. Once he understood what had happened, he stopped eating those products and was able to keep both diseases at bay. But his story doesn't end there. Clarence's diabetes had resulted in a very low testosterone level. He had assured his wife, who was forty-two, that he was infertile, so they no longer bothered with birth control. But when he cured himself of diabetes by cutting down on sugar and animal protein, his testosterone level rose, and lo and behold, his wife became pregnant. This was not a pleasant surprise for a couple whose other children were heading off to college. Fortunately, they are now happy with their surprise addition to the family—and with Clarence's improved health.

Grains and Weight Gain

THINK GLUTEN AND your first association is likely to be wheat. Although barley, rye, and sometimes oats also contain gluten, no grain is nearly as omnipresent in the American diet as wheat. As I mentioned earlier, the weight-promoting properties of wheat prompted us to choose wheat over other less "weighty" grains ten thousand years ago. Although wheat may be our favorite grain, it is not your friend, regardless of whether or not you have been diagnosed with celiac disease or nonceliac sensitivity to wheat.

Wheat is addictive, acting like an opiate in your brain. Like most people, you tolerate its ill effects because you are addicted to it. In addition to its addictive properties, wheat presents another huge problem for us—it actively promotes weight gain. You will learn how this happens in chapter 5, but meanwhile, consider this: to fatten a steer or other animal for slaughter, the farmer feeds it grains (and soybeans and other legumes), along with low-dose antibiotics. Grains with a side of antibiotics have the same effect on humans, plumping us up and playing a major role in accounting for our horrifying health statistics. According to the Centers for Disease Control, 70.7 percent of American adults are overweight, and of those almost 38 percent are obese.[14] Twenty years ago, less than 20 percent were obese. Sadly, being overweight is the new normal, and lectins play a large role in this obesity crisis.

And remember, our wheat intake doesn't just come from the grains we eat directly. Since we feed animals that wind up on our dinner table both grains and beans *and* antibiotics, that toxic stew also winds up in us, creating the perfect storm. And the storm becomes even more dangerous when we overuse broad-spectrum antibiotics ourselves.

The Most Dangerous but Avoidable Lectin in Wheat? It's Not Gluten

GLUTEN HAS BEEN the bad boy in the nutrition world for the last few years, escalating the interest in low-carb diets advocated by Dr. Robert Atkins and Dr. Arthur Agatston (creator of the South Beach Diet). Dr. William Davis, author of *Wheat Belly,* and Dr. David Perlmutter, author of *Grain Brain,* continue to eschew grains and have brought wheat addiction to the fore in their books, but both focused on the gluten in wheat. In actuality, gluten is just a small piece of the puzzle.

You've already met a stealth villain lurking in wheat: wheat germ agglutinin (WGA). Just to be clear, WGA is not associated with gluten; rather, it is found in bran. This means that white bread contains gluten but not WGA, while whole wheat bread contains the double whammy!

Wheat germ agglutinin is an especially small protein compared with most other lectins, which are relatively large. So even if the gut mucosal barrier has not been compromised, WGA can pass through the walls of the intestine more easily than other lectins can. But this is just one of many ill effects caused by consuming WGA. It also:

1. Behaves like insulin, disrupting normal endocrine function by pumping sugar into fat cells, where the sugar soon turns to fat, resulting in weight gain and the development of insulin resistance.
2. Blocks sugar from getting into muscle cells, creating still more body fat, and starving muscles of nourishment.
3. Interferes with the digestion of protein.
4. Promotes inflammation by releasing free radicals, which can thin the mucosal lining of the gut.
5. Cross-reacts with other proteins, creating antibodies that can induce autoimmune responses. These antibodies are distinct from those formed by a reaction to gluten.
6. Crosses the blood-brain barrier, taking with it other substances to which it has bonded, and causing neurological problems.
7. Kills cells, without distinguishing between normal and cancerous cells.
8. Interferes with the replication of DNA.
9. Causes atherosclerosis, the hardening of arteries from a

buildup of plaque (which is never mentioned in conventional medicine).

10. Enables entry of influenza and other disease-causing viruses into the body from the gut by bonding to the sialic acid in the mucosal lining.

11. Contributes to the development of nephritis, or kidney inflammation.[15]

So how do you avoid WGA? Simply steer clear of whole-grain bread and other whole-grain products.

The Whole Story on Whole Grains

ALTHOUGH WHOLE GRAINS have been considered health foods only for the past few decades, it's worth recalling that a few thousand years ago, once grinding technology made it possible to remove the fibrous parts of wheat and other grains, the privileged classes opted to eat "white" bread. They relegated whole grains such as brown rice and brown bread made with whole grains to peasants. The goal was to refine grains so they were easier on the gut, as well as to make bread whiter. Of course, the rich didn't know it at the time, but whole grains are considerably higher in lectin content than grains that have been stripped of their fiber, which explains why they were easier on their tummies. Greeks and Romans even debated over which country had the whitest wheat. FYI, Egypt won that contest.

Today, everyone "knows" that brown rice is healthier than white rice, yet the four billion people who use rice as their staple grain in Asia have always stripped the hull off brown rice to make it white before they eat it. Stupid? No, very intelligent; the hull has the lectins and these cultures have been removing it for thousands of years. Although I once believed that any white grain was inferior to any brown (whole) grain, I have since changed my stance. Traditionally, the Chinese, Japanese, and other Asian people have not been plagued with obesity, heart disease, diabetes, and other conditions that are so common in the United States.[16] I will go so far as to say that if you're overweight, there's a good chance that it's because you're a believer in the myth of "whole-grain goodness." Distressingly, the renaissance of whole-grain products has reintroduced WGA and a host of other lectins back into our diet.

This current obsession with "whole-grain goodness" is totally counter to what our forebears had been trying to do with grains, but it is not the first time this fad has surfaced. Back in 1894, Dr. John Kellogg, a physician and superintendent of a sanatorium, was unsuccessful in his efforts to get his patients to eat whole grains. (He was obsessed with "regularity," which he saw as the key to good health.) When his patients refused to eat them, he and his brother, Will Keith Kellogg, came up with a way to disguise whole grains, in this case corn, in what became Kellogg's cornflakes. And so started a change in what constituted a "healthy" breakfast, namely cold cereal, and the genesis of a billion-dollar industry. That industry soon moved on to wheat as the "perfect" breakfast cereal, reintroducing WGA and a host of other lectins into our diet. Just so you realize how recent a phenomenon cold cereal is in human diets, no European or Asian had ever eaten it until 1945 when American troops stationed abroad introduced it after World War II. I have many patients who emigrated from Eastern Europe or the Middle East and had never eaten cereal until the 1960s or '70s.

But the wider interest in whole grains took root only in the last fifty years among hippies, food faddists, and some nutritionists. Now the whole-grain movement has gone mainstream, with breakfast cereals, bread, and other baked goods touted as health foods and often marketed with seductive words such as "whole-grain goodness." However, this trend has actually wrought damage on our collective gut and opened the door to other health problems. The increased consumption of both whole-grain foods and processed foods translates into a double whammy of lectin exposure.

You may have heard of the French paradox, which refers to the fact that the French are able to eat baguettes (made with white flour), drink red wine, and enjoy butter without gaining weight or suffering the ill health effects, specifically heart disease, that plague Americans. In her book *French Women Don't Get Fat*, published a decade ago, author Mireille Guiliano, who was born and raised in France and now lives in the United States, brought the French paradox to our shores, revealing how she enjoyed all these supposedly unhealthy foods while maintaining her trim figure and good health for decades. And the French paradox doesn't apply just to the fairer sex. Middle-aged French men experience roughly half the rate of heart disease that American men do and live an average of two and a half years longer.[17] But the real reason that both French men and women are more likely to keep their shape and have fewer heart problems than Americans is that they are not consuming WGA. It's also why Italians eating their own version of white bread and only small portions of pasta made with white flour—in Italy, pasta is a first course, not the main dish Americans make of it—don't get fat, or at least not as fat as Americans. I travel extensively in Italy, studying their food and culture, and the sad news is that they too have been influenced by the American trend: whole wheat pasta is beginning to appear on menus in cities frequented by tourists.

Skip Both Wheat *and* Glucosamine

The lectin WGA has a particular affinity for attaching to joint cartilage and stimulating our immune system to attack our joints. Both the inflammation and resulting pain can be temporarily alleviated with an over-the-counter nonsteroidal anti-inflammatory drug (NSAID) such as aspirin (Bufferin, Anacin, or Ecotrin), ibuprofen (Motrin or Advil), naproxen (Aleve, Anaprox, Naprelan, and Naprosyn), or ketoprofen (Orudis KT). Or a physician may prescribe an NSAID such as Celebrex, Zorvolex, Indocin, or Feldene, among others.

All these drugs may provide short-term relief, but they have deleterious side effects on your gut (see pages 79–84 for a detailed discussion). Glucosamine occurs naturally in your body and is found in the fluid that surrounds and cushions joints, where it serves its role as one of the building blocks of cartilage. Glucosamine binds to WGA, relieving or eliminating the inflammation and therefore the pain. Taking glucosamine sulfate in supplement form has a salutary effect for many, but not all people. The reason it is effective is not because it magically relieves joint pain, but because it binds WGA and other lectins in the gut, which are then eliminated before they can enter your body. To break the vicious circle of taking NSAIDs to reduce the side effects inflicted by WGA, simply omit wheat and other lectin-containing foods from your diet. You'll be shocked and delighted to see what happens.

Natural and Manipulated Lectins

UNTIL THE 1950s most people followed organic gardening methods, fertilizing their crops with manure and using mulch to protect roots and the microbes in the soil from extreme cold. By the middle of the twentieth century, thanks to petrochemical fertilizers, a remnant of the munitions manufacturing for World War II, and the development of refrigerated railcars, heirloom produce began to give way to hybrid varieties developed by seed companies to satisfy the needs of commercial growers. A major factor was the need to grow produce in Southern California, Florida, and other warm parts of the country that could be shipped in a refrigerated truck or railcar for distribution across the country. Hybrid vegetables and fruit that could withstand the journey and arrive in good shape meant that, regardless of whether you lived in South Carolina or South Dakota, you could find out-of-season produce year-round. Hybrids that made the cut were deemed desirable and varieties that couldn't meet the shipping test fell out of favor.

However, shippable hybrids haven't had hundreds of years to develop the natural ability to deal with inclement weather and insects and other plant predators, as well as to compete with weeds. Because these plants lacked such natural defenses, commercial farmers began to rely on heavy use of biocides (pesticides, insecticides, and herbicides). The next step in the process of making modern farming more efficient and profitable was genetic modification. In bioengineered plants, lectins are artificially inserted. Scientists selectively add foreign genes into a plant's basic genome to command the plant to manufacture specific lectins that enhance the plant's ability to resist insects and other pests. This is one form of genetically modified organisms (GMO).

Not only do the food staples we eat today contain far more lectins than did the vegetables and fruits our grandparents ate, they also are more likely to be GMOs. And remember, these fruits are picked unripe, leaving their lectin content intact. Finally, and let me emphasize this point: just because the produce you are eating is grown organically doesn't mean that you were designed to eat that plant. Lectins are naturally concentrated in the leaves and seeds of all plants, regardless of whether the plant is grown organically or conventionally. This means that while you can avoid GMO foods, you cannot avoid lectins. The solution then is controlling which ones (and how much of them) you consume.

Hormesis and the Lectin Paradox

Without question, plants can mess with your body, but at the same time, they contain compounds that can be beneficial. Their toxic nature actually educates the innate immune system (the nonspecific immune system passed down from mother to infant at birth) to assist you in fighting off pathogens such as pneumonia and viruses. Other lectins are antimicrobial. One lectin inhibits the growth of the HIV virus. Lectins in garlic, bitter melon, and other herbs possess healing properties. Researchers are currently investigating the potential of some lectins to treat cancers, because they bind to cell membranes. Nonetheless, if you are lectin sensitive, the fact that lectins initiate chronic inflammation likely offsets the benefit of any anticancer action.

To understand the lectin paradox, that certain foods can be both good for you and bad for you, it helps to understand the concept of hormesis, which refers to the fact that compounds that are bad for us in quantity are often simultaneously good for us in moderation. This concept is often expressed as "the dose makes the poison." Eating such foods educates and mildly stresses the immune system and cells in general, and therefore increases the likelihood of a longer life span. In the case of lectins, a little bit of the toxin can be protective. For example, bitter plants warn you to eat just a little of them. In general, long-lived cultures have a history of eating bitter greens and herbs. As I said in my first book: more bitter, more better!

Hormesis is actually an argument for eating a varied diet. We humans evolved as a traveling species. There is evidence that our hunter-gatherer forebears ate about 250 plant species on a rotating basis. Most humans don't even eat a tenth of that number, which in my opinion is an excellent argument, which we will get to later, for why we need to take supplements.

The Gluten Distraction

LET ME RETURN to the particular lectin called gluten for a moment. Like a guy whose car was hijacked by bank robbers and used to commit a crime, gluten is just a minor player, and not the primary culprit in the debate surrounding the healthfulness of eating grains. In fact, in countries that depend on gluten as a major source of protein, people do just fine. Seitan, for example, a dietary staple in Indonesia, contains no WGA, just gluten. For most people, going gluten-free is like throwing out the baby (the protein) with the bathwater (the gluten). In fact, a lot of people who struggle to give up gluten actually continue to eat foods that are more problematic, thanks to the other lectins they contain. Many people assume so-called gluten-free foods are grain-free. Not so. Wheat, rye, and barley may be eliminated in gluten-free foods, but a look at the list of ingredients reveals that these grains have been replaced with corn, rice, or teff, each of which contains multiple forms of glutenlike lectins, including zein, oryzenin, panicin, kafirin, and penniseitin. These products also often include soy or other bean flours, which of course also contain lectins. And again, sugar in one form or another frequently appears high on the list of ingredients.

There is another reason that people may mistakenly think that the problems they have with bread and other baked goods stem from sensitivity to gluten. Since 1950, commercial bakers in the United States have replaced the rising agent of yeast with transglutaminase, which is also a binding agent. When I do eat bread in the United States, it makes me feel bloated, but I have no such reaction with white bread made with yeast when I am in Europe. That's because yeast ferments and destroys the lectins in wheat, taming their effects. And guess what? In France and Italy, where bread is produced by traditional yeast-rising techniques, almost all the bread is white, not whole wheat. It contains gluten, which has been digested by the yeast, but no WGA. Would it surprise you then to learn that sourdough bread, made by fermenting wheat with bacteria and yeast, consistently ranks as one of the safest and least injurious breads, in terms of blood sugar spikes? The bacteria and yeast together "eat" the lectins and a good deal of the sugars!

And here's the kicker: Most "gluten-free" baked products are also treated with transglutaminase to make them fluffier and more appealing. Transglutaminase is also used to bind together ground meat and seafood (fake crabmeat is one example), which is why it's often referred to as meat glue. Unfortunately, transglutaminase can pass the blood-brain barrier and act as a neurotransmitter disruptor, making it extremely harmful and often responsible for the condition known as gluten ataxia, which is similar to Parkinson's. Nonetheless, transglutaminase is FDA approved and does not need to appear on product labels.

It is important to note that transglutaminase also sensitizes us to glutens even if we're not gluten-sensitive. Read that last sentence again. This means that if you assume you are sensitive to gluten because you have certain symptoms after eating store-bought bread and other products made with wheat, you may instead actually be reacting to transglutaminase.

Finally, when whole grains are used in processed foods, including bread and breakfast cereals, it is necessary to add dangerous preservatives such as butyl hydroxytoluene (BHT) to block the oxidation of the polyunsaturated oils in those whole grains. I'll get to BHT and its cousins soon, but for now, let's just say that you might as well be spiking your bread or cereal with estrogen. These oils reside in the germ of the grain. Unlike a saturated fat such as coconut oil, polyunsaturated fats are always on the lookout for oxygen atoms with which to bond, and when they do, the fat can become rancid. Rancid bread or crackers taste, well, rancid. A few years ago, I was lecturing in France and had to catch a very early flight back to the United States. I asked if breakfast could be delivered to my room at about 4:00 a.m. The front desk manager assured me that they would be happy to provide breakfast at that hour but said they could not deliver any croissants, since those would not yet have been made. When I suggested that leftover croissants would be fine, he became apoplectic, assuring me that they would never do that, as they would be unfit to eat.

Remember this story when you peruse the sell-by date of any commercial bread or cracker or snack product. If the date isn't the day it was manufactured, then the product for sure contains BHT or another similar deadly preservative. There are many reasons you want to avoid BHT—among them the fact that it is a major endocrine disruptor, acting like estrogen. This is the last thing in the world you want your kids to be consuming, because estrogen prompts fat storage; it also promotes early puberty in girls and "boobs" on seven-year old boys.[18] And if you need further incentive to avoid this preservative, know that BHT is used in embalming fluid, among other commercial uses. I kid you not!

Patient Patterns

BEFORE I REALIZED that lectins are largely responsible for our poor health and excess pounds, I observed specific patterns in the health of my patients—and then in the benefits they derived from my diet program. When I shifted the focus of my medical practice to restorative medicine (sometimes referred to as functional medicine), many of my first patients were overweight men with heart disease. In the most basic terms, "restorative medicine" refers to medical practices that enable the body to heal itself rather than just treat the symptoms of disease. Usually my overweight patients were dragged in to see me, kicking and screaming, by their slim wives. Each woman wanted me to "fix" her husband. Changing habits is a team sport, so in addition to the various sophisticated blood tests and genetic markers I would draw from the husband, I usually asked the spouse to have the tests taken as well as a new patient. I also took a complete medical history from them both.

Much to my surprise, these thin, supposedly healthy women had a number of health issues in common with one another. A shocking number were hypothyroid, most due to Hashimoto's thyroiditis, an autoimmune disease supposedly of unknown cause. (Not so, as you'll learn.) A great number of them also had arthritis, often with very tender nodules in their finger joints. To relieve the pain, they typically took one or more of the NSAIDs, and most of them had also been using a stomach-acid reducer such as Prilosec, Prevacid, or Nexium for years. In addition, a huge number of them relied on antidepressants. Many would tell me, "If you were married to my husband, you'd be on them, too!" But that's not all. Often, they were also taking one or more drugs for osteoporosis and had been told that they had IBD (irritable bowel disease). In fact, my average (supposedly healthy) female patient was on seven medications!

This compilation of hypothyroidism, arthritis, acid reflux, osteoporosis, bowel issues, and depression (and the drugs they took to relieve them) formed a pattern in these slim women. I started looking for other things they had in common. What were they eating? If you guessed "healthy" foods, you're right! They dined on whole wheat pasta, whole wheat bagels with fat-free cream cheese, egg white omelets, and salads with dressing on the side. They avoided fats like the plague. And yet, most of them were on a statin drug like Lipitor or Crestor to reduce their cholesterol levels, as well as the fistful of drugs for ailments that they considered "normal." It seemed that the "healthier" they ate, the unhealthier they became.

And what of their husbands? Almost to a man, they followed a now familiar pattern: the use of medications to reduce high blood pressure, acid reflux, and cholesterol, to relieve arthritis and other forms of pain, and to induce sleep. The medicine cabinets in these households must have been a regular pharmacopoeia!

When the results of these specialized tests came back, certain markers of inflammation and immune cell activation also emerged with remarkable consistency: the immune systems of my patients and their wives were in full attack mode. But once I put them on a two-page food list I had modified from the one in my earlier book, *Dr. Gundry's Diet Evolution*, and advised them to remove certain household and personal grooming products from their homes, I consistently witnessed their body's natural ability to heal itself.

Word gets around. Soon women with similar health issues were turning up at my office on their own, minus a portly husband. But this time, a significant number of these women were either overweight or obese. Many told a similar story: that their often vague complaints would be tossed aside by their doctors as "female issues": hormone disorders, depression, or anxiety. Most of them had tried every diet under the sun, having gone to Weight Watchers, Lindora, Medifast, etc. Many had made a genuine commitment to exercise programs and yet here they were: fat and miserable. They carried with them the same cluster of prescriptions as my skinny women. They came because they knew something was wrong and their friends had said that I could "fix" them. And sure enough, the same dietary prescription that I gave my other patients fixed these folks as well.

Then other patients appeared with autoimmune diseases, such as rheumatoid arthritis, lupus, and multiple sclerosis, and immune-system diseases, such as lymphomas or multiple myelomas, Crohn's, and ulcerative colitis. I soon became known as the Fixer. Next, stage 3 and 4 cancer patients arrived. You'll be shocked to hear this, but not only did these autoimmune and cancer patients match similar patterns, most got better by following my food list.

Lectin Detection

FROM THERE, HOW did I specifically identify lectins as a primary cause for so many patterns of health problems in my patients? Good question. It actually happened in a roundabout way. In my thirty-plus years of practicing medicine, I have come to the conclusion that the problems we have with our health are actually caused by very small things. This is particularly true of big health problems. Once more with feeling: Very small things (like lectins) can cause huge health problems. And it was a simple observation by one of the earliest adopters of my original dietary program that started me down a path that resulted in this book.

The tests I order on all my patients reveal many patterns that have helped me understand what is happening to our collective health, but it wasn't until I worked with a patient by the name of Tony that I experienced my eureka moment. Tony was a strikingly fit, energetic, mostly vegetarian—he called himself a flexitarian—man in his early forties who had fully adopted my principles. As a result, he was eating lots of greens, and banishing grains and pseudo-grains, potatoes and other starches, as well as beans and other legumes. He had also dramatically cut back on fruit and seeded vegetables (which as you now know are botanically fruits). Tony had also upped his intake of fish, shellfish, fish oil, olive oil, avocados, and macadamia nuts.

Like all of my patients, Tony experienced improved vitality and athletic performance shortly after starting the program, and he lost ten pounds. But Tony suffered from vitiligo, a skin condition in which pigmentation is lost. (That's why Michael Jackson, who suffered from the same problem, became paler and paler over the years.) Vitiligo is caused by the gradual destruction of the pigment-producing cells of our skin called melanocytes, which are modified nerve cells that migrate to our skin in the embryonic stage of development. Why these nerve cells die in people with vitiligo was unknown at the time, but an autoimmune process was suspected.

The term "autoimmune process" is a catchphrase used to describe how the body's immune system gets confused and begins attacking its own cells. Patients with autoimmune disease are told that their immune system is making a mistake. In Tony's case, his melanocytes were being treated as if they were foreign invaders and had to be killed, leaving him with patches of unpigmented skin. And, to be sure, his immune system was doing a good job of killing the cells it had misidentified.

Now, I've seen just about everything in my years as a physician, and I like to think of myself as pretty unflappable—but I was shocked to see and hear what happened when Tony started on my diet. Within weeks, he saw the pigment return to his skin. That's right: His vitiligo vanished—or more properly reversed itself—and his skin pigmentation returned to normal. How did that happen? Frankly, I didn't know at the time. I did know that my dietary protocol was highly anti-inflammatory, but that didn't explain the resolution of Tony's vitiligo. Thousands of years ago, Hippocrates, the father of modern medicine, had described the body's ability to heal itself, which he called *veriditas* (green life force). He believed that the physician's job was to identify which forces were keeping the patient from healing himself and then remove them. *Veriditas* would take it from there. Clearly, Tony's new eating habits had removed the roadblocks to his body repairing itself. There was *veriditas* in action, right before my eyes!

So back I went to the review of my research—specifically, my xenotransplantation research as a pioneering surgeon in the art of heart transplants. What was in my program (or what wasn't in his new diet) that made Tony's body stop attacking his melanocytes? Had he added something, or had he removed the external force that was preventing his body's natural process of self-healing? Based on my transplant knowledge, I picked door number 2, the removal of an external force. But what was the external force?

A word of explanation is in order. Most people with various health problems believe that certain foods or supplements are anti-inflammatory, meaning that they dampen inflammation. What I was looking for is the actual *cause* of inflammation, which, if Hippocrates is right (and he is), would stop inflammation in its tracks. In other words, it wasn't that my diet was quelling the inflammation in Tony's body, which most healing diets purport to do. It was, in fact, that my diet was removing the root causes of inflammation, and once those were removed, his body was capable of healing itself without the need for any anti-inflammatory compounds. This seemingly small discovery will change how you think about how your body functions.

Clearly, inflammation was causing Tony's problem, but where did the inflammation come from? Strange as it seems, what I discovered was that there was inflammation in his melanocytes because they look suspiciously like lectins to the immune system. Tony's immune system had been attacking his melanocytes because, through no fault of their own, they bore a striking resemblance to lectins. And because my diet had purged lectins, the cause of the inflammation was removed.

Over hundreds of millions of years, plants have evolved a strategy of creating proteins (like lectins) that bear a striking resemblance to critical structures in their predators. When lectins get through the gut wall, they activate the immune system, which starts shooting without first asking questions—and that means it may shoot both at the lectins and also at the critical structures that resemble the lectins. Don't forget that one of the original purposes of lectins is to prompt an immune response on the nerves of an insect to paralyze it. In this instance, Tony's melanocytes—remember, they are modified nerve cells—were being misidentified as foreign. It was a case of mistaken identity, or what scientists call molecular mimicry—and it led to my eureka moment. Once Tony eliminated lectins, normalcy returned. I now knew lectins were causing this problem. But how did they get into Tony's body from his gut in the first place?

Pattern Matching

PATTERN MATCHING, a term borrowed from the computer science field, refers to the act of checking a sequence of items to find the constituents of a pattern. It happens every time you search for information on the internet using Google, Bing, or Ask. As you enter each keystroke, the search engine pattern matches and offers up what you appear to be looking for. The more information you type in, hopefully the better the match. But, as you know, the search program often mismatches, sometimes in frustrating or humorous ways. For example, perhaps you are planning a wedding and start to enter the words "white flowers," but the search engine jumps the gun and offers up content on white flour. That wasn't quite what you had in mind!

You will recall that I had found strikingly common patterns in all my female patients' medical complaints, as well as in their eating habits. And many of the findings that I presented in *Dr. Gundry's Diet Evolution* came from observing patterns in blood tests, particularly for triglyceride and cholesterol levels, that matched people's food choices. These patterns were predictable each and every time, and in every person. This observation is so important that I am repeating it here (and you will understand the full implication when you get to Part II). The patterns followed simple time-of-year food availability and predicted whether the body was in a "store fat for the upcoming winter during the summer" mode or "burn fat to survive the winter" mode. The choices of food, even the sweetness of food, communicated with our cells, via pattern matching, about which season it was, and we responded accordingly, either by gaining weight (summer) or burning calories in the form of fat for energy (winter). Pattern matching is the secret to how every living organism—no matter how small or large—operates. And by using those sophisticated blood tests, I came to realize that pattern matching and my ability to measure their effects on my patients underlie most positive or negative health states.

Immune System Scanners on Patrol

WE'VE COME TO know only in the last few years that your immune system uses quite simple scanning systems that look for and match patterns. I mentioned these systems in chapter 1 when discussing the second of the three strategies lectins use to fool your immune system. As a reminder, these scanners are known as TLRs; that stands for toll-like receptors, but I like to think of them as tiny little radars. They are found in all cell membranes of your body (and that of every animal).

Every protein, whether it is a virus, lectin, or cell wall, possesses a unique bar code. The TLRs in your body and on your white blood cells of your immune system behave like a Star Wars early warning system, looking for patterns that indicate foreign invaders, mainly bacteria and viruses. The TLRs constantly scan and "read" the molecular "fingerprints" or bar codes of whatever protein enters your body, just as a scanner at the checkout counter reads and interprets the UPC bar code on each product you purchase, identifying it and determining its price. Once the TLRs ascertain whether a particular bar code represents friend or foe, they decide how to respond, either by letting the protein pass without a challenge or by turning on alarms and air raid sirens to alert your body and immune system that an invasion is under way.

Now envision another set of receptors, which act like a USB port on a computer, that literally scan incoming hormones, enzymes, and cytokines for instructions about what those hormones and enzymes want the cell to do. This second set of receptors, known as G-protein coupled receptors—let's call them G-spotters—serve as docking ports on all cells, similar to those on the space station. When an incoming shuttle wants to unload its cargo and information, its docking mechanism must fit the mechanism on the space station, just as you can only use a charger with a compatible plug to recharge your iPhone 7. Likewise, only if a hormone or enzyme fits into the receptor can information be exchanged.

If this communication system within your body sounds fantastical, consider that we take for granted that our cell phones operate using invisible electrical pulses emanating from satellites or cell phone towers. Our bodies' cellular communication works in much the same way.

In other words, your immune system's job is to scan for friend or foe patterns, and to sound the alarm whenever it encounters recognized patterns of foreign proteins. It then shares the knowledge of the foreign protein patterns with the rest of the body, so that troops can be more easily rallied against the enemy in the future. This is what happens when you get a flu shot. A protein from the outside surface of the flu virus is injected into your arm. Your immune system sees this protein, reads its bar code as foreign, attacks it—and then it makes scanners on white blood cells and immune-signaling proteins that will be permanently on the lookout for the flu protein bar code. If the real flu virus gets in your system, wham, your body is ready. The TLR scanners—remember them as tiny little radars—recognize the incoming missile as a foe, they send out messages to alert the body, the missile defense system is launched, and white blood cells attack the foreign protein like a smart bomb. Result: no more flu virus. Victory!

The Search for Patterns

THE DESCRIPTION OF these scanners won the Nobel Prize for Medicine in 2011. A year later the discovery of the receptors (G-spotters) was awarded the Nobel Prize for Chemistry. Together, these discoveries allowed me to connect the final dots between patients who had what initially appeared to be completely unrelated problems.

As I discovered, the cause of all my patients' problems was that their cells' TLRs and G-spotters were scanning for patterns, detecting patterns, turning on alarms, or activating cellular machinery. That's because their TLRs and G-spotters were receiving information from input sources that never existed fifty years ago, thanks to a fundamental alteration in the foods people eat and the drugs and personal care products they (and you) use. In short, you have been hacked. And as a consequence, this process had devastated the health of my patients—and is almost certainly responsible for your health problems as well.

How can I know for sure that this is what is happening, and that the constant scanning is largely responsible for an array of health problems? After all, these lethal events are unfolding within you at the cellular, molecular level without your knowledge. The compounds that trigger these receptors are so small, so invisible, that they seem insignificant. But thanks to the inflammatory hormone measurements and tests that I use, I've been able to track them for the last few years.

The information I have gained from working with my patients has helped me find patterns in the immune system and the inflammation it generates that until now have been hidden from view. And what I've found is that lectins, and perhaps other foreign proteins, play a big role in disrupting communication between cells. Because lectins are master pattern mimickers, much of the information they communicate to cells is inaccurate. And the cause of *all* of my patients' problems is that their TLRs were inappropriately turning on alarms or that their receptors were receiving inappropriate information. Regardless of my individual patients' health issues, the common denominator was a disruption in messaging. The patterns being detected by their immune system had set off an immunologic and hormonal firestorm within each and every one of them, devastating their health. These conditions resolved when proper communication was restored. And the good news? It's all about making simple changes in your diet and lifestyle.

A Deadly Case of Mistaken Identity

WHEN YOU WERE a kid and got a sore throat, your mother probably worried that it was caused by a bacterium called *beta-hemolytic streptococcus*, known colloquially as strep throat. If you have kids of your own, you have the same concerns. Strep throat can lead to rheumatic fever, a very severe illness. But rheumatic heart disease, which is what happens after surviving rheumatic fever, is what interests heart surgeons like myself. This condition used to be the primary reason for heart-valve replacement, because survivors' valves were almost always destroyed later in life.

How valve destruction happens in rheumatic heart disease is important to you, even if you've never had strep throat. The cell wall of the streptococcus bacteria is made of fats, sugars, and proteins and is identified by its characteristic bar code. If you've been infected with this particular strain of streptococcus, your immune system makes scanners that patrol your bloodstream, ever on the hunt for the same bar code. Unfortunately, this bar code looks remarkably like the ones on your heart valve's cell wall surface.

Imagine the streptococcus scanner's surprise as it floats past your heart valves and comes across what it perceives is a streptococcus bar code! The scanners send messages to attack and kill what it mistakenly identifies as streptococcus. Then your immune system goes into full attack mode, day after day, year after year, silently and painlessly attacking your heart valve. Finally, the valve is so damaged that it stops functioning, and I'm called in to replace it.

As I remove that valve, I notice that the contents of the valve look a lot like the crud inside of the coronary arteries on which I do bypasses. That's another clue to the puzzle: modern coronary artery disease looks just like the immune system attack that causes rheumatic heart disease. I'll tell you what causes that immune attack on your coronary arteries a bit later, but be prepared. Scanner confusion in response to apparently similar bar codes results in unwarranted attacks, and it is the underlying cause of most of our current diseases and health issues.

Dangerous Impostors

EACH PROTEIN HAS a unique bar code, but as you just saw with streptococcus bacteria, many bar codes are remarkably similar. And some lectins are specifically designed by the plant to resemble compounds that are considered harmful by the body—such as lipopolysaccharides (LPSs), which are molecules that make up the cell walls of certain bacteria in our microbiome. I'm not one for swearing, but I can't resist calling them "little pieces of shit," because that's exactly what they are! LPSs are fragments of bacteria that are constantly being produced as bacteria divide and die in your gut. They travel through your gut wall and out into the body by riding on and hiding in saturated fats.

Your immune system cannot tell the difference between a whole bacterium and a fragment of one, so it treats LPSs as a threat, just as though a true bacterial infection was present in your blood or elsewhere in your body. Your immune system then summons your white blood cells—I think of them as fighter jets and troops—into the attack, causing inflammation. But the extra bad news is that our immune cells, which are ever on patrol for these foreign bodies, can mistake the pattern of lectins for the pattern of LPSs and attack them, as though bacteria were loose in your system—further inflaming your body as a result.

But the most dangerous trick pulled by lectins, which I now see on a daily basis in my patients, is that they bear an uncanny similarity to the proteins on many of our important organs, nerves, and joints. Now, in an abundance of caution, your immune system doesn't want to make a mistake in defending your body by not attacking something important. In the days before antibiotics, you would have been in big trouble if bacteria were present in your body, which is why your immune system is hypersensitive to anything that even remotely resembles a bacterial cell wall or other foreign protein.

My colleagues in rheumatology call this response autoimmune disease, but it is actually "friendly fire." If an animal eats something containing lectins and gets sick, doesn't feel well, or doesn't thrive, it rapidly figures out that eating that particular plant seed or product isn't a good idea. Remember, a weakened enemy is the best kind of enemy from a plant's standpoint. And if you can get your enemy to shoot himself in the foot, you're ahead of the game. When a plant predator (including a human) attacks itself with an immune reaction, it becomes less likely to eat the plant (and therefore its "babies"). Equally as important, it is less likely to reproduce and create more plant predators, again helping ensure the survival of the plant species.

A God Learned How to Cure Himself

My good friend Tony Robbins called me about five years ago, looking for help. An eminent guru, a holy man considered a "god" to twelve million people around the world, was in a hospital in India, awaiting an urgent five-vessel coronary artery bypass grafting for severe coronary artery disease. Could I intervene and help him avoid surgery? My answer was a resounding yes! It's not every day that I meet a god.

The sixty-two-year-old guru's blood work did not look promising. Not only did he have severe coronary artery blockages, he was also terribly diabetic, with HbA1Cs—a marker of sugar and protein intolerance—of greater than 9.0 (normal is less than 5.6), and advanced kidney failure. When he consulted me via Skype, I asked him if he was indeed a god, and he replied that people call him a god because he performs miracles and cures people. I responded by asking, why he doesn't just cure himself, if he performs miracles. His reply? "You know how this god thing works; I can cure anyone else, but I can't cure myself! That's what I need you for." We hit it off immediately.

The guru was being treated by an ayurvedic physician, and he ate a traditional Indian diet heavy on rice, legumes, and naan, a kind of flatbread. He had a classic "Delhi belly," aka a beer belly. When I made it clear that the foods of his faith were the cause of his diabetes, heart disease, and kidney failure, he was shocked. These were the foods recommended by all the gods before him. How could they be so unhealthy? My reply was the same as it is to anyone else who eats "healthy": How's all that healthy eating working out for you if you have all these diseases?

As Einstein was fond of saying, the definition of insanity is doing the same thing over and over and expecting a different result. I put the god on the Plant Paradox Program, and within a few weeks his chest pain was gone and his blood sugar level started to decline. Things were going well for about three months, until his blood tests results were suddenly terrible again. When we next Skyped, I asked him what happened. Apparently, every three months there is a festival to worship him and all the monks, and his followers shower him with foods for the gods, which he is obliged to eat. This pattern repeated itself for about two years; two steps forward, one step back every three months when another festival occurred.

Finally, on a Skype call a few years in, I couldn't take it anymore. "Aren't you god to your followers?" I asked. "Yes," he replied. "Well, doesn't god make the rules about what god likes to eat and what pleases him?" I asked. "I never thought about it like that," he said. "I will tell my monks and my followers that we must all eat Gundry style to please me." And that's just what he did.

Today, the guru's skin has a radiant glow of health. His stress tests on his heart are normal, and his kidney failure is history, as is his diabetes. Without medications, his HbA1C is an acceptable 5.5 and going down. Oh, and one more thing: His ayurvedic doctor now also eats Gundry style!

Each one of us has the power, the green life force energy, to heal from within once the external forces that prevent that natural ability are removed. The god had the power to heal himself, after all. As he and I agreed, I can show you the path, but it is you who must walk it.

Patterns Causing Problems

ANOTHER IMPORTANT LESSON I've learned from my patients is that your immune system reacts to lectins to a greater or lesser degree depending on who you are—meaning your family history and genetics—and, more important, whether those lectins are getting past your previously intact intestinal barrier. It seems simple, right? Not so. In the next chapter, we'll look more closely at our current health crisis and specifically the rising tide of obesity and related diseases. Most important, we'll look at how to reverse it. Because as it turns out, the ability of lectins to mimic other proteins and confuse the body's messaging plays a major role in many, many conditions. By using the forthcoming principles and my updated dietary program, I have seen patients resolve the following health problems:

- Aching joints
- Acid reflux or heartburn
- Acne
- Age spots, skin tags
- Allergies
- Alopecia
- Anemia
- Arthritis
- Asthma
- Autoimmune diseases (including autoimmune thyroid disease, rheumatoid arthritis, type 1 diabetes, multiple sclerosis, Crohn's, colitis, and lupus)
- Bone loss (including osteopenia and osteoporosis)
- Brain fog
- Cancer

- Canker sores
- Chronic fatigue syndrome
- Chronic pain syndrome
- Colon polyps
- Cramps, tingling, and numbness
- Decline in dental health
- Dementia
- Depression
- Diabetes, prediabetes, insulin resistance
- Exhaustion
- Fat in the stool (due to poor digestion)
- Fibromyalgia
- Gastroesophageal reflux disease (GERD), Barrett's esophagus
- Gastrointestinal problems (bloating, pain, gas, constipation, diarrhea)
- Headaches
- Heart disease, coronary artery disease, vascular disease
- Hypertension
- Infertility, irregular menstrual cycle, miscarriage
- Irritability and behavioral changes
- Irritable bowel syndrome (IBS)
- Low counts of immunoglobulin G, immunoglobulin M, and immunoglobulin A
- Low testosterone
- Low white blood cell count
- Lymphomas, leukemias, multiple myeloma
- Male-pattern baldness
- Memory loss
- Migraine headaches
- Nutritional deficiencies due to malabsorption—e.g., low iron levels

- Parkinson's disease
- Peripheral neuropathy
- Polycystic ovary syndrome (PCOS)
- Skin rashes (including dermatitis herpetiformis, eczema, and psoriasis)
- Slow infant and child growth
- Unexplained bouts of dizziness or ear ringing
- Vitiligo
- Weight loss or weight gain

Okay, okay. I know what you're thinking: I've cited just about every illness and health complaint out there! How can one thing cause them all? Believe me, twelve years ago I myself would have tossed this book out the window if you had suggested that everything on this list was caused by consuming lectins, in collaboration with chemical and other disruptors that have infiltrated our bodies. However, my experience with tens of thousands of patients is proof that this is in fact the case—and that following my protocol will heal what ails you.

What Has Changed?

IF WE'VE KNOWN about lectins for more than a century and we eat lectins daily in a huge variety of foods—you'll find a complete list on pages 203–204—why isn't everybody being attacked by lectins? Well, maybe they are. Or, if they weren't attacking us in the past, why are they attacking us now? And what has changed? I have uncovered how lectins are infiltrating our bodies, and we'll look at those disturbing factors in the next two chapters.

Your Gut Under Attack

You've absorbed some complex and surprising concepts in the last two chapters—and there's more to come, so consider this fair warning. Amazing as it may sound, everything I am about to tell you is backed up by peer-reviewed published research by scientists from prestigious universities around the world, as well my own research at my Center for Restorative Medicine. Let me also remind you that the problems you have with your health (and perhaps your weight) are actually caused by very, very small things. You'll understand what I mean by that as we begin to explore the fascinating world that is your gut.

You and Your Holobiome: Best Friends Forever

WITHIN YOUR INTESTINAL tract and mouth and on your skin—and even in a cloud around you—live hundreds of trillions of different minute microbes: bacteria plus a good number of viruses, molds, fungi, protozoa, and even worms. One of our biggest health misconceptions comes from our collective lack of awareness of who we really are. The *real* you—or the *whole* you—is actually what you think of as "you," plus those multitudinous microbes. In fact, 90 percent of all the cells that constitute you are nonhuman. To go a step further, 99 percent of all the *genes* in you are nonhuman.

At first glance, the multiple life-forms with which we coexist may seem like an alternate reality. Yet you and your microbes are literally in this life together. Your health is dependent on them—as theirs is on you. At the most basic level, you are not alone. Most of us think that we are totally in charge of the decisions we make and the things we do. Your microbes—or "bugs," as I fondly call them—would vigorously disagree. You may recoil at the thought that minute nonhuman organisms or even simple nonliving molecules exert so much power over you. Yet, we know that this is true.

You can think of it this way: you and your bugs can be seen as a country composed of trillions of inhabitants, human and nonhuman cells alike. The nonhuman cells are the legal aliens performing work for the country as a whole in a guest worker program. These aliens are housed on their side of the tracks: on our skin and in our intestinal tract (and even in specific "work zones" within the intestinal tract).

This multiplicity of microbes has collectively been called the microbiome, although scientists are now using the term "holobiome" as more descriptive; holobiome includes not just the microbes in your gut, but also those on your skin and even in the cloud of bacteria surrounding each of us (much like Pig Pen in the Peanuts cartoons). Whichever term you prefer, you provide a home for these microbes, and they provide services in return. Yes, they rely on you to feed and house them, but what is initially harder for most of us to accept is that we are equally dependent on them. Without our microbes, we could not live and function. We know this from experiments with germ-free mice, studies that initiated the research on the interaction between a host organism and its microbes. Germ-free mice, which are raised without a microbiome, are shorter and smaller, live shorter lives, and are more susceptible to disease because their immune system never develops properly.[1] As a result, we know how vital it is that you keep your holobiome well fed and happy.

I can't resist sharing a quick story: I entered the state science fair as a fifth grader in 1960, and based on the research from the time into what is now called the holobiome, my project was to build a germ-free-mouse environment. Little did I know that decades later I would be writing about the synergy between human hosts and microbes. As I've said, this isn't my first rodeo.

Hard at Work in Your GI Tract

NOW LET'S TAKE a closer look at what is going on in your gastrointestinal (GI) tract. For many of the "guest workers," your gut is where they reside and do their job, breaking down and digesting plant cell walls and extracting energy and shipping it in the form of fats to you. Like all other animals, we are totally dependent on these microbe workers to do this crucial job. Even a termite cannot "eat" wood; bacteria in its tiny gut actually do the work to digest the wood and convert it into energy. If they weren't there, the termite would starve.

One of the workers' two main jobs is to extract energy from plants that are eaten by their host. The other is to act as a sentinel for the host's immune system. Because there is so much genetic material in the holobiome, some scientists believe, as do I, that we have "outsourced" much of our immune surveillance, almost like putting our genetic material in the cloud. The prevailing theory is that we have outsourced the initial jobs of detecting friends or foes and of deflecting foes to our holobiome.

Where these guest workers reside varies by species, but there are generally three sites for animals to house their workers and break down plant material: for cows and other ruminants, it is the stomach or multiple stomachs; for gorillas and other great apes, it is the small intestine; for humans, it is the large intestine (colon).

To understand where we are going, let's pause for a short anatomy lesson. Your GI tract, which extends from your mouth all the way down to your anus, is actually your skin turned inside out. The inside contents of your intestines are actually outside of you. That's right, the contents of your intestines are every bit as much a part of the outside world as the world that you see around you. Whoa! How can that be? If it's inside of you, how can it be outside?

Think of a highway tunnel under a river. Cars entering the tunnel are outside the river when they go into the tunnel as well as when they come out. As they pass through the tunnel, they're not *in* the river, are they? Of course not. They're still outside the river, but they happen to be inside a passageway that contains air rather than water. Even though they appear to disappear into the river and emerge from the other side of it, they never were actually "in" the river. So, too, most of the food you swallow, along with your guest workers, appears to be inside you but is actually outside of you, even though it passes *through* you. Your intestinal wall serves as a border fence to separate the guest workers from the rest of you.

Meanwhile, your skin is the home to trillions of skin flora (microbes), and it has two primary functions: first, to protect you from the outside world; and second, to absorb and get rid of materials. The first of these jobs is the more important (or so we thought).

The lining of your intestines is your skin turned inside out and has the same two jobs as what you think of as your skin. However, in this case, the more important job is to absorb materials in the form of food. As a reminder, coiled within your belly, your intestinal surface has the same surface area as a tennis court! But here's the problem. As you now know, the wall that lines your intestines is only one cell thick. These cells are bonded together by tight junctions, which are supposed to prevent anything "foreign" from breaching the border into your body's tissues and bloodstream. The objective is to keep the contents of your intestine, including your holobiome, where they belong, outside of you. If they get inside of you, all hell breaks loose.

Strange but True: A Gift from Mom

You inherited your initial collection of bugs from your mother. By design, when you exited the birth canal, you were inoculated with her set of microbes to constitute your initial holobiome. This collection of bugs was essential to educate your newborn immune system and its cells, a process that actually starts well before birth. *Lactobacilli*, the type of bugs that thrive on milk sugar (lactose), don't normally live in your mother's vagina, but during the last three months of pregnancy, they migrate there. Would it surprise you to hear, then, that a mother's breast milk contains complex sugar molecules (oligosaccharides) that her infant cannot digest, but that are necessary for the health and growth of her infant's bugs? And did you know that without a normal set of microbes from your mother, your immune system couldn't develop properly? In fact, if you were born by cesarean section, it takes fully six months to build a normal set of microbes and a functioning immune system—just because you didn't journey down Mom's birth canal!

Everything in Its Place

FIVE POUNDS OF organisms—those bacteria, worms, protozoa, fungi, molds, and viruses, collectively known as your holobiome—live in your intestine, your skin, and the air around you and they help make up the whole that is you. Researchers have identified well over ten thousand different organisms found in the holobiome to date, and the number climbs every year, as the Human Microbiome Project expands.

Why are those five pounds of microbes associated with you? Well, your holobiome plays a major role in your immune system, nervous system, and hormonal system—the whole enchilada of you—and communicates to human cells how things are going in the "outside" world. The microbes in your GI tract are there to digest things you cannot digest and pass that digested food into you, but they are also there to do battle with things you swallow that are meant to do you harm—including the plant proteins called lectins.

How the Gut Wall *Should* Work

EVEN THOUGH THESE nonhuman cells that make up your holobiome are essential to your health and well-being, your human cells think these "other" cells belong outside of you. It's fine to receive messages and nutrients from your microbes, as long as they stay on their side of the fence. As the poet Robert Frost famously wrote in "Mending Walls," "Good fences make good neighbors." Your bugs are your close neighbors, but they need to stay on their side of the fence, meaning outside your skin and the lining of your gut.

Let me use the example of a nuclear power plant to help you understand how crucial this "fence" is between your microbes and the rest of your body. Controlled nuclear fission is an important yet extremely dangerous source of power. Uncontained, it represents the atomic bomb, but compartmentalized and controlled, it can power electrical generators and produce nonpolluting electrical energy. Supposedly impenetrable containment structures keep the radiation in check, but the danger is so great that all personnel wear radiation detectors, which serve as scanners. Other scanners are positioned around and outside the main reactors. If radiation is detected, the alarms sound, signaling an imminent threat to health. And as the 2011 meltdown of the Fukushima nuclear plant tragically illustrates, the escape of this toxic nuclear material will damage the area surrounding the plant, perhaps permanently.

Though obviously on a much smaller scale, think about how most of your microbes are housed in your GI tract. Those contents should be contained by the intestinal lining, which acts like the containment vessel of a nuclear reactor, to protect you from contamination. Your gut bugs are akin to the nuclear energy. As long as they know their place and remain confined in the "outside world" of your gut, these organisms are essential for you to function. But in reality, your intestinal wall is being breached on a daily basis—causing numerous and serious issues throughout the rest of your body.[2] Is it any wonder that many days you feel like you're suffering a "meltdown"?

Keeping intestinal microbes in their place is difficult because the intestinal barrier has two somewhat contradictory jobs. Not only must the cells that line your intestines keep lectins out, they must simultaneously let nutrients in. That's a daunting task. Again, you have only a single layer of locked-together mucosal cells (called enterocytes) in charge of preventing unwanted inhabitants of the GI tunnel from escaping and getting into you.

SUCCESS STORY

The Typical Vegan Diet Doesn't Cut It

An eighty-year-old cookbook writer specialized in vegan cookery, meaning that her diet had a heavy reliance on grains and beans. She had collaborated with Dr. John McDougall, who was one of the first proponents of an all-plant diet. When I met the writer, she was extremely thin and had severe arthritis in her hands. Tests revealed that she also had severe lupus as well as celiac disease, classic manifestations of lectins breaching the gut wall. I placed her on the Plant Paradox Program, and the lupus and celiac markers quickly resolved. Despite her newfound health, my patient decided to retry her old way of eating what she called a "normal" vegan diet of grains and beans. The reaction was a tenfold increase in lupus markers, diminished kidney function (lupus nephritis), and increased congestive heart failure. This time the writer saw the light and returned to my program, with the happy result that all her issues once again resolved. Please remember this story when we talk about reintroducing lectins in Part II.

What Should (and Should Not) Pass Through the Gut Wall

ONLY TINY SINGLE molecules of digested food *should* pass through the intestinal wall. So how does the good stuff in that salad and bowl of soup you had for lunch ultimately get through your intestinal wall? Simply put, in order to cross the border checkpoint from your GI tract into you, all food has to be broken down into individual amino acids (from protein), individual fatty acids (from fat), and individual sugar molecules (from sugars and starches). These small, single molecules provide energy (calories) and nutrients. Acids, enzymes, and yes, your microbial guest workers do all that work of digesting big molecules for you.

Your mucosal cells then literally bite off a single molecule of amino acids, fatty acids, and sugar, pass it through the body of the cell, and release it into your portal veins or lymph system abutting the back of these cells. These tiny molecules go through the system without ever having to break through the "locked arms" of the tight junctions of mucosal cells. When all is working well, the big molecules remain outside where they belong because they are literally too big for the cells of the intestinal wall to "swallow" them. How come? First, your mucosal cells can't bite off more than they can chew. Second, if everything is functioning properly, big molecules should not get through; if they do appear across the border, your immune system concludes that a foreign invader is lurking and sounds the alarm.

Breaching the Gut Wall

THIS IS A great system, except when it isn't. As you might suspect, things don't always work the way they are supposed to. Thanks to changes in what we eat, how foods are grown, and other causes—like consuming over-the-counter painkillers, particularly nonsteroidal anti-inflammatory drugs (NSAIDs)—lectins and lipopolysaccharides (LPSs) now breach the intestinal border on a daily basis. With the exception of WGA, lectins are big proteins, and you now know that big proteins can't normally get through the intestinal wall without difficulty. But lectins are adept at prying apart the tight junctions between the cells that make up your intestinal mucosal border. This breach also allows larger molecules to pass though into the body, where they too wreak havoc. And when lectins, LPSs (remember, I think of these cell walls of certain bacteria as little pieces of shit, which they literally are), or both escape from your gut and into your body, your immune system perceives this as an attack, goes on high alert, and signals your body to store fat and supplies for the "war" effort. Simultaneously, lectins bind to and block the border crossings of each intestinal cell so that vitamins and other nutrients can't be absorbed.

If lectins cause all the problems listed on pages 68–70, why haven't other health-care practitioners told you about this? My only answer is "You can't see unless your eyes are open!" Most doctors and nutritionists are completely unaware of lectins and their effects, which is why to them it would appear that most people are able to eat lectins, including gluten, and not experience any ill effects. The key word in that last sentence is "appear."

SUCCESS STORY

Cured of Crohn's Disease

I met Jill W. on Skype a couple of years ago. A twenty-year-old college junior, she was on a full scholarship provided by the foundation one of my patients had started to encourage students to go into careers that study immunology. My patient had suffered from Crohn's disease, a disabling autoimmune disease of the bowel, which is treated with transplant antirejection drugs. I put her on the Plant Paradox Program, and within three months she was cured of Crohn's, and as a side effect had lost fifty pounds. Needless to say, she was delighted with the turn of events, so she shared the two-page Plant Paradox Program food list with

Jill, her scholarship student, who also suffered from Crohn's. An eminent professor of gastroenterology at the Mayo Clinic was treating Jill at the time. My patient asked if I would talk with her, and I said yes, of course.

Jill began our conversation by telling me that when her sponsor had sent her the Plant Paradox list, she was suspicious. She had been on every diet for Crohn's without success. Moreover, her professor (and doctor) had assured her that Crohn's was genetic—that was his area of research—and that diet had nothing to do with it. With a sheepish look on her face, she told me that to humor her sponsor, she began the Plant Paradox Program. Then her face lit up on the video monitor: "After two weeks, I had the first normal bowel movement of my life, and they have been normal ever since. But two days ago, I called my doctor at the Mayo Clinic with the exciting news that my Crohn's was cured by the diet. He told me that it was a placebo effect, because diet has nothing to do with Crohn's and that my 'cure' was all in my mind.

"I was so upset," she continued, "that I got off the phone and went into the kitchen where my mother was baking Christmas cookies. I ate two of them. A few minutes later, it was like a bomb went off in my stomach. That night, the cramps and diarrhea returned. I immediately went back on the Plant Paradox Program and all is well now. But, Dr. Gundry, why didn't my doctor believe that it was the food all along that was causing my Crohn's? How can he not see that?"

I told her, as I'll tell you again: Your doctor can't see unless his eyes are open! First of all, there's no way to know that lectins are causing problems if you don't even know what lectins are. Second, even an awareness of lectins doesn't mean you understand the implications of what they do.

Read on to see how my eyes were opened. Soon your eyes will be as well. And I'll also provide you with the tools to repair your gut lining and restore your health. Remember, much of what goes on in your body is undetectable by conventional means. What if lectins are doing harm but it's not obvious—or not immediately obvious? My patients' blood work certainly suggested that damage was occurring, suggesting that lectins or something that looked remarkably like them were getting through the locked-arm mucosal barrier. But how could lectins suddenly get through, after eons during which they couldn't? What had changed?

A Clue Emerges

I WAS PERPLEXED, to say the least. Then, about twelve years ago, I ran into the head of pathology in the hall of my hospital. He said, "Hey, you trained as a general surgeon before becoming a heart surgeon. What do you know about intestinal webs?" I told him that I had never heard of them. Neither had he, he replied, and proceeded to tell me about a woman in her fifties who had come in with intestinal obstruction and was immediately rushed into the operating room where a large part of her small intestine, which was swollen and blocked in several areas, had to be removed. When the pathologist opened the bowel, he discovered "webs" of tissue, like washers on the fitting of a garden hose, which almost completely blocked the entire interior of the tube. Only pinhole openings remained. The pathologist had never seen anything like it.

Intrigued, I asked where the webs had come from. He didn't know yet, but he researched it, and sure enough, it's actually quite common in people who regularly use NSAIDs, such as Advil and Motrin, both brands of ibuprofen, or Aleve, Naprosyn, Mobic, Celebrex, and aspirin. All but aspirin were introduced in the early 1970s for pain and fever relief and as an arthritis medication in lieu of aspirin. Prolonged use of aspirin was clearly associated with damage to the stomach lining, but because other NSAIDs did not damage the stomach, drug companies heralded them as nothing short of miraculous.

My next question to my colleague was how these NSAIDs cause intestinal webs to form. His reply was that he didn't care, now that he knew what the webs were. But, being the curious type, I started investigating, and in doing so, I opened a Pandora's box and have never looked back. In brief, NSAIDs do not damage the stomach lining, which we can view with a gastroscope; instead, they damage the lining of the small intestine, which is beyond the reach of a scope. Because we could not see their ill effects, NSAIDs have done extreme damage to the barrier that keeps not just lectins, but also LPSs, out of you.

Who Let the Dogs Out?

"FRIENDLY" BACTERIA, WHICH populate the innermost layer of cells in the gut (the mucous layer, right next to the intestinal cell border), thrive on complex resistant starches called fructooligo-saccharides (FOS). These beneficial bacteria not only live in mucus, they also stimulate mucosal cells to make more of this good stuff. Mucus then acts as a moat to trap lectins and block them from passing through the intestinal border. The more mucus you produce, the more resistant you are to lectins—unless you're regularly taking NSAIDs. (Mucus isn't confined to your gut. It turns up as the snot in your nose, where it likewise traps foreign proteins and keeps them out of your body. Yup, snot is good!)

Copious research published over the last half century reveals that gulping down apparently harmless NSAIDs is like swallowing a live grenade. These drugs blow gaping holes in the mucus-lined intestinal barrier. As a result, lectins, LPSs, and living bacteria are able to deluge the breaks in your levee, flooding your body with foreign invaders. Inundated by these foreign proteins and other invaders, your immune system does what it does best, producing inflammation and pain. This pain in turn prompts you to down another NSAID, promoting a vicious cycle, which can ultimately result in your seeking out prescription-level pain relievers. In other words, that harmless Aleve or Advil is the pharmaceutical industry's gateway drug,[3] as you will discover in the next chapter. A course of antibiotics, stomach-acid reducers, or even changes in our food supply also allow bad bacteria to move in and take over, just as NSAIDs do.

Increased intestinal permeability from lectins and LPSs, as well as the regular use of NSAIDs and acid-reducing drugs, produces what is commonly called leaky gut syndrome. Although, along with others, I originally thought that leaky gut was an isolated condition affecting a few unfortunate individuals, now I am convinced that leaky gut underlies all our disease issues, just as Hippocrates posited. Adding insult to injury, consuming the lectins in whole-grain products and other baked goods—including even gluten-free varieties made with the rising agent known as transglutaminase (see pages 51–52)—independently makes the intestinal permeability worse. Remember that for centuries, the bran from these grains was discarded, making whole grains a relatively recent addition to our diet—and a recent problem as a result.

The *Real* Cause of Autoimmune Diseases

NOW LISTEN CAREFULLY. What I'm about to tell you will shatter your current beliefs about conditions commonly called autoimmune diseases. If you suffer from Crohn's disease, ulcerative colitis, microscopic colitis, hypothyroidism (or Hashimoto's thyroiditis), lupus, multiple sclerosis, rheumatoid arthritis, Sjogren's syndrome (dry eyes and mouth), scleroderma, systemic sclerosis, psoriasis, Raynaud's syndrome, dermatomyositis, fibromyalgia, osteoarthritis (that's plain old arthritis), or any other—that's right, *any* autoimmune disease—the good news is that you can eliminate it without using drugs! I get to see it happen every day. And the answer lies in healing your leaky gut, which we will discuss in Part II.

Modern research has confirmed Hippocrates's belief that all of these diseases begin in the gut and can be cured by healing the gut. Strictly from word-of-mouth recommendations, 50 percent of my practice for the past ten years has involved the treatment and cure of autoimmune diseases. And based on copious and rigorous measurements of laboratory and clinical markers of disease activity at my institute, I (along with others) am now convinced that *all* autoimmune diseases are caused by alterations in the good bugs and the bad bugs that live in your gut and your mouth and on your skin, along with a change in the permeability of your gut wall and mouth and gums.

What impacts that permeability? As we learned above, NSAIDs, antibiotics, acid-blocking drugs such as Nexium and Prilosec, and the biocide Roundup all change your gut flora and the mucous layer of your gut. This compromises the barrier wall of your intestines on a daily basis, thereby allowing lectins in. And this confluence of forces prompts your immune system to unleash an attack on you, in a classic case of mistaken identity caused by molecular mimicry.

As a reminder, molecular mimicry is caused by our immune cells attacking proteins on cells or organs that resemble the patterns on lectins and LPSs.

The spectrum of deleterious effects from leaky gut initially occurs out of sight, but when the damage to your intestinal wall becomes so severe that you lose the absorptive part of your intestine, it makes its presence known by less protein showing up in blood tests. Much as a sponge or chamois cloth can absorb liquids, under normal circumstances the intestine is capable of taking up large amounts of proteins, fats, and sugars—until it can't. To understand just how insidious this is, think of how smoking cigarettes can silently destroy the oxygen-exchanging surface of the lungs long before a diagnosis of emphysema or chronic obstructive pulmonary disease (COPD) is made. Likewise, lectins can silently savage the absorptive layer of your intestine. In both situations, by the time the damage is apparent, it is thought to be too late for repairs. In my practice, I often see skinny people who cannot absorb nutrients no matter how much they eat. In fact, much of what we assume is a normal part of the aging process is actually the cumulative effect of lectin toxicity. But unlike COPD, this damage can be repaired! When a city is bombed in wartime, the residents flee and the city cannot be rebuilt until the bombing ceases and the people return. Think of lectins as incoming bombs. In order to repair the damage, you must stop eating lectins—and I am going to show you how.

A Symbiotic Relationship

THE MAJOR ROLE your microbes play in essential jobs such as digestion, elimination, and gut health is just the tip of the iceberg. Microbes are also the main defenders of your health. They constitute a complex ecosystem and are in constant communication with your brain and the rest of your body, sending and receiving messages.[4] Long before instant messaging became a way for us to communicate via our electronic devices, these microbes have been transmitting messages back and forth to control our hormones, our appetite, and our preferred foods, among other functions.

You and your microbes coexist in what biologists call a mutually symbiotic relationship. Your existence depends upon them and their existence depends upon you. The animal kingdom offers many examples of symbiosis. For example, a water bird known as a plover picks food off the teeth of a crocodile. The bird gets its dinner and the croc gets clean teeth, which enables it to keep hunting. Other birds, such as the oxpecker, or tickbird, ride around on the backs of large African mammals, consuming the annoying insects that flock to them. As just one example of the symbiotic relationship with your holobiome, certain microbes on your skin will fight to the death to heal a wound and protect you from other microbes that would harm you. The "good" microbes defend you because you and they are in a symbiotic relationship. The deal is that you feed them and they protect you.

As such, your gut buddies are invested in the care and upkeep of their home. They even communicate their happiness by making most of the feel-good hormones, such as serotonin, for you. (If you are taking an antidepressant, let me assure you that your gut buddies have left the building!) However, if you alter this relationship, the roles can change. Drive off the good bugs or let the bad bugs in, and it's as though gang members have taken over a pleasant neighborhood. They have no interest in the care and upkeep of you; they are only out for themselves. They also hijack the ancient communication system between the normal gut denizens and your brain, making you crave the foods that *they* need; namely sugars, fats, junk foods, and fast foods. This hijacking operation is just another reminder that it's not your fault that you're tired, sick, or overweight.

This complex system normally enables the various inhabitants and cells of your holobiome to communicate and coexist. As strange as it may seem, these single-celled organisms are intelligent beings, which act just as you (or any other complex multicelled organism) do. Have the right bugs within you, and give them what they want, and not only does no one get hurt, but you and they also thrive. But let the bad ones take over, and you get taken over as a consequence. Although it is hard to believe, "they" control most of you. And in just the last fifty years, numerous factors have changed dramatically, resulting in an untoward disruption of the normal communication systems within your body and its microbes.

In the next chapter, I will introduce you to what I call the Seven Deadly Disruptors, which with your broken gut have conspired to allow lectins, LPSs, and other foreign invaders into your gut. At the most basic level, that's why you feel you aren't in sync with yourself.

The Brain-Gut Messaging Path

The vagus nerve, also called the sympathetic nervous system, is the largest nerve coming from the brain to the gut. It communicates orders to all the various organs in your body. Recently, exciting studies have shown that lectins reach the brain not only through the blood but, shockingly, also by climbing the vagus nerve from the gut into the brain.[5] It turns out that for every fiber leading from the brain to your heart, lungs, and your abdominal organs, there are nine times as many fibers leading up to the brain from the gut. There are actually more neurons in your gut than in your entire spinal cord. You truly have a second brain within your gut, and that brain is controlled by your holobiome. Unlike what I and most other doctors were taught in medical school, the vagus nerve exists to get information to the brain from the gut, not the other way around. I tell my patients that when they have a gut instinct, they are absolutely right!

A Shift in the Balance of Power

AS LONG AS the good bugs are in the majority, you should be in good shape, but when the bad guys dominate, problems prevail. Fostering the right mix of microbes is essential to restoring health and preventing disease. You must feed the good microbes what they need to thrive, while simultaneously eliminating sugar and other foods on which bad microbes feast. Like any host, you must feed your guests as well as yourself, and in this case, in order to nourish yourself, you must first nourish the good microbes.

That seems simple enough, and it is why many well-meaning health gurus ask you to take probiotics and eat fermented foods. But not so fast. Even good bugs need to stay on their side of the intestinal border. If you have good bugs and you take an Advil or Aleve, or swallow some acid blockers, or eat lectins that you aren't designed to interact with, your intestinal wall is breached, and the nuclear meltdown occurs—despite having plenty of good bugs!

Ultimately, though, due to changes in the food supply, over-the-counter and prescription drugs, and environmental factors that have occurred imperceptibly over the last half century, most of your ancestral personal microbes have been destroyed, enabling others to dominate.[6] Regardless of how aware you may have been of your holobiome, the fact is that it has been disrupted. And the reason you, like so many other people, are not enjoying perfect health is that your relationship with your microbes (along with a number of environmental triggers) has changed. If you are overweight, likely the same forces are at work. Instead of working symbiotically with you, your microbes are incapable of providing valuable information—and worse yet, they may convey false information, much as a virus can take over your computer, inserting new data that leaves your system vulnerable.

Don't despair. There is light at the end of the tunnel. Once you understand the root causes of your health problems, including the tendency to pack on extra pounds, I'll reveal the details of the program proven to repair your damaged gut and restore your body to health and vitality.

From Ninety-Eight-Pound Weakling to Champion

The parents of Michael V., an emaciated thirteen-year-old, brought him to see me. Michael's father was a wrestling coach, but his son was skin and bones and clearly needed help. They had heard that I could cure Crohn's disease, which he had suffered from thanks to having taken antibiotics much of his life to treat a chronic tonsil infection. The immunosuppressant drugs he was taking for the Crohn's were not helping, and the diarrhea and bloody stools were clearly taking their toll.

The boy was ready to try anything, including giving up the foods any teenager loves. We dove in and together we banished lectins from his diet and rebuilt his gut wall with high-dose vitamin D_3, prebiotics, and probiotics. Within three months, Michael's bloody diarrhea and cramps were gone, and he started gaining weight—he even started training with his dad.

Even though it was hard for the boy to stay on the program, whenever he cheated, he immediately felt it in his gut, making it easier to stay on track. The peer pressure was tough, but he kept telling me that feeling well never tasted so good. With each visit, we tapered his immunosuppressant cocktail until it was gone. By that point, he was in high school, and he had joined the wrestling team.

Michael is now a vigorous, muscular, handsome young man. Last year, father and son came to my office. His dad was carrying the sports section of the local paper. It featured a lead story about his son, who had nearly wasted away five years earlier—and was now a division winner of the California State Wrestling Championship. He is now off to college with a sports scholarship.

Beating Back the Gut Busters

IN THE NEXT chapter, you'll learn how to identify and then avoid or eliminate the Seven Deadly Disruptors, which have opened the door to lectins and other gut busters. These disruptors are playing a major role in changing you and your gut microbes, and they have been controlling you for some time now—feeding you and your holobiome information via the food you eat, the beverages you drink, the personal care products you use, the household cleaners you use, and even the containers that hold your food and beverages. All have altered you (or your parents) and our microbes over the last fifty-something years. All are subtle, invisible, and undetectable. And all have allowed lectins through your gut wall, making you the victim of ongoing autoimmune attacks and hormonal disruptions.

As we'll soon see, proper diet and certain supplements are key components of what will become your gut protection and repair strategy. And effective as this dietary approach is, it needs to be accompanied by certain lifestyle changes.

Know Thy Enemy

The Seven Deadly Disruptors

There is an infamous experiment you've probably heard of. Drop a frog into a pot of very hot water, and it will jump right out. But put it in a pot of lukewarm water and slowly raise the temperature, and it will blissfully sit there until it boils to death. The difference in the two outcomes is simply because the change in temperature is so gradual that it is imperceptible to the frog's temperature receptors, or pattern matchers.

Like that frog, so subtle have the changes within your body been that you, too, have barely noticed. All these big things that have profoundly altered you arise from very small things. Each negative alteration of your body impacts your health, which, in turn, means that you crave more unhealthy foods and/or need more drugs or medical procedures. We have become dependent on many of these products and procedures, which *appear* to improve our health and standard of living, but actually make us sicker and potentially hasten our death. Meanwhile, the most heavily funded healthcare system in the world is collapsing from the resulting financial burden, aggravated by the needs of an ever increasing number of patients.

Living Longer but Not as Well

THERE IS A misconception that our collective health has improved significantly in recent decades. (If that is indeed the case, then why are we so overweight as a nation?) Much of that idea is based on the fact that the average life expectancy has increased over the last five decades. In 1960, average life expectancy for American men was 66.4 years; by 2013, it was a full ten years longer.[1] For women, the average ages were 73.1 and 81.1, respectively. But you have to understand that this data is heavily weighted by dramatic reductions in recent decades in the prevalence of infectious diseases, which disproportionally impacted infants and children. This phenomenon is the real reason life expectancy appears to have risen dramatically over half a century. Vaccines now protect youngsters from killer epidemics of measles, German measles, mumps, diphtheria, typhoid fever, scarlet fever, whooping cough, influenza, and other infectious diseases. Antibiotics have saved millions more lives from conditions that once often proved fatal. Infant mortality has also dropped significantly, thanks to improvements in prenatal care and childbirth practices. In 1935, fifty-six of every thousand children did not survive their first year. By 2006, this number was down to fewer than six kids per thousand,[2] although black children are still far more likely than white children to succumb to disease. Moreover, the United States still lags behind twenty-five of the other richest countries in its infant mortality rate.[3]

Life expectancy is a critical gauge of any society, of course, but equally important is what I call health expectancy. Even if we are living longer, are we living better? These days, for most people, a vast amount of their later life is spent in a state of progressive decline. Despite the belief that "fifty is the new forty" and other such hopeful claims, we are collectively far less healthy than our parents were at a comparable age. A new study reveals that from about fifty onward our health begins to decline, far earlier than was previously assumed.[4] However, unless you are fortunate enough to be a "canary," you are likely outwardly unaware of this decline.

We also take a lot more medications. When my patients first come to me, they are on an average of seven different drugs. Is this any way to live? I have a better idea: Die young—at a very old age. Or as Liping Zhao, a Chinese holobiome researcher, puts it, "Eat right. Stay fit. Live long. Die quick." I believe that this is what most people want for themselves.

How do we compare with the rest of the world's population? Globally, the United States doesn't fare very well in the life expectancy department, ranking thirty-fifth. Japan, on the other hand, ranks second. But then things get interesting. Americans spend on average of $8300 per person annually on health care, but only $2200 for food. The Japanese spend $3300 and $3200 on health care and food, respectively.[5] What does that say about our priorities?

Over the last half century, we have artificially but effectively propped up life span with a host of medical procedures, drugs, and treatments. A person with dementia might live for decades if s/he is well cared for, but is that living well? As a heart surgeon, I have done my part to extend the lives of thousands of individuals, and the devices I've invented make heart surgery safer, so patients are more likely to survive an operation and go on to live for years more. Meanwhile, the number of people living with type 2 diabetes and other serious health problems has also increased geometrically. The period of senescence, of growing old, has extended significantly, with huge increases in health-care costs for older people. Just to be clear, I'm not advocating letting people die when medical intervention can prolong their lives; however, I am making a distinction between quality of life and years of life.

By the way, to puncture another myth, there have always been people who were fortunate enough to avoid or survive the diseases that once killed so many children and adults and live well into their nineties. Just visit a churchyard in one of the original thirteen colonies and you will see the evidence engraved on their gravestones.

Invisible but Insidious Damage

MOST OF YOU will be surprised to learn that substances you use every day, eat every day, and drink every day—substances that you have been told are good for you—have been altered such that they can completely change the way your cells communicate with not only other human cells, but also the organisms that make up the "other you." And these changes have largely come about within the last fifty years.

Could it be that we're just like that frog sitting in the pot of water? What if each of us is being attacked every day, but the assault is virtually imperceptible—imperceptible, that is, until the water is boiling? Well, if you have any of the conditions listed on pages 68–70, guess what? The water is already boiling. But who lit the fire?

I have startling evidence that at least seven subtle changes that have occurred in the last fifty or so years have completely, and potentially irrevocably, altered your health. We have been subjected to new patterns in food and, even more recently, new ways of processing food, and to new personal care products that mimic a whole different set of compounds. At the same time, environmental toxins and electric lights have utterly changed our environment. Thanks to these disruptors, or rogue pattern matchers, you really aren't "yourself" anymore. You've already learned about two other disruptors: whole grains and transglutaminase. As a reminder, whole grains directly introduce lectins, particularly the protein wheat germ agglutinin (WGA) into your gut. They both initiate the intestinal leakage of LPSs into your bloodstream and incite hormone mimicry. And consuming transglutaminase sensitizes you to glutens even if you're not gluten-sensitive.

SUCCESS STORY

The "Healthy" Hoax

When she came to me, seventy-six-year-old Jennifer U. had rheumatoid arthritis and elevated inflammation markers, which we abolished and returned to normal numbers by following the Plant Paradox Program. This was all good news until Jennifer started eating Dave's Killer Bread. She assumed it was healthy because it was made with a variety of whole grains and promised to "rock your world." (One loaf contains no less than twenty-one grains and seeds!) Almost immediately, all her inflammation and rheumatoid markers skyrocketed and she reexperienced the severe joint pain that had gone away. Not surprisingly, when I had her eliminate the well-named bread, all her markers returned to normal.

Not only do these disruptors, along with the seven that follow, wreak havoc on your health, they also predispose you to gain weight. They feed you information via the food you eat, the beverages you drink, the medications you take, and even the food containers and personal care products you use. And that information transforms you unwittingly into a weight-gaining machine, no matter what you do.

DISRUPTOR 1: Broad-Spectrum Antibiotics

Over the last fifty to sixty years, our culture has experienced a number of momentous changes in health and disease prevention, but medical improvements can be a double-edged sword, akin to the plant paradox. Like plants, they keep you alive, but they can also kill you. A sterling example of such a medical advance is broad-spectrum antibiotics, which were initially considered miracle drugs. Developed in the late 1960s and early 1970s, broad-spectrum antibiotics are capable of killing multiple strains of bacteria simultaneously. (Most antibiotics used these days are this type.) Indeed, they have saved and continue to save countless lives from diseases such as pneumonia and septicemia. However, these antibiotics effectively allowed doctors to carpet-bomb an infection without worrying about exactly which bacterium was the culprit. We doctors were so impressed with these antibiotics that we used them, and sadly still do, even in situations where our best guess is that a virus, which isn't killed by antibiotics, is the culprit.

Little did we know at the time that we were also carpet-bombing ourselves. How so? Every time you take a course of Levaquin, ciprofloxacin, or another broad-spectrum antibiotic for a urinary-tract or another infection, you kill most of the microbes in your gut. Shockingly, it can take up to two years for them to return. Many may be gone forever. Even worse, each time a child takes antibiotics, the likelihood increases of him or her developing Crohn's disease, diabetes, obesity, or asthma later in life.[6]

Today, there is a greater understanding of bacteria than there used to be. Many species we once regarded as bad are now considered beneficial. Think of it this way: Your holobiome is like a mature rain forest, an incredibly complex ecosystem where one species' existence is dependent on several others for survival. Now imagine that you just burned that rain forest to the ground with napalm, Agent Orange, or a carelessly discarded match. Even if you immediately replanted seeds for all the trees and plants—the same way that people try to reseed their guts with probiotics—do you really think you will have a mature rain forest in a few weeks? Now imagine that every time your rain forest started to grow back, you hit it again with another round of napalm—comparable to taking a broad-spectrum antibiotic just because you have a cold that gave you an annoying cough. There is an ongoing scorched-earth pattern where there should be a luxuriant green forest. Don't get me wrong, targeted antibiotics can be lifesaving; but you should be very cautious about taking broad-spectrum antibiotics for anything other than a life-threatening infection.

And our consumption of antibiotics doesn't just come from filling a doctor's prescription. Almost all American chicken or beef contains enough antibiotics to kill bacteria in a petri dish! You can bet that it indiscriminately kills the friendly bacteria in your gut. Until recently, it was perfectly legal to give organic free-range chickens aresenic, producing a "healthy" pink blush. Wait, isn't arsenic a poison? Right you are. Besides being a poison and an antibiotic, arsenic is also a hormone disruptor that mimics the action of estrogen. A bill to ban the use of arsenic in chicken feed in Maryland was once defeated by a generous grant from Monsanto, which makes arsenic, to the campaigns of Maryland state senators.[7] The bill did later pass, and in 2013 the FDA banned the use of three of the four forms of arsenic nationally.[8] However, the fourth form, nitarsone, was exempted. As this book goes to press, it appears the FDA will finally ban this form as well. In addition, both soybeans and corn are used in chicken feed, and both of these products also contain estrogenlike substances. Ultimately, that "healthy" chicken breast boasts the equivalent of one birth control pill's worth of estrogenic substances!

The Risky Business of Diminished Efficacy

I was in medical school in the 1970s when *Clostridium difficile,* which had been a relatively marginal microbe found in the colon, suddenly began to kill lots of people. The reason was that broad-spectrum drugs had come along and wiped out all sorts of microbes, including protective ones, in our intestinal tract. And when the good guys were gone, a gang member like *Clostridium difficile* stepped up and overran the colon. We should have realized that carpet-bombing would have such consequences, and indeed today, bacteria known as superbugs are resistant to these antibiotics, creating a potentially life-threatening situation for certain individuals. An epidemic, widespread resistance to certain antibiotics could have disastrous consequences.

More recently, the heavy use of Baytril (Cipro's sister drug) to treat poultry against *E. coli* and a bacterial infection associated with respiratory disease has resulted in increased resistance on the part of humans who are given Cipro to combat a bacterial infection.[9] The FDA has acknowledged that human resistance is troubling. But a turkey farmer is not going to dose a single sick turkey with Baytril; instead, he adds the antibiotic to the water supply for the whole flock. And the problem doesn't stop with Baytril, which is one of a class of powerful drugs known as fluoroquinolones.

The FDA, physicians, and consumer groups are all concerned that Baytril's heavy use on animals could make humans resistant to Cipro, which is used to treat salmonella, campylobacter, and other food-borne diseases (as well as anthrax) in humans. This means that if a person consumes bacteria in inadequately cooked meat or handles such meat improperly and becomes ill, s/he may not respond to treatment with Cipro. In fact, the urology team at my hospital has found that at least 50 percent of all women with urinary-tract infections carry bugs that are resistant to Cipro.

Broad-spectrum antibiotics make pigs, chickens, and other animals grow faster, larger, and fatter. And if they have that effect in animals, it's unsurprising that they'd do the same to humans. Believe it or not, a single dose of antibiotics taken by a woman during pregnancy can make her children fat. A single round of antibiotics given to a child can make him or her obese. By altering your intestinal flora, which communicate with your immune system, antibiotics cause your body to go into a war state, increasing fat storage so your immune cells have all the fuel they need to fight off these invaders. And antibiotic residues from the flesh and milk of animals only magnify the effect when a person also takes broad-spectrum antibiotics.

SUCCESS STORY

Antibiotics Induced Crohn's Disease

Sara Y. is a seventy-one-year-old woman who was given repeated antibiotic doses for six weeks for a recurrent urinary-tract infection. She began to develop severe abdominal pain, followed by bloody diarrhea and severe joint pain and arthritis. Despite no previous history of gastrointestinal problems, a colonoscopy revealed Crohn's disease. Then, rather than connecting the dots, her doctor referred her to a rheumatologist who advised treatment with immunosuppressants (you see such drugs advertised daily on television). Thankfully, Sara refused a drug-based medical treatment and instead sought my help. By eliminating lectins from her diet and rebuilding the "rain forest" in her gut with the Plant Paradox Program, she cured herself in six months.

DISRUPTOR 2: Nonsteroidal Anti-Inflammatory Drugs (NSAIDs)

Known by the pharmaceutical industry as "gateway drugs" to more powerful painkillers, ibuprofen (Advil and Motrin), naproxen (Aleve), Celebrex, Mobic, and other nonsteroidal anti-inflammatory drugs (NSAIDs) were introduced in the early 1970s as an alternative to aspirin, which was known to damage the stomach lining. However, we now know that NSAIDs damage the mucosal barrier in the small intestine and colon, allowing lectins, LPSs, and other foreign substances to pass through the intestinal wall, initiating a war within your body. Evidence of the war is increasing inflammation, which you feel as pain. And the more pain you have, the more NSAIDs you take.

How could we not have known this? Actually, the pharmaceutical companies did,[10] but because our gastroscopes didn't reach that far, we doctors initially had no methods of seeing damage in the small intestine. It wasn't until we had camera pills you could swallow that we realized what was really happening, and by then NSAIDs were ubiquitous. Remember that poor woman with the intestinal webs? NSAIDs had so destroyed the walls of her gut that massive amounts of scar tissue had formed. That whole process opens up pathways to more invaders, while setting up a vicious cycle: the more LPSs that escape, the more pain; the more pain, the more you use NSAIDs—until you graduate to the big boys, the prescription painkillers. NSAIDs are both the number-one pharmaceutical seller and the number-one health menace. So, remember this: Swallowing one Advil or Aleve is like swallowing a hand grenade. Also remember: The precursors of Advil and Aleve, ibuprofen and Naprosyn, were recognized as so dangerous when they were introduced in the 1970s that they were available only as prescription drugs.

SUCCESS STORY

The Student Who Came in from the Cold

An avid rock climber and college student in Colorado, Emily J. had injured her ankle in a fall about six months earlier. Her orthopedist had treated her with high doses of Motrin and Aleve, but after about a month into this therapy, she noticed that her hands and feet were turning blue and that cold weather seemed to intensify the problem. This condition, known as Raynaud's syndrome, is now believed to be an autoimmune problem. Soon, Emily couldn't even hold a pen and had to leave college. Hoping that the warm climate would provide relief, she came to spend the winter with her grandmother in Palm Springs. When things didn't improve, she sought the help of a local yoga master and massage therapist, who referred her to me. When I met Emily, her hands and feet were cold and blue. Once I had heard her story, I knew that her gut barrier had been breached by NSAIDs the orthopedist had prescribed, and that lectins and LPSs were on the loose in her system. Blood work confirmed these assumptions, as well as a telltale low level of vitamin D, despite the fact that she was taking a large amount daily. We instituted the Plant Paradox Program, started her on probiotics and prebiotics, and pushed her blood level of vitamin D to 100 ng/ml. Two weeks later, her hands and feet were changing color and within six weeks had returned to normal. Emily resumed her studies in Colorado and has never looked back, except to say thank you.

DISRUPTOR 3: Stomach-Acid Blockers

Let me count the reasons acid-blocking drugs such as Zantac, Prilosec, Nexium, and Protonix are to be avoided at all costs. Most of these drugs are proton pump inhibitors (PPIs), which reduce the amount of stomach acid. However, as long as it stays where it belongs, stomach acid serves an important function.

The acid in the stomach is so powerful that only a few important bacteria can tolerate it as their home; as a result, many of the bad bacteria that you swallow never make it out alive. (By the way, unless they are in spore form or enteric-coated, most of those expensive probiotic bacteria products you consume never make it out of your stomach alive either!) Acids from the stomach normally confine bacteria to the large intestine through a process called the acid gradient. As the contents from the stomach move farther down the intestine, more alkaline fluids from the bile and pancreas gradually dilute the acid, but it is only when food reaches the colon that the acid is finally sufficiently diluted. Bacteria in the colon, where most of our gut bugs live, typically like an oxygen-free, low-acid environment.

Now here's the problem: without stomach acid to kill "bad" bacteria, these pathogenic (disease-producing) bacteria can overgrow, further altering normal gut flora. Moreover, lacking stomach acid, bad bacteria and even good bacteria can easily crawl up from their designated home in the colon into your small intestine, where they don't belong. There they either disrupt the gut barrier, the condition generally called leaky gut, or cause a condition called SIBO (small intestine bacterial overgrowth). Once in your small intestine, where they are *not* supposed to live, the bacterial cell walls (LPSs) and lectins have easy access into your circulatory system. This in turn stimulates your immune system to combat the incoming threats from LPSs and lectins with—you guessed it—inflammation! And with that comes weight gain, as your body stores fat to fuel your white blood cells' battle with the enemies.

The use of PPIs, such as Prilosec and Nexium, doesn't just interfere with the proper functioning of your stomach acid. PPIs not only stop stomach acid production, but also can kill off your mitochondria's ability to produce energy in every cell in the body via their own proton pumps. Remarkably, these PPIs cross the blood-brain barrier and poison your brain's mitochondria. One study showed a 44 percent increased risk of dementia among 74,000 people aged seventy-five and older who had used these drugs, compared with those who did not.[11] Other studies have linked the use of PPIs to chronic kidney disease for the same reason.[12] We have been systematically poisoning the energy-producing organelles in every one of our cells just to have another piece of pepperoni pizza. Because of these risks, all these over-the-counter drugs, as well as their prescription counterparts, come with a warning that you should never take them for more than two weeks. Nonetheless, many people toss them down for years, resulting in serious damage. When these acid blockers were introduced in the 1980s, they were considered so dangerous that they had to be prescribed by a physician. Seeing a pattern here?

The use of acid reducers also prompts a totally new population of intestinal bugs—those which are normally killed off by our stomach acid and are extremely foreign to our immune system—to grow in place of our normal bugs. People who use acid blockers have three times the likelihood of getting pneumonia,[13] which these foreign bugs cause, than those who don't use such drugs. If that isn't bad enough, acid-blocking drugs also foster incomplete protein digestion. Since lectins are proteins, acid blockers therefore allow more lectins into the gut.

Finally, because stomach acid is necessary to break down dietary protein into amino acids before they can be absorbed in your gut, we have produced an entire generation of senior citizens who are protein malnourished. That's not because they aren't eating enough protein; instead, it is because they have no stomach acid to digest it! When protein can't be broken down and absorbed, it leads to muscle wasting, called sarcopenia, a health crisis among the elderly. In fact, regardless of age and the reason they are in the hospital, most patients admitted to the hospital have very low levels of protein, not because they aren't eating sufficient protein—in fact, they are eating too much, as I'll explain soon—but because they cannot turn it into the amino acids that can be absorbed, thanks to their regular intake of PPIs.

SUCCESS STORY

A Precancerous Condition Disappears

Elena J. was sixty-seven years old and had suffered from severe heartburn most of her life. A few years before Elena consulted me, her gastroenterologist had done a routine scope of her esophagus and taken some biopsies. The results confirmed that she had Barrett's esophagus, a precancerous lesion of the lower esophagus. She was treated with double doses of PPIs, but the more of these drugs she took, the weaker she became and the more her belly hurt. When she came to see me, Elena's blood work revealed classic lectin intolerance, and a low protein level—without acid in her stomach, she couldn't digest protein. I recommended that she follow the Plant Paradox Program and immediately stop taking Nexium and Protonix. "What about my gastroenterologist's advice and the Barrett's?" she asked. I assured her that as a cardiothoracic surgeon, I dealt with the esophagus daily and that we could handle any problem that came along. She dove in to the program, and to her surprise, her heartburn vanished and her stomach stopped hurting. Within six months, her protein levels had returned to normal. One year later, during her scheduled follow-up esophageal scope, her gastroenterologist was delighted to tell her that all signs of the Barrett's esophagus were gone, and her biopsies were negative. "Aren't you glad you took two different acid reducers?" he asked. She nodded politely, but hasn't seen him since. When I asked Elena why she didn't tell him what she had really done, she just sighed and said, "Do you really think he would have believed that?" She's right, but perhaps you will!

Forbidden Trojan Horses

I call the deadly disruptors "Trojan horses" because the enemy is hidden inside, just as problematic lectins lurk sneakily in many foods. Equally important to the dietary changes you will make in the Plant Paradox Program is the removal of products that are Trojan horses. In addition to eliminating broad-spectrum antibiotics (with your physician's permission, of course), you want to omit the sources of other deadly disruptors and replace them with neutral substitutes. Consult the lists below.

- **PAIN-RELIEVER ENEMIES:** Generic ibuprofen or Advil, Aleve, Naprosyn, Celebrex, Mobic, and other NSAIDs.
  - **Friendly Substitutes:** Boswellia or white willow bark.
- **ACID-REDUCER ENEMIES:** Zantac, Prilosec (omeprazole), Protonix, Nexium, and Imeprazole.
  - **Friendly Substitutes:** Rolaids are a low-sugar source of calcium carbonate. Also chew DGL wafers.
- **SLEEP-AID ENEMIES:** Ambien, Restoril, Lunesta, and Xanax.
  - **Friendly substitutes:** My favorite combination of sleep aids is in Schiff Melatonin Ultra, or buy time-release melatonin and take 3 to 6 mg before bed.

DISRUPTOR 4: Artificial Sweeteners

Products such as sucralose, saccharin, aspartame, and other non-nutritive artificial sweeteners alter the gut holobiome, killing good bacteria and allowing overgrowth of bad ones. Believe it or not, a Duke study showed that a single Splenda packet kills 50 percent of normal intestinal flora![14] And again, once the bad guys take over, you gain weight as a defense mechanism to ensure supplies for your army of defenders. Ironically, although such products are supposed to aid in weight loss, they do just the opposite.

In addition, sweet tastes, once available only in summer from ripe fruit and perhaps the occasional honeycomb, signal the body that it's time to store fat for winter, regardless of the actual season. (We now effectively live in endless summer with fruit and sweet treats made with real or fake sugar available year-round—and around the clock.) Taste buds for sweetness actually occupy two-thirds of the surface of your tongue. They are there to make sure that when high-caloric fruit or honey was available, your ancient ancestors were certain to eat it. Your taste buds don't actually taste sugar; rather, when a sugar molecule (or any other sweet substance) attaches to their receptor by fitting into the dock, they taste "sweet." The nerves from your tongue transmit this "sweet" information to your pleasure receptors (docks) in your brain, which is your reward center. It in turn urges you to get more of this great stuff because you just won the fruit tree lottery and you are going to be the big winner when winter arrives and there isn't much food around.

It's the Sweetness, Not the Sugar

Now here's the problem with artificial or even natural (think stevia) noncaloric sweeteners. Your body can't distinguish between the sweetness of sugar or other caloric sources and these calorie-free sweeteners. That's because the molecular structure (pattern) of the calorie-free sweeteners fits into the sugar-docking port on your taste buds and prompts the same pleasure signal to your brain that real sugar prompts. Then, when the calories from real sugar (glucose) don't arrive in your bloodstream and are not detected by glucose receptors in your brain, your brain feels cheated. It "knows" you are eating sugar because it "tasted" sugar, but it's really angry that the sugar didn't arrive and prompts you to get some more. Back you go, looking for more sweet tastes. That's why, despite drinking eight Diet Cokes a day—they were practically glued to my hand—I was once seventy pounds overweight. An avalanche of research proves that instead of aiding in weight loss or weight maintenance, nonnutritive sweeteners actually cause you to gain weight.

Listen to Your Internal Clock

Nonnutritive sweeteners and sweet tastes are also endocrine disruptors (discussed below) and disrupt the circadian rhythms of your body's internal clock, another trigger for weight gain. How so? All of your cells operate on a circadian clock; there's even a clock gene. Anyone who has traveled across time zones knows what jet lag feels like, and it happens because your circadian rhythm is disrupted. Almost all bodily functions operate in circadian fashion. Even your holobiome has circadian rhythms. Just as there are twenty-four-hour clocks, there are also moon cycle clocks (believe me, emergency room visits for crazy behavior follow full moon cycles) and seasonal clocks. These seasonal clocks are controlled not only by day length, but also by seasonal food availability. In the not-too-distant past, sweet tastes were not a year-round event. Instead, they correlated to fruit season, which always preceded winter, when food was of limited availability. Regardless of whether winter is a dry season, a wet season, or a cold season, there is cyclically less food in winter and more in summer. So when you eat sweet foods year-round, even if it is natural sugar from fruit, you disrupt this ancient rhythm and continually gain weight. As you will soon learn, the year-round availability of fruit is one of the largest contributors to our obesity crisis.

Artificial Sweetener Trojan Horses

- **THE ENEMY:** All artificial sweeteners, specifically saccharin (Sweet'n Low, Sweet Twin, and Necta Sweet), aspartame (Equal and NutraSweet), acesulfame K (also in Equal and NutraSweet), sucralose (Splenda), and neotame. Also steer clear of soft drinks or sports drinks, any health or protein bar that contains any of these sweeteners, as well as any form of sugar, including corn, agave syrup, or pure cane sugar. Ditto for any processed foods with such sweeteners.

- Friendly Substitutes: Stevia (SweetLeaf, which contains inulin), Just Like Sugar (made from chicory root), the sugar alcohols xylitol or erythritol (Swerve), yacón syrup, and inulin. Use all in moderation, particularly sugar alcohols, which can create gassiness and diarrhea.

- SPOILER ALERT: Any sweet taste, even from stevia, stimulates an insulin response that makes you want more, as discussed above.

DISRUPTOR 5: Endocrine Disruptors

Also called hormone disruptors, these low-dose estrogenlike agents are a diverse group, encompassing chemicals found in most plastics, scented cosmetics, preservatives, and sunscreens, and other products as diverse as cash register receipts, along with dichlorodiphenyldichloroethylene (DDE), which is a metabolite of dichlorodiphenyltrichloroethane (aka DDT), the insecticide lindane, and polychlorinated biphenyls (PCBs).[15] All regularly play havoc with our hormones. According to the Endocrine Society's second statement on endocrine disruptors, exposure to these powerful agents has been found to affect individuals and test animals (as well as their descendants) in multiple ways, some of which may not show up for years.[16] Problems include:

- Obesity, diabetes, and other metabolic diseases
- Both female and male reproductive issues
- Women's hormone-sensitive cancers
- Prostate problems

- Thyroid problems
- Impaired development of the brain and neuroendocrine systems

Problematic Preservatives

Many of the compounds in this class of agents are used as preservatives or stabilizers; a prime example is butyl hydroxytoluene (BHT), which is used in processed foods, including whole-grain products. With the advent of "healthy" whole-grain flour, the previously discarded omega-6 fat in the bran oxidizes and goes rancid unless there's a stabilizing agent like BHT to prevent spoilage. Bisphenol A (BPA) is used in lightweight plastic water bottles to make them tough and heat-resistant—and even in babies' teething rings![17]—as well as in the thin plastic lining of most canned goods to keep the metal from corroding and contaminating the contents. Parabens in cosmetics and sunscreens serve a similar purpose. Methylparaben, an estrogenlike compound, is also a major allergen, and is used to preserve most drug solutions in multiuse containers. If you thought that you were allergic to the painkiller novacaine at your dentist's office, it was actually the methylparaben in the bottle.

Recent research suggests that tert-butylhydroquinonet (tBHQ), a synthetic food preservative, may be responsible in part for the recent increase in food allergies.[18] The additive is used in numerous processed foods, including bread, waffles, crackers, and other baked goods, as well as nuts and cooking oil. The presence of tBHQ in a product need not be listed on the label. It seems that consuming tBHQ stimulates our T cells, which are key to our immune system, to release proteins that can stimulate an allergic response to foods such as wheat, milk, eggs, nuts, and shellfish. Under normal conditions, T cells release cytokines, which protect the body from invaders, but the presence of tBHQ constrains the normal action of T cells.

You probably know that antibacterial chemicals such as triclosan, found in hand sanitizers, soaps, deodorants, toothpaste, and countless other personal care products, destroy "good" microbes in your mouth and gut and and on your skin. However, you may not know that they also promote obesity by changing gut flora, as well as by acting like estrogen. And let me assure you that you need normal bugs in all of these places—including your mouth. These good bugs in your mouth are responsible for taking compounds that you exhale and converting them into a potent chemical that dilates your blood vessels and promotes normal blood pressure. The use of mouthwashes, which kill mouth bacteria as they give you that "minty clean" breath, dramatically increases blood pressure.[19] If you use mouthwash and have been told you need to take medication to lower your blood pressure, ditch the mouthwash ASAP. Triclosan in hand sanitizers and toothpaste has also been shown to produce bladder cancer and to stimulate precancerous cells to proliferate. The next time you enter the supermarket, step away from the sanitizer dispenser and no one gets hurt—especially your gut bugs.

Depletion of Vitamin D

Sunscreens prevent the absorption of vitamin D. But all the compounds discussed above, whether in sunscreens or other products, also lower your liver's ability to convert this critical vitamin to its active form. This prevents the regeneration of new cells in your protective intestinal wall barrier, allowing more lectins and LPSs through, along with other foreign bodies. Men with prostate cancer have very low levels of vitamin D. Despite the fact that my practice is in Southern California, I have found that almost 80 percent of my patients have low levels of vitamin D in their blood. In fact, anyone in my practice with leaky gut or autoimmune diseases has low levels. Lacking sufficient vitamin D, and in the face of repeated assaults on the walls of the intestine and the lack of ongoing repair to keep out lectins and LPSs, the body constantly senses that it is at war. It's not surprising, then, that most of my overweight and obese patients are also very deficient in vitamin D.[20] Such a deficiency also impedes the generation of new bone, setting the stage for the development of osteoporosis. My thin female patients with osteopenia and osteoporosis also have low levels of this critical vitamin when they first come to see me.

The Fat-Storage Hormone

Most hormone disruptors mimic the action of estrogen, whose main purpose is to tell cells to store fat in anticipation of an upcoming pregnancy. Now, 365 days a year, we store fat for an upcoming pregnancy regardless of our age or even our gender! Is it any wonder, then, that girls are coming into puberty at age eight or that guys have "man boobs" and a gut that looks suspiciously like they are about to give birth? Instead of hooking up to a receptor and then leaving, the way regular hormones do, estrogenlike compounds attach to a receptor and remain permanently switched on, disrupting normal messaging. The cumulative effect of these minute amounts of estrogenlike compounds is actually more powerful than the hormone itself would be.[21] BPA is banned in Canada and Europe, but in 2015 a lawsuit in the United States attempting to force the FDA to ban BPA was defeated, thanks to a large grant to congressional campaigns by the American Chemical Council, which opposed the bill.[22]

Fear Those Phthalates

If you find your tongue tripping over the word "phthalates," take it as a warning. These synthetic compounds, which began to appear early in the twentieth century, are ubiquitous. They are used to soften plastics—think wall coverings, vinyl flooring, the gloves you wear when washing dishes, the trays used to package meat and fish, the plastic wrap you cover leftovers with, even the toys your children play with, and on and on. Thanks to plastic wraps and plastic containers, phthalates are omnipresent in our foods. Phthalates also act as solvents in perfumed items, turning up in hair sprays, lubricants, insect repellents, and thousands of other household and personal care products. Specific chemicals in the phthalates family include equally difficult to pronounce names such as dicyclohexyl phthalate (DCHP), di-2-ethylhexyl phthalate (DEHP), di-n-octyl phthalate (DnOP), and bisphenol S (BPS).

Animal and human studies have associated phthalates with many examples of endocrine disruption, including smaller than usual testicles in rats.[23] The presence of highly concentrated phthalate metabolites in men's urine has been associated with damage to the DNA in sperm.[24] Being exposed to these chemicals at a young age may be associated with premature breast development in girls.[25] Babies whose umbilical cords reveal higher exposure to phthalates are more likely to have been born prematurely.[26] These compounds are major hormone disruptors, locking onto estrogen receptors in the fetal brain, as well as in you and your children. They also permanently attach to the thyroid hormone receptors on cells, blocking the real thyroid hormone from delivering its message. Think of a plane blocking the Jetway that you want to use.

Studies have been conducted in Europe, Canada, and China in an effort to establish how much of this class of chemicals is in their food supply, but the first American study did not take place until 2013.[27] It looked at a relatively pristine upstate New York population, and found that the major sources of phthalates in humans were obtained from (in order of rank) grains, beef, pork, chicken, and milk products. So, if you are tired and fat and your hair is thinning, and you are eating whole-grain foods and boneless skinless chicken breast, and your doctor assures you that your thyroid hormone levels are normal, so you can't be hypothyroid, think again. You may be *making* thyroid hormone, but it can't get into the gate and off the plane to talk to each of your cells because phthalates are blocking the way. These phthalate-laden "healthy foods" are some of the very items you will be omitting (or severely restricting) on the Plant Paradox Program.

Arsenic in Our Food—No Kidding

You'll recall that arsenic, which can be found in chicken, is a not just an antibiotic and a poison, but also a hormone disruptor. Chicken has become a large part of the standard American diet, replacing beef, lamb, pork, and other meats. But here's something to stop you in your tracks: The more chicken a pregnant woman consumes, the smaller her baby boy's penis[28] and shorter his attention span. Arsenic and phthalate contamination also influence his choice of toys and his behavior.[29] Research on rats suggests that greater chicken consumption, and therefore increased exposure to arsenic and phthalates, exposes the brains of male babies to estrogen mimetics in utero (in addition to the mother's real estrogen), which impacts sexual imprinting and potentially gender identity.

Another Reason to Avoid Bread

Would you want to eat your yoga mat? Well, azodicarbonamide, an endocrine disruptor that is employed as a foaming agent in the manufacture of synthetic leather products, carpet underlayment, and yoga mats, is also used to bleach flour and condition dough.[30] Most fast food restaurants, including Wendy's, McDonald's, Burger King, and Arby's, use it in some or all of their bread products. The use of azodicarbonamide in bread has been banned in Europe[31] and Australia. In this country, Subway has voluntarily eliminated it from its products.[32] Exposure to azodicarbonamide has been shown to provoke asthma and allergies,[33] as well as to suppress immune function,[34] particularly when it is heated or baked. Additionally, this chemical has been shown to break down gluten into its individual proteins, gliadin and glutinin, making them more immediately available and therefore more immediately irritating.

Endocrine Disruptor Trojan Horses

These powerful disruptors are in countless products. The following are just the tip of the iceberg.

- **ENEMIES:** Any food that uses BHT as a stabilizing agent, particularly commercial baked goods. Hint: It is likely that BHT has been added if the food comes in a wrapper or has the words "whole grain." (Don't forget that any cracker, bread, cookie, or "crunchy" bar probably also contains transglutaminase.) Food manufacturers are not required to list this chemical on the packaging.
  - **Friendly Substitute:** Homemade baked goods using approved flour substitutes (see page 201).
- **ENEMIES:** Teflon, the brand name for polytetrafluoroethylene (PTFE), and similar products used on nonstick cookware, as well as on stain-resistant fabrics and carpeting. Perfluorooctanoic octanoic acid (PFOA) is also used in some nonstick cookware.
  - **Friendly Substitute:** Use conventional cookware or those with a ceramic coating that are certified to contain no PTFE or PFOA made by T-fal, Amoré, Culina, and other manufacturers.

- **ENEMIES:** Containers made of BPA plastic.
  - **Friendly Substitutes:** Buy products (and store leftovers) in glass or stainless steel containers, which are nonreactive. Purchase canned foods only in BPA-free cans. Some bottled water is sold in non-BPA plastic, but it is debatable that these plastics are any safer. Just when you thought it was safe to get back in the water—pun intended—it turns out that BPS causes the same if not more problems as BPA.[35] Purchase a stainless steel or glass water bottle (one with a protective wrapper) and use your own tap or filtered water instead.
- **ENEMIES:** Plastic wrap and plastic bags.
  - **Friendly Substitutes:** Old-fashioned wax paper works, or reusable cloth sandwich bags (sold on Etsy).
- **ENEMIES:** Store and bank receipts printed with thermal paper, which may or may not contain BPA.
  - **Friendly Substitutes:** Have your bank receipt emailed to you. If you need the receipt from a store in case you have to return something, ask the salesperson to put it in the bag. When you get home, use kitchen tongs to remove it. Wash your hands after touching receipts. Photograph receipts with your smart phone and then get rid of them. Encourage vendors you use often to switch to BPA-free paper such as that made by Appleton.
- **ENEMIES:** Sunscreens with parabens, such as methylparaben. Avoid all sunscreens unless the active ingredient is titanium oxide. Also avoid scented products.
  - **Friendly Substitutes:** Check the Environmental Working Group (EWG) website for its Guide to Sunscreens, which includes some products without parabens: www.ewg.org/sun screen/.

- **ENEMIES:** Makeup with parabens.
  - Friendly Substitutes: The EWG also has a database of more than 62,000 cosmetic products without parabens: www.ewg.org /skindeep/.
- **ENEMIES:** Deodorants and antiperspirants that contain parabens or aluminum.
  - Friendly Substitutes: Again, EWG has analyzed and rated deodorants and antiperspirants as part of its cosmetics database: www.ewg.org/skindeep/browse/antiperspirant;deodorant. Acceptable brands include Be Green, Purely Great, and Penny Lane Organics.
- **ENEMIES:** Hand sanitizers with triclosan and all antibacterial soaps. Aside from all their health risks, there is no need to use such products. Soap and hot water are all you need.
- **ENEMIES:** Toothpastes with triclosan and its cousin triclocarban. Triclosan is also in certain mouthwashes and antibacterial toothbrushes. For a long list of other personal care products with this chemical, see http://drbenkim.com/articles/ triclosan-products.htm. Pass them all by. You also want to avoid toothpaste that contains sodium lauryl sulfate (SLS).
  - Friendly Substitutes: Jason, Face Natural, Desert Essence (Natural Tea Tree Oil or Neem flavor), and Trader Joe's Antiplaque No Fluoride All Natural (Peppermint or Fennel) toothpastes contain neither triclosan nor SLS. Ditto for my new favorite (despite its unappealing name): The Dirt's Natural Organic Fluoride Free Toothpaste with MCT Coconut Oil.
  - Tom's of Maine products contain no triclosan, and its Botanically Bright line offers two SLS-free products.

DISRUPTOR 6: Genetically Modified Foods and the Herbicide Roundup

Herbicides, insecticides, and pesticides are different forms of biocides. Herbicides kill weeds, allowing a crop plant to grow without having to compete for water and nutrients with other species. Insecticides have helped reduce the number of victims of mosquito-borne diseases, while pesticides have improved crop yield and provided food for billions who would have likely otherwise died of starvation. But the unintended consequences of biocides are just as momentous. They have introduced powerful poisons into our systems from the food we eat, even the produce we touch, and sadly, the animals we eat. These poisons hack in via our intestinal tract or our skin, unleashing genetic programs within us, as well as in other animals and plants. The compounds are rogue pattern matchers that turn genes on or off within our cells, fundamentally changing the signaling within the body.[36]

The herbicides Roundup, made by Monsanto, and Enlist, made by Dow Chemical, both contain 2,4-D (an ingredient in the notorious Agent Orange) and glyphosate. Traces of both these major disruptors are found in the meat and milk of animals that are fed grains and beans, as well as in crop plants and products made with them.

A brief history is in order here. Genetically modified organisms (GMOs) were created by inserting foreign genes into plants, with the objective of making the plant either produce more of its own insecticides (lectins) or produce resistance to Roundup. In theory, Roundup would kill the weeds around the crop, leaving the GMO plant protected. Sounds logical.

Short-term studies suggested that the residual Roundup on the grains or beans would cause no harm to humans, as we lack what is called the shikimate pathway, or the plant pathway that Roundup uses to paralyze weeds, thus leading to their death. As a result, Roundup was approved as safe by the FDA. So what's the problem? First, the GMO plant produces novel proteins and/or lectins that our bar-code scanners recognize as foreign, causing inflammation when we eat them. Second, when Roundup is sprayed on a GMO crop, the crop can withstand the chemical onslaught while the nearby weeds wither and die. However, industrial farmers now routinely apply Roundup as a desiccant to non-GMO crops as well. A dried-up dead plant makes it easier to harvest wheat, corn, soybean, beans, and canola on a fixed schedule, saving time and money with a single sweep of the field.

Now, if you naïvely think that Roundup is washed off the harvested grains before they are processed, I've got some oceanfront property here in Palm Springs to sell you. That glyphosate remains on the grains and beans and is fed to our livestock in feed lots and incorporated into their fat, meat, and milk, which you then eat or drink. Almost all grains and beans fed to industrial farm animals are also GMO. These altered genes have been found not only in the meats of these animals, but also in the milk of nursing mothers and the umbilical cord blood of their infants! But, worse, since Roundup is used to harvest almost all non-GMO grains and beans as well, you consume it directly via these "healthy" foods, because the outer part of the grain, once routinely stripped away in processing, is now left on for "whole-grain goodness."[37] Roundup is then delivered into your gut where it does its real damage.

Just like plants, gut bacteria utilize the shikimate pathway, and they do so to make three essential amino acids: tryptophan, tyrosine, and phenylalanine. Since animals lack this pathway, our only source of these essential amino acids is via our gut bugs. Tryptophan and phenylalanine make serotonin, the essential "feel good" hormone, while tyrosine and phenylalanine are essential for thyroid hormone production. But when we eat GMO foods or conventionally grown foods harvested with Roundup, the shikimate pathway is blocked and our gut bacteria are unable to produce these essential amino acids.

Let me reiterate this critical point: Because non-GMO foods are now routinely harvested by spraying Roundup on them, and given the fact that all livestock and poultry are fed these grains and beans, you get a double whammy of Roundup even if you avoid GMO crops. Is it any wonder my skinny whole-grain-eating female patients were on antidepressants and thyroid medication? The glyphosate in whole grains, soybeans, and other beans had poisoned these women's own production of serotonin and tyrosine. This not only paralyzes the shikimate pathway and hinders our supply of those three amino acids, but also alters the composition of our normal gut flora by causing good gut bugs to die off.

That's a lot to take in, but here's the worst part. Our normal gut bugs have evolved to eat gluten. If you kill these guys off by eating gluten-containing foods, beans, or soy that has been sprayed with Roundup, you suddenly lose your main defense that made gluten harmless for the vast majority of us. That means you, too, become gluten-sensitive. On top of that, Roundup also bonds with gluten, making it antigenic (capable of inducing an immune response) even to people who aren't sensitive to gluten itself.[38] But wait, I'm not done yet. Roundup also paralyzes key liver enzymes (cytochrome P450 enzymes) that convert vitamin D to a form that your body can use to recycle cholesterol—meaning Roundup effectively raises your cholesterol! Plus, you need that vitamin D to foster repair of your now-damaged gut wall.[39]

Again: you are what you eat, and what the things you are eating, ate.

Frightening Results

In 2015, the International Agency for Research, the cancer agency of the World Health Organization, declared glyphosate, the active ingredient in Roundup, a "probable human carcinogen."[40] As a result, the Organic Consumers Association (OCA) and the Feed the World Project (now the Detox Project) teamed up to offer the public the opportunity to have their water or urine tested for glyphosate, the active ingredient in Roundup. The response was so overwhelming that testing has temporarily been suspended, pending construction of a larger lab. But the results of the first 131 individuals who submitted specimens are staggering. According to results released in May 2016, 93 percent of the urine samples tested positive for glyphosate, with children showing the highest levels. (No glyphosate turned up in water samples.) People who lived in the western and midwestern states generally had higher levels than individuals in other parts of the United States. Presumably, because the OCA partnered this program, the test subjects were more likely to consume organic foods than the general public, meaning that either organic food has been contaminated or there are other as yet unknown sources of glyphosate. A laboratory at the University of California San Francisco did the testing, the first such comprehensive and validated project conducted in this country.

The organizers of the testing program are hoping not only to inform the public of the risks of glyphosate, but also to persuade the U.S. Environmental Protection Agency to ban the chemical, which is currently under review. Meanwhile, the U.S. Department of Agriculture (USDA) does not currently test food for glyphosate residues, citing the high cost as a deterrent. However, the FDA announced in early 2016 that it would begin testing foods such as soybeans, corn, milk, and eggs at some unspecified future date.[41]

(The OCA and Detox Project are now offering food testing to non-governmental organizations and commercial companies only for $176 per sample.)

The United States lags behind other countries in examining and addressing risks posed by glyphosate. In 2013, El Salvador banned this endocrine-disrupting agent because it was linked to the deaths of thousands of agricultural workers from chronic kidney disease. And the European Union continues to ban the use of Roundup in EU countries, a position diametrically opposed to that of the United States.

The permit for continued use of glyphosate is up for renewal in 2017 in the United States, amid fierce debate on its risks and merits. There are some efforts to ban the use. A growing number of scientists are risking attack by the biotech industry by releasing studies that link glyphosate to cancer, kidney and liver failure, birth defects, infertility, increased risk of allergies, and digestive issues, among other chronic illnesses.[42] Sealed documents reveal that Monsanto has been aware of the devastating health effects of the chemical for forty years.[43]

According to Ronnie Cummins, the international director of the OCA, in a press release announcing the program for testing water and urine for Roundup, "We hope that at the very least, states—and eventually the federal government—will require mandatory labeling of foods containing genetically modified organisms, 84 percent of which are grown with glyphosate and likely contain residues of the chemical. But ultimately, this dangerous chemical must be banned."[44]

Ironically, the use of GMO crops was supposed to increase production levels of crops and reduce the use of herbicides. But according to an in-depth examination by the *New York Times*, using data from the Food and Agricultural Department of the United Nations, the Union of Industries of Plant Protection (France), the U.S. Geological Survey, and the USDA's National Agriculture Statistics Service, these promises have not been realized.[45]

In actuality, crop yield per acre in Canada and the United States has indeed increased over the last twenty years, after GMO crops were introduced. However, they have also increased, and often at a higher rate, in Western Europe, which banned GMO crops and relies solely on conventionally grown agriculture. Moreover, in the last decade, the use of the herbicides, including the weed killer Roundup, has increased dramatically in the United States in this time frame. Meanwhile, France has reduced its herbicide use dramatically.

Glyphosate and GMO Trojan Horses

- **ENEMY:** Roundup and similar products.
  - **Friendly Substitute:** Mix a gallon of white vinegar with a cup of salt and a tablespoon of liquid dishwashing soap; spray that mixture on weeds. There are a number of variations on this recipe, including lemon juice instead of white vinegar and Epsom salts instead of salt.
- **ENEMY:** GMO foods.
  - **Friendly Substitute:** Organic foods.

Become a Code Breaker

Once you are attuned to the following terms, you will find them on a remarkable number of food products. Don't be fooled by their positive or at the very least innocuous-sounding implications.

You want to stay away from all products with these labels. Here are the real meanings of these coded messages:

Coded Message	Translation
"All vegetarian feed"	Contains grains, pseudo-grains, and/or soy, all likely GMO. Often found on poultry products.
"Free-range"	According to a 2007 federal law, chickens labeled free-range (or cage-free) can be crammed inside a warehouse and fed corn and soy-beans as long as a door to a small patch of grass is left open for at least 5 minutes a day. Of course, under crowded conditions, most chickens never see the light of day.
"Gluten-free"	More sugar and lectins than the gluten-containing product it re-placed.
"All natural"	So are hurricanes, tornadoes, earth-quakes, and arsenic! This is a mean-ingless term, as neither the FDA nor the USDA has defined it.
"No cholesterol"	The fats that replace cholesterol are actually full of bad omega-6 fats.
"No trans fats"	Again, there are mostly bad omega-6 fats in this product.
"Partially hydrogenated"	There are *really* bad omega-6 fats in here.
"No artificial ingredi-ents"	There is nothing "artificial" in rat droppings, either! At best, this is meaningless.

"Heart healthy"	Big Food and Big Pharma want you to eat this! And by the way, one product certified as "heart healthy" by the FDA is Froot Loops! However, avocado, salmon, and nuts don't pass muster by the FDA. Go figure.
"All organic ingredients"	Buyer, beware. Arsenic is organic and it is legal to feed it to so-called organic chickens. It is a major antibiotic and endocrine disruptor. GMO crops, if raised organically, can be also labeled "organic."

Finally, please don't be misled by the organic, free-range label when it comes to poultry. I cannot emphasize enough that it means that these birds were kept in a warehouse (with access to the outdoors, although they have likely never actually ventured out), and were fed organic corn and soybeans. And if the label says "fed an all vegetarian diet," put the package down and step away from the meat counter. Chickens are insectivores, not grain eaters. In addition, if the label on your fish says it is organic Scottish, Norwegian, or Canadian salmon, put it back. This means that it was fed organic grains and soybeans. Do you really think they followed the salmon around to see if they were eating "organic" seaweed? Likewise for organic beef—if the label does not specify that the animal was grass-fed and grass-finished, suspect a trick. All cows at some point in their life eat grass. Therefore, in theory and in practice, all beef can be—and is—labeled grass-fed, even though that cow spent most of its life eating grains and beans in a feedlot.

DISRUPTOR 7: Constant Exposure to Blue Light

For millennia, we and all other animals have acquired food in response to changes in daylight, and specifically to the blue wavelength spectrum of daylight. Long days and short nights stimulate your body to eat as much food as possible to prepare for upcoming winter. Conversely, short days and long nights stimulate us to seek less food, which is scarce, and instead burn the fat we've acquired in summer as fuel. Hunting or foraging for food when little is available makes no sense when you would expend more calories than you are likely to find.

So, in winter, instead of seeking food, we are designed to burn the fat we've acquired. The hormone leptin, which makes us feel full, turns on this signal. This seasonal cycling between the use of glucose for fuel and the use of fat for fuel is termed metabolic flexibility. And the instructions for this cycling are mediated by the blue spectrum of light.

Modern life is dominated by blue light, creating an unnatural and practically nonstop exposure to this wavelength. Televisions, cell phones, tablets, other electronic devices, and even certain energy-saving lightbulbs emit light in the blue range of the spectrum, which is known to interfere with sleep. Blue light suppresses the production of melatonin, the hormone that helps you fall asleep, and sleep deprivation is associated with obesity.[46] Blue light also stimulates ghrelin and cortisol, which are, respectively, the "hunger" and "awake" hormones. And because our genetic programming associates blue light with daylight, this constant exposure tricks our bodies into thinking we're perpetually in the season with longer daylight hours (summer). This prompts us to constantly pack on pounds in anticipation of the shorter daylight hours of upcoming winter, which never arrives, thanks to electric lights. Now that this ancient rhythm has been completely disrupted, we live in 365 days of "endless summer." For all these reasons, I recommend that you minimize your exposure to blue light in the evenings.

Blue Light Trojan Horses

- **ENEMY**: Constant exposure to blue spectrum light.
  - **Friendly Substitutes:**
    - Download an app (justgetflux.com) to change the blue light emitted from any device's screen to an amber tint when the sun sets, by simply typing in your zip code. Utilize the yellow screen option on your iPhone or Android. The new iOS has an easy-to-use "Night-Shift" function.
    - When the sun goes down and you use your cell phone or other electronic devices, wear amber-tinted, blue light-blocking glasses, which are made by Uvex, Solar Shield, Pixel, and many other companies. A wraparound style blocks blue light coming from the side as well as that from directly in front of you.
    - Replace the bulbs in your bedroom (if not all rooms) with blue-blocking bulbs. I particularly like the Good Night Biological LED Lamp made by Lighting Science (www.lsgc .com), which was originally developed for NASA astronauts.

In Cahoots with Lectins

HOW DO THE Seven Deadly Disruptors come together with lectins to make us fat and sick? The damage we have sustained from lectins makes us all the more vulnerable to the additional assaults caused by the disruptors. When LPSs and lectins breach the intestine's containment walls, your body goes on the defensive. In order to have sufficient calories to fuel the white blood cells (your immune army) fighting the war within your body, your muscles become insulin- and leptin-resistant. We're insulin-resistant and leptin-resistant (often called metabolic syndrome) *not* because we're fat; instead, *we're fat because we're saving calories for the war effort*, as the following chapter elucidates.

Thanks to the combination of hormonal confusion and circadian rhythm confusion caused by these disruptors and the ongoing release of lectins and LPSs into our bodies, we have unleashed a total shock to our normal operating system. In the next chapter, we'll dive deeper into this very subject to help you understand why we have become fatter, sicker, and less fit over the last half century. You'll also learn why these problems are not your fault. Now, let's understand where that fat is stored and why it's there.

How the Modern Diet
Makes You Fat (and Sick)

You are probably still unsure whether that long list of conditions (including being overweight) on pages 68–70 can be resolved by following the Plant Paradox Program. But as has been shown in peer-reviewed medical journals, simply changing your diet and making some lifestyle changes can effect amazing changes in your overall health. As the sixteenth-century British naturalist and physician Thomas Muffet wrote, "Men dig their graves with their own teeth and die by those fated instruments more than the weapons of their enemies." Five centuries later, his words still ring true, as does Hippocrates's famous declaration: "Let food be thy medicine and medicine be thy food."

Now, my belief in these complementary statements is not just a matter of faith. It stands on the bedrock of evidence: my research, the research of others, and the thousands of people who arrived in my office complaining of a variety of ailments and have since cured themselves by following my eating plan. Many of my patients initially were also carrying around excess pounds. Once they began the program, weight loss was almost inevitable, usually without major effort.

A Healthy Weight

I KNOW THAT many of you are eager to get to the weight-loss part of this book, but hold your horses just a bit longer. It's important to first understand that any tendency to pack on extra pounds and any difficulty slimming down are not because you are a lazy or undisciplined person. If you are carrying around extra baggage, the likely reason is because you are eating the wrong foods and/or not eating the right foods. In my experience, what the Plant Paradox Program removes from your diet is more important than what it adds. That's my first point. But second, disease issues and weight issues are often inextricably linked, which is why this chapter deals with both.

Another key point that is not on most people's radar is the role that our gut bugs play—not only in health and disease, but also in maintaining a normal weight. Some microbes help keep you slim and healthy. Other gut bugs contribute to weight gain. Still other bugs that make you sick may interfere with the absorption of nutrients and make it difficult to maintain a healthy weight. You could be stuffing yourself with food, but if your gut bugs aren't facilitating proper digestion, you may be missing out on both calories and micronutrients. Celiac disease is just the tip of the malnutrition iceberg; numerous other conditions can interfere with proper digestion and nutrient availability as well.

<hr>

SUCCESS STORY

Usher Loses Pounds and Gets the Role

My assistant got a call from a Mr. Raymond who wanted to thank me personally for what I had done for him with the Plant Paradox Program. I was puzzled since I didn't know anyone by that name and didn't recall ever giving a Mr. Raymond my two-page list of foods to eat and avoid; but I was intrigued, so I picked up the phone. Usher Raymond IV was on the line. Yes, that Usher. It seems that he had been cast to play Sugar Ray Leonard in the movie *Hands of Stone*. When the real Sugar Ray met Usher, the boxer sized him up and said he was too fat to play him! Now, if you have ever seen Usher, "fat" would not be a description that you would use. Seven percent body fat is not fat. But there it was; Usher was too fat to play Sugar Ray. So Usher went on the Paleo diet, then a gluten-free diet, and finally a raw vegan diet. He also worked out for five or six hours a day. Nothing worked. Did he need to exercise more, or cut more calories? He was so frustrated he nearly gave up.

Around this time, Usher's agent was visiting a girlfriend in New York who had been following the Plant Paradox Program with great success. The agent took a copy of the food list off the refrigerator and went back to Usher. Fifteen dropped pounds later, Usher was on the phone with me. He was now Sugar Ray! He had been eating everything he wanted from the "good" page and avoided everything on the "bad" page. By following this two-page list, he had lost the weight he needed to. Miraculous? Not at all—just the perfect functioning of a perfectly designed system. Now Usher wants the world to know about the plant paradox.

I know how frustrating diets and exercise can be in attaining an elusive goal. What if that goal was just waiting for you to attain it? What if perfect weight and health was the natural consequence of allowing your own nature to thrive, once the obstructions from "healthy" foods and "all-natural" products were removed from your life? That is what the Plant Paradox Program can do.

The Weight War—and More

BEING OVERWEIGHT (or underweight) is a clear signal—but only one—that there is a war being waged within your body. If you are reading this book, I can assume that you are concerned about the state of your health—and likely your weight. You are in good company. In hindsight, something started to go awry with our collective health in the mid-1960s. You'll recall that today, 70.7 percent of American adults are overweight. Of those, almost 38 percent are obese, up from less than 20 percent two decades ago.[1] Additionally, there has been a huge increase in the incidence of diabetes, asthma, arthritis, cancer, heart disease, osteoporosis, Parkinson's disease, and dementia. One in four people now has one or more of the dozens of autoimmune diseases. Despite the fact that most of us now work only seven- or eight-hour days and are better fed than our grandparents, many of us suffer from low energy. There's also a dramatically higher incidence of allergies. There are now even EpiPens, syringes filled with adrenaline, marketed to worried parents for their kids to carry to school so they can inject themselves in case some other kid opens a package of peanuts. Peanuts didn't kill us back in 1960.

We've blamed the Western diet, the environment, and inactivity for our poor health and excess pounds. Although the current advice on each of these subjects may contain a grain of truth, each misses the big truth. Not that these actions or inactions don't also contribute to poor health, but they are not the *primary* cause of our health crisis. That's why a diet or an exercise program may work for a few weeks, or maybe even a few months—but then it all falls apart, and you're back to square one. Sound familiar? The reason none of these "solutions" produces lasting change is that they do little or nothing to end both the battle of the bulge and the related battle within your body.

The Artist Who Couldn't Make Art

The sister of a seventy-seven-year-old Japanese sculptor brought him to see me. Hobbled and stooped over, walking with a considerable limp, he reached out his gnarled hand and I was shocked to see the arthritis that wracked his body. He spoke little English, but his sister recounted the sad story about how this revered sculptor of massive wood carvings could no longer create his art. He was unable to hold a hammer and chisel, a carving knife, or a brush (he also painted, usually on large canvases). On the advice of his orthopedic surgeon, the sculptor was chewing Motrin, Advil, and Aleve like candy, and he was scheduled for a knee replacement, to be followed by a hip replacement. He had come to me for cardiac clearance for the operations. I suggested the Plant Paradox Program and he agreed. With a little help from his sister, I showed him the two-page list and the foods to avoid. He also stopped the NSAIDs immediately.

Four months later, the sculptor returned, this time with no limp. He jumped out of the chair and shook my hand vigorously. Then, acting like he had a paintbrush in his hand, he waved it on an invisible canvas, smiling and saying, "Paint, paint, paint!" While doing this, he was literally prancing about the exam room. "What about the knee operation?" "No," he replied. "Knee good! No operation!"

That was two years ago. I saw him and his sister recently and he brought in a cover story from the *Los Angeles Times* on an exhibit of his collected works at the Hammer Museum. Many of his finest and largest were done in the last two years. No longer wracked with pain, he was enjoying presenting his great talent to the world.

Amazing but True: Smaller Bodies and Brains

Based on ancient skeletal remains, we know that twelve thousand years ago humans averaged six feet in height. However, by 8000 BCE, the average human had shrunk to four feet ten inches—that's a whopping fourteen inches in just a few thousand years! Our ancestors became much shorter after the agricultural revolution, which is when grains and legumes became staples of the diet. And prior to that time, there is no evidence of arthritis in skeletal remains. In contrast, all skeletons of modern people, except those who don't eat many lectin-containing foods, have arthritis. (You'll recall that the mummified remains of ancient Egyptians revealed that they suffered from arthritis a mere two millennia after starting to cultivate grains.) And it doesn't stop there: the size of the human brain was 15 percent larger twelve thousand years ago than it is today! And we call that progress?

The Failure of "Diets" and the Exercise Conundrum

AN INDICATION OF our concern with our health and weight is our obsessive focus on weight-loss diets, despite our ongoing failure to convert that concern to lasting results. "Diets" are among the myths that have distracted us from the real issues regarding our health. But weight-loss diets are doomed to fail because they don't address the underlying sabotage of our foods and other products we come in contact with. The recent revelation that most of the "winners" on *The Biggest Loser* reality show had regained most of their weight after their original "success" was ballyhooed on TV should come as no surprise to most "dieters." If you have come to the conclusion that 99 percent of all such weight-loss programs are useless in the long run, I commend you for seeing the harsh light of day.

End the war within your body and you will find your weight normalizes as well. An integral part of self-healing is achieving the weight your body "wants" to be. You'll also significantly increase your longevity odds. But dieting to slim down and then reverting to your past habits is never a real fix. On the other hand, changing your way of eating and other habits once you understand the effects of certain foods (and certain products) on your system is a whole different ball game. And that is the game plan I will be presenting to you. *Diet,* as in a way of eating, is the key to success.

Numerous studies show that exercise doesn't help you lose weight. One problem with exercise is it makes you hungry. Another is that for the vast majority of people who are significantly overweight, it hurts to exercise so they don't stick with it. But this is not to say that exercise, as in living an active lifestyle, is pointless. A huge study shows that regular exercise (and not just as a workout at the gym, but an overall commitment to being active) can be a valuable aid in helping you *maintain* your weight.[2] Moreover, staying physically fit has numerous other benefits, including improving cardiovascular health, moderating your blood pressure, boosting your HDL ("good") cholesterol, and lowering your triglycerides. Both aerobic exercise and weight-bearing exercise also improve your balance (so you are less likely to injure yourself in a fall), lift your mood and alleviate stress, up your energy level, and enhance the quality of your sleep. And that's just for starters.

What Research Is All About

EVER SINCE DEFENDING my thesis on the biological and social factors driving human evolution for my graduation requirements at Yale University, I have been fascinated with the effect of food and the choices of food on human evolution and population growth. I used this knowledge and the subsequent human research studies I performed at my institute to develop the program that resulted in *Dr. Gundry's Diet Evolution*. However, this was just a stepping-stone to what I have learned in the years since. Just as humans have evolved as a species, my research has resulted in an evolution in my thinking—and it started with a visit to Metagenics, a major nutriceutical manufacturer. I had been asked to address its scientific team about the principles of my book. At that time, I was a full-bore carbophobic—a code word for one who believes that carbohydrates (sugars) are evil and the cause of all disease. I had severely restricted them in my dietary plan. After I presented my data and hypotheses, one of the Metagenics researchers stood up and asked, "How do you explain the Kitavans?"

Those darn Kitavans! This South Pacific tribe is the bane of existence to low-carb, fat-is-king researchers. Kitavans smoke like fiends and get approximately 60 percent of their calories from carbohydrates and 30 percent from coconut oil. Despite this, they don't have heart attacks, strokes, or other indicators of cardiovascular disease and they are remarkably thin, all the while living long and disease-free lives with little need for medical care. Low-carb advocates, my former self included, have long dismissed the Kitavans as exceptions to the rule, citing (without evidence, I might add) that their remarkable health is secondary to eating a calorie-restricted diet, with its known positive effects on health and longevity. Case closed, right?

Not so fast. The primary duty of a researcher is to constantly test your hypothesis. Indeed, the actual purpose of research is to prove that your hypothesis is wrong! Only if you *cannot* prove it wrong can it possibly be right. So, after initially waving off the Kitavans as calorie-restricted freaks of nature, I went back to my research from Yale and beyond, looking for the driving forces behind any culture's food selection. And I discovered, thanks to the work of Staffan Lindeberg, that despite the fact that they consume a large number of calories, the Kitavans are very skinny. The calorie is a calorie (calories in equals calories out) argument seemingly doesn't apply to Kitavans. Research (re-search) means to look again, and so I did. This chapter is the result of that second look, and of observing what happened to my patients when I applied these new insights.

The Real Reasons for a Choice

WE HAVE ALREADY discussed how approximately ten thousand years ago, most humans traded a nomadic hunter-gatherer existence for an agriculture-based lifestyle. The foods previously consumed were primarily seasonal fruits (available only once a year), seasonal big game, and fish and shellfish, along with a significant reliance on starches in plant tubers, which could be utilized by roasting after mankind discovered how to harness fire about one hundred thousand years ago. Although this regimen would have provided abundant calories, the number of humans on the planet remained minuscule. Then, suddenly, calories began to come from the grains of grasses, legumes, and—in the case of all cultures except Asians—milk from cows, sheep, and goats.

The traditional theory of why our forebears transitioned to these foods was that these crops could be stored and the animals herded. You could grow grains and beans in one season, but once dried and properly stored, they would not wilt or rot. Cows and other bovines could be milked, and the milk could be used immediately or turned into cheese (which could also be stored). Because these foods could be consumed throughout the year, it allowed populations to remain in place, despite changes in weather and even times of crop failure. That's the theory that I was taught and accepted. But suppose that there was another "hidden" reason that the first farmers chose grains, beans, and milk.

Whenever I get into an argument about the benefits of exercise with a long-distance runner, I point out that, by definition, the most successful animal is the one that finds the most calories for the least amount of effort. That is the genetic definition of success. But the corollary that was staring me in the face was this: The most successful animal is the one that stores the most amount of fat from any available calorie. Perhaps we had gotten it all wrong. Maybe our ancient ancestors didn't opt for grains, beans, and milk because they could be stored. Suppose if, instead, it was because they discovered that this trio of foods had the unique ability to literally turbocharge fat storage for any given calorie, relative to any other foods?

Good-bye to Diabetes and Thirty Pounds

I see a lot of Hispanic patients, and they often share the same confluence of health problems as my other patients. They, too, have diabetes, autoimmune issues, and excess weight, in this case in large part attributable to the replacement of their ancestral diet with modern substitutes, and with moving from an agricultural society to an urban lifestyle. Maria S. is representative of many such patients. She was forty-seven years old and had severe diabetes and was on insulin injections when I first saw her, with an HbA1C (a marker of diabetes) at 7.9—when the upper limit of normal is 5.6. Within a year, Maria had cut her positive markers for autoimmune disease in half. Her HbA1c is now 5.9, approaching normal. Her fasting blood sugar level has dropped from 146 to 109 and she is now off all medications, including insulin. As a bonus, Maria has lost thirty pounds. The wonderful thing is that although she speaks no English, she was able to follow the Plant Paradox Program, thanks to her children acting as translators.

The Best Way to Fatten Up

IF I'VE HEARD it once, I've heard it ten thousand times from my patients: "Whole grains and beans are key to a healthy diet." But I am here to tell you that the evidence with animals is exactly the opposite. I grew up in the 1950s and 1960s in Omaha, Nebraska, which at that time boasted the world's largest stockyard. In our stockyards, as any Cornhusker knows, we fattened our beef on corn! Why truck cows from all over the midwest to Omaha to fatten them on corn? Because cows don't get fat eating hay and grass—every farmer knows that. As early as the nineteenth century, pigs raised in the Ohio River Valley were fattened with corn before being herded to slaughterhouses in Cincinnati. The farmer could make more money walking corn-fattened pigs to market than putting the corn on barges to send to pig farms. The popular expression of the day was that you drove your corn to market in a pig.

This may surprise you, but a pig is not normally a fat animal. Wild boars and feral pigs are lean, sleek, muscular animals. You Arkansas Razorback fans know what I mean. But you may not know that a pig has the identical digestive system and cardiovascular system to a human, which is why I use pig valves to replace defective human valves. Think about that next time you are accused of eating like a pig! And as with pigs, eating corn fattens up us humans.

A number of my patients seek my treatment for weight loss, but at least half of them see me for the relief of autoimmune diseases. Many of those folks are of normal weight. As I mentioned earlier, one of the happy side effects of my program is returning to a normal weight, regardless of the patient's original reason for seeing me. But over the years I've had a small group of patients who, once they make the food changes that I ask for to cure their autoimmune disease, keep losing weight and can't keep it on. Early in my new career, I asked them to eat more fat, particularly avocados, but that didn't help. As the years passed, patient after skinny patient would return three or four months later carrying some additional pounds. Invariably, they had added bread, pasta, corn, or beans to their diet. Yes, when all else failed to restore their lost weight, grains and beans did the job. But to everyone's chagrin, it also elevated the markers of inflammation in their blood. My more recent and effective solution to this problem is to have them eat large amounts of macadamia nuts.

There it was again, the plant paradox in action: the very foods that promoted our ancestors' ability to gain weight and survive a harsh winter, making them more likely to produce a new genetic copy (aka a baby), were the same ones that would hasten their eventual demise—and ours. If you've read my first book, then you know that our genes will always choose this route: maximize calories from food in order to reproduce, then assure the destruction of the parent after the child is grown so that there is sufficient food for that child or grandchild.

Here, then, is the reason grains and beans took over the world. It wasn't because they were "healthy." It wasn't because they could be stored. No, it was merely because such foods promoted greater fat deposits per calorie than any other food source. That was good then, but it certainly isn't now. Nor is the fact that such a diet also does a better job of shortening the postreproductive years.

You'll recall that it isn't just grains and beans that turbocharge fat storage, but also milk products. Lactating animals use milk for one thing: to promote rapid growth and weight gain in their offspring. All milk is loaded with insulinlike growth hormone. Sadly, multiple studies show that another component of milk, casein, and in particular casein A-1, becomes the lectin beta-casomorphin, which encourages fat storage by promoting inflammation. Remember, inflammation indicates a state of war, and the war effort requires fuel for the troops, stimulating the storage of more fat for fuel.

Unbelievable but True: The Power of Poop

If you take feces from obese rats and feed it to skinny rats, presto change-o, the skinny rats become fat! The reverse is also true: a skinny rat's poop makes fat rats thin. Yes, you are interpreting that correctly: the organisms in your intestines control how skinny or fat you will be. Recent studies have shown that feces from fat humans given to skinny rats will make them fat; it works even better if you throw in some "fertilizer" in the form of sugars and fats! Still not impressed? Consider this: In the 1930s, institutionalized patients with severe depression were given laxatives to clean out their colon, and then given fecal enemas from happy people. You guessed it: the depressed individuals became happy.

As a student at the Medical College of Georgia in the 1970s, I witnessed cure after cure of a severe infection of the colon called *Clostridium difficile* colitis, which had occurred in patients given newly introduced broad-spectrum antibiotics. Again, the method was to give patients fecal enemas, in this case made with the poop of healthy medical students. In fact, once a week, the "honey pot" was passed around to all of us medical students to make a deposit, in order to have fresh poop available to treat this horrible disease. Little did we know then that the antibiotics had disturbed the intestines of these patients, and that the microbes in our feces restored them to health.

The Lectin Link to Obesity and Ill Health

I HAVE ALREADY introduced you to wheat germ agglutinin (WGA), and explained that it is implicated in celiac disease and also bears a striking resemblance to the hormone insulin. Now let's take an in-depth look at the actions of insulin and problematic effects that occur when WGA mimics insulin.

Normally, when sugar enters the bloodstream from our gut, the pancreas secretes insulin into the bloodstream, and the insulin then travels to three main places: fat cells, muscle cells, and neurons. Insulin's primary job is to open the door to any cell to allow glucose to enter and provide fuel, particularly to three important types of cells.

1. **IN FAT CELLS**, insulin attaches to a docking port on a fat cell membrane and flips a switch that tells the fat cell to convert that glucose to fat and store it. When insulin has done its job, it separates from the docking port and no more sugar can enter the cell.

2. **IN MUSCLE CELLS**, insulin unlocks the door to the cell and ushers in glucose to be used as fuel.

3. **NERVE CELLS** (neurons) also require insulin to admit glucose through their cell membrane. The fact that neurons require insulin to get glucose is a relatively new finding, and we now know that insulin resistance also occurs in the brain and nerves—it is called type 3 diabetes.

Once insulin docks in the appropriate ports and releases information, the fat, muscle, or nerve cells tell the hormone that the message has been received. The hormone then backs out of the docking port, leaving it ready and available for the next hormone to attach.

Problems arise when lectins mimic insulin and bind to those docking ports on cell walls instead. The lectins either give the wrong information or block the release of the correct information. To understand the consequences, imagine that you are a passenger on a plane after a long flight, and another plane is still sitting at your Jetway at the terminal. You can't get off the plane (release your information) until that plane moves. But suppose it never moves! Now what? As long as lectins occupy the "Jetway," the proper messaging is interrupted or silenced—indefinitely.

Now let's look at what happens when the lectin WGA fits into each type of insulin receptor docking port:

1. In the case of a fat cell membrane, WGA locks on for good and continues to instruct the cell to make fat from any sugar floating by—ad infinitum. Think about it: if you were living eight thousand years ago, any plant compound that could enhance your ability to store fat from the meager calories you obtained would be a great plant. But that's no longer a great benefit—and lectins such as WGA and a host of others in every grain do far more just to potentiate fat storage directly into fat cells.

2. If WGA attaches to a muscle cell, it likewise permanently locks on to that insulin receptor—but in this case, the opposite effect results. WGA blocks the real insulin from docking, just as another plane sitting at your arrival gate means you cannot deplane. The result is that the muscle can't get glucose; instead, it is shunted to a waiting fat cell, where WGA continuously pumps in sugar. Would it surprise you to learn that early man was far more muscular before the advent of grains and beans? Take a look at any ancient Egyptian frescoes and statues: these were skinny, nonmuscular people. As it turns out, insulin mimicry is the true cause of the muscle wasting as we age! The more lectins we eat, the more the receptors for insulin on our muscles are filled with WGA and other lectins, and the more muscle we waste.

3. When WGA and other lectins lock on to the insulin receptor in nerve cells and neurons, they block the entrance of sugar there as well. With no sugar reaching its neurons, the hungry brain demands more calories. If you block insulin receptors with WGA, you get a hungry human—one who will eat more and hopefully be a big winner when winter arrives. This may have

been fine in the short term, promoting mankind's early survival; but if this process continues, more WGA and other lectins bind to insulin receptors in the brain and nerves, causing brain cells and peripheral nerves to die, resulting in dementia, Parkinson's, and peripheral neuropathy.

The cumulative result is less muscle mass, starved brain and nerve cells, and plenty of fat. Sound familiar?

Recently, it has been found that lectins climb the vagus nerve from the gut into the brain and can be deposited in the substantia nigra,[3] the switching center in the brain, damage to which causes Parkinson's disease. This explains why, according to a large Chinese study, patients who have had a procedure called a vagotomy back in the 1960s and 1970s (in which their vagus nerves were surgically cut to treat ulcers) have a 40 percent lower incidence of Parkinson's compared to age-matched controls.[4] Lectins weren't reaching the brain as readily, and therefore weren't able to cause as much harm. It also explains why Parkinson's is more prevalent among vegetarians, as they consume more plants (and therefore more lectins). Remember, the plant is just doing its job: ridding the world of unwanted pests, including you!

To summarize, in ancient times when food was scarce, weight gain from consuming the lectins in grains and beans was a huge benefit, but today, the same result works against us. Now let's move to the second way lectins work for us and against us.

Preparing for War

I MENTIONED ABOVE that my patients who needed to replace lost weight had resorted to grain- and bean-based foods, but in doing so, most of them found that their inflammation markers had begun to rise. Was inflammation also promoting their weight gain? Remember, LPSs and lectins act like foreign invaders, which cause TLRs to alert the body that it is under attack and to go into "war mode." During a war, the troops must be well nourished in order to fight the enemy, so food is often rationed for noncombatants. White blood cells and the immune system serve as the troops, while the muscles represent the civilians at home. By making muscles and the brain resistant to the effects of both insulin and leptin (the hormone that makes you feel full), calories are shunted away from the muscles and the brain, ensuring there are sufficient calories to fuel the white blood cells on the battlefront. Moreover, if there is a war going on, your body sends signals to encourage you to find more calories for the war effort. The more lectins you ingest from grains and beans, the hungrier you are.

This is a key point: You are insulin- and leptin-resistant not because you are overweight; rather, you are overweight because your body is at war and is saving calories for the war effort. This is the complete opposite of the common wisdom of why we bulk up. However, if the body senses that there is no war because no lectins and no LPSs are getting into the body, there is no reason to hoard calories, by either conserving food or seeking more food. Weight loss is a "side effect" of ending the war. No wonder almost everyone was slim fifty years ago, back when our bodies weren't constantly at war!

Fat Storage

YOU'VE PROBABLY BEEN told that if you store fat around your midsection, it is the dangerous fat pattern known as apple-shaped, but if you store fat on your buttocks or hips, what is called pear-shaped, you are okay. There is a lot of truth to this finding. To understand why fat is stored in the gut, let's return to our war analogy. The troops need fuel and it needs to be near the front lines, where the troops are battling the lectins and LPSs. And where is the war? Right, it is at the wall of your intestines, in your gut, where lectins and LPSs have broken across the border. Fat is not the culprit; rather, it is a sign of the battle being waged in your belly. It's not called "belly fat" for nothing.

As a heart surgeon, I have known for years that when I open up a patient to do a coronary artery bypass I will find a large amount of fat surrounding these arteries on the surface of the heart. That fat is really thick and hard, and it's there even if you are skinny. If there is a lot of fat, I know that a war is being waged nearby and that the call for supplies is constant. The war is in your arteries, and I am doing a bypass because you lost the war. In fact, multiple studies show that pericardial fat (fat on the arteries) directly correlates with the amount of disease inside the blood vessels.[5] What are the implications? Wherever we find excess fat, that means there is a war being waged. Fat in your gut signifies not only that there is a war going on in your intestines, but that sadly it is spreading to your heart and brain, much like terrorist sleeper cells.

SUCCESS STORIES

An Alternative to Surgery

Surgery or a different diet—that's the choice I give many of my patients. Although I am a heart surgeon, if the patient is a good candidate for my dietary approach and indicates interest in this alternative, I always discuss the Plant Paradox Program with him or her. As long as someone adheres to the diet, the results are remarkable. Offering patients this option has earned me the nickname No More Mr. Knife Guy! Here are just a few of the many people who have avoided major surgery with simple lifestyle choices.

BLOCKED NO LONGER. When Vincent P., a sixty-seven-year-old theatrical producer, developed chest pain while exercising, an angiogram showed a narrow lesion in his right coronary artery, which had been previously treated by implanting a stent. His cardiologist referred him to me for dietary treatment of several other arterial lesions, which were 60 percent blocked and not eligible for stents (but still of concern). After following the Plant Paradox Program for ten months, Vincent had another angiogram, which showed that all of the remained blockages had been resolved, making surgery or other stents unnecessary. Six years later, Vincent takes no medication, routinely passes his stress tests, and recently opened an off-Broadway show.

A PROMISE KEPT. Sonja R., a fifty-eight-year-old farmer and severe diabetic, was scheduled for an emergency triple bypass after having a heart attack. Five of her arteries had severe blockages. In the pre-op room, she asked whether any other option was possible. After I told her about my dietary approach, she said she would be my best patient if I would not operate on her. She kept her promise: three years later she has lost forty pounds, is no longer a diabetic, takes no medications, has no chest pain, and has a normal response to my cardiac stress tests. Sonja now raises pastured chickens and goats, makes goat yogurt, and hauls wheelbarrows of manure and soil daily.

GOODBYE TO DIABETES. At sixty-nine, Howard L. was obese and took eight medications daily for diabetes and other conditions. He had suffered a heart attack and was scheduled for an emergency five-vessel bypass surgery. In the pre-op room, I could tell that he was extremely anxious. After we spoke for a while, Howard told me he didn't think he was going to make it through surgery and asked whether there was another option. When I offered him my diet, he jumped at the chance. Now, five years later, his diabetes and chest pain are history, he takes no medications, he has lost thirty pounds, and he regularly passes his annual stress tests.

An Abundance of "Successful" Diets

WHY ARE THERE so many diets? And why do so many of them work (at least temporarily)? Do they have anything in common? Step back and tick off a few of the most successful and popular diet philosophies of recent years: low-carb, high-protein (Atkins, Protein Power, South Beach, and Dukan, to name a few); low-carb, high-fat, high-protein (Paleo, ketogenic-Paleo); low-fat, high-carb (Ornish, McDougall, Fuhrman, Esselstyn). Each of these approaches can lay claim to immense success among its followers. Alan Levinovitz, Ph.D., recently parodied the popularity and success of these totally different diets in *The Gluten Lie and Other Myths About What You Eat.* The book presents a fictional UnPacked diet, which is based on eliminating plastic wrappers (I kid you not). He cites websites to visit, pretends to sell products, and provides testimonials from patients. After you avidly read the multiple arguments Levinovitz makes in support of his program, you are suddenly confronted with the fact that he carefully cherry-picked his data, used other diet gurus' own words, and stole testimonials from most of the wildly different programs listed above about the great results. The joke is seemingly on us. (But what Levinovitz misses is the fact that all the data he quotes about the dangers of plastics are actually true, as you learned in the last chapter.)

I have had the privilege of treating a number of patients who were firm adopters of each of the above-mentioned programs. They may have controlled their weight, yet they continued to have troubling medical issues, including advancing coronary artery disease and autoimmune disease, to name just two. Let's dig deeper into what really happens on these diet programs.

The Problem with Most Low-Carb Diets

A LOW-CARBOHYDRATE DIET—think Atkins or South Beach—often works well in the short term. Heck, it worked well for me initially. However, if and when you return to eating significant amounts of lectin-containing carbohydrates, those lost pounds usually make a comeback. Even if you stick with the program, your weight loss typically stops or slows significantly at a certain point. All low-carb plans are inherently high-protein diets, and thus restrict carbohydrates, all grains, and legumes—and with them, their lectin load. When the South Beach and Atkins diets reintroduce grains and beans in the maintenance phase, and people invariably start to gain weight, what is suggested? You guessed it: go back to the first phase and cut out grains and beans!

The Paleo concept takes the high-protein diet a step further and is based on the faulty assumption that early man dined on buffalo and other large animals on a regular basis and that's what made us healthy. In all likelihood, such kills were hardly a regular occurrence. Instead, our forefathers likely subsisted mostly on tubers, berries, nuts, and animal protein sources such as fish, lizards, snails, insects, and small rodents. Now, don't get me wrong—our "ancestral diet" was designed to do what any diet does: ensure that you grow up, reproduce, and then get out of the way. Your genes designed the ancestral diet to make you an ancestor, if you get my drift. Enabling you to live long is counterproductive to maximizing the number of humans being born, just as making cars that last forever is counterproductive for the automobile industry. I hate to break it to you, but any success you may have experienced on the Paleo diet or another low-carb plan, whether as weight loss or improved health, was *not* the result of restricting carbohydrates and eating lots of protein and fat. Rather, any positive response was the result of—guess what?—eliminating most lectin-containing foods. Don't forget that the Paleo concept is defined by what our Stone Age ancestors supposedly ate 100,000 years ago.

Finally, my Paleo colleagues somehow don't realize that all our ancestors were originally from Africa and never encountered any lectin-containing food from the Americas. Sorry, folks, but tomatoes, zucchini "noodles," bell peppers, goji berries, peanuts, cashews, sunflower seeds, and chia or pumpkin seeds are not ancestral foods—and they are loaded with lectins.

Another Approach to Restricting Carbs

A KETOGENIC DIET, which is traditionally prescribed to help people, including children, with diabetes moderate their blood sugar and insulin levels, is also a low-carbohydrate diet—but with a significant difference. Instead of replacing most carbohydrates with protein, a true ketogenic diet also limits protein, relying instead on certain fats for the majority of calories. (Ketosis refers to burning fat rather than glucose from carbohydrates for energy.) If you limit certain animal protein intake, as the Plant Paradox Program does, you will almost certainly lose weight. And when I limit it even more with a modified ketogenic version of the Plant Paradox Program, I see remarkable success not only with patients with diabetes (or who are extremely insulin-resistant) but also with those suffering from cancer, dementia, Parkinson's disease, autoimmune disease, and a number of gut diseases. (Chapter 10 addresses this modification.) The question is: are most people on a ketogenic diet in ketosis, and is that why they are losing weight? The answer from my patients' laboratory assessments is a resounding no! So, why the weight loss? Once more, removal of the vast majority of lectins from their diet, not the addition of fat, made the difference.

Hold the Fat and Push the Whole Grains

DO PEOPLE LOSE weight on low-fat, whole-grain diets such as those from Ornish, Esselstyn, and T. Colin Campbell (*The China Study*)? Indeed they do. I've seen a lot of them as patients because although they did lose weight, these diets failed to halt the progression of their coronary artery disease. But why the weight loss? I think it is the result of four factors:

1. They remove the lectin-containing fats so prevalent in our American diet, namely soy, peanut, cottonseed, sunflower, and canola—all of which not only contain lectins but are also extremely high in polyunsaturated omega-6 fats, which are used by our TLRs to incite the inflammatory cascade. Inflammation equals war equals store fat near the war zone—in the coronary arteries.
2. Because they have eliminated fats, low-fat diets do not allow LPSs, which have to travel on long-chain saturated fatty acids

to sneak through the gut wall, where they would cause inflammation. That is a good thing, but the well-meaning physicians who had once demonized all fat and championed low-fat diets have come to realize that all fat is not the same. Fish oil is now an integral part of Dr. Dean Ornish's program, and Dr. Joel Fuhrman has made fatty nuts an important part of his diet.[6] Luckily, neither of these regimens allows lectins to cross the gut barrier, so they are "safe."

3. They use whole unprocessed grains, not ground-up "whole grains." Now, I feel a little like Mark Antony here, when he said, "I come to bury Caesar, not to praise him." So why am I defending whole grains? First, most whole-grain "foods" are not actually whole grains, but are ground-up versions. Do you ever actually see a lot of "whole grains" in that piece of bread or cracker? Their lectins have already been released, and, as a double whammy, their fats are treated with BHT to prevent oxidation.

4. These physicians have correctly focused on organic grains, which are far more likely to be untouched by Roundup and the resulting death of the normal gut bugs. As a result, the diets enable the gut to handle gluten and prevent gang members from moving into the void created by that herbicide.

And then there's this sad fact: these diets are generally intolerable, so you don't eat much. Even the Kellogg brothers couldn't get their sanatorium guests to eat whole grains, hence the birth of Kellogg's cornflakes (ground-up grains). A review of Dr. Esselstyn's original study shows a 50 percent dropout rate. It's not a diet you can live with, so any positive results in terms of weight loss may be short lived.

Why have the followers of these programs who became my

patients found that their coronary artery disease had progressed? The WGA in wheat continued to bind to the endothelial lining of their coronary arteries, which their immune system attacked. If you ever wondered why the southern Chinese, Japanese, and Koreans (all of whose staple grain is rice) have lower heart disease rates than Americans, remember this: rice contains no WGA. Nor does the taro root the Kitavans eat in abundance. Likewise, the millet, sorghum, and yams that are African staples contain no WGA.

What We Share with Elephants

WANT ONE MORE shocker about grasses and grains? In the wild, where they dine only on the leaves of trees (like our forebears), African elephants have no known coronary artery disease. Due to habitat destruction, however, herds of elephants now graze on grasslands or are fed hay and grains. These animals have a 50 percent rate of severe coronary artery disease, thanks to the lectins they were never designed to eat, which bind to their arteries and incite an attack.

It is now time to reveal which sugar molecule the WGA and other lectins are after. As it turns out, there's a particular sugar molecule that elephants—and humans—possess that causes this problem. This lectin-binding sugar, called Neu5Ac, sits on the lining of blood vessels and the absorptive cells on the gut wall known as enterocytes. Most mammals have a sugar molecule called Neu5Gc on the lining of their gut wall and blood vessel walls. But humans lost the ability to make this molecule at the time our species diverged from chimps and gorillas eight million years ago. Instead, we make the lectin-binding Neu5Ac, a characteristic shared with shellfish, mollusks, chickens, and elephants. (Yes, strange bedfellows!) Lectins, and particularly grain lectins, bind to Neu5Ac but cannot bind to Neu5Gc. This explains why captive chimps eating a human grain-based diet don't get atherosclerosis (hardening of the arteries) or autoimmune disease, but the poor grass-eating elephants do get coronary artery disease. The chimps lack the lectin-binding sugar molecule, but elephants and humans possess it—and it gives us heart and autoimmune diseases in spades when we eat lectins in grasses and seeds.

The Anti-Aging Approach

REMEMBER, YOUR GOAL is to eat a life-enhancing diet, not just one that will help you shed excess pounds and keep them off. A serious problem with any low-carb or "ancestral" dietary approach is that consuming significant amounts of certain animal protein, particularly red meats, is known to be a major trigger of aging, as well as of atherosclerosis and cancer. How so?

Back to our old friend Neu5Ac. Stay with me, as it gets more complex before I can simplify it. Cattle, pigs, and sheep all carry Neu5Gc, which your immune system recognizes as foreign when you eat their meat. Now, Neu5Gc looks a lot like Neu5Ac (the bar codes are nearly identical). There is significant data suggesting that when our immune system is exposed to the foreign sugar molecule Neu5Gc from red meat, we develop an antibody to the lining of our own blood vessels, which has Neu5Ac. This causes the antibody to attach to the lining of our blood vessels, mistaking our own naturally occurring Neu5Ac for the Neu5Gc we've consumed, and calling in a full-fledged attack from our immune system.

This is the perfect example of friendly fire, and it provides further proof why shellfish, mollusk, and fish eaters have better heart health than meat eaters. Furthermore, it has been shown that cancer cells use Neu5Gc to attract blood vessel growth toward them, via production of a hormone called vascular endothelial growth factor (VEGF), which I measure in all my patients. VEGF production is promoted by an immune attack on Neu5Gc. Cancer cells even use Neu5Gc to hide from our immune cells, essentially cloaking themselves in an invisible shield. What's more, human tumors contain large amounts of Neu5Gc, despite the fact that we have no genes to manufacture it. That means the tumor cells got it from that beef, pork, or lamb you ate, and nowhere else.

In plain English, the reason to avoid red meats is to avoid an autoimmune attack that promotes heart disease and cancer, all because of a genetic mutation of a lectin-attracting sugar molecule that's found in humans.

A diet low in any animal protein has been shown to extend life, as will be discussed in chapter 9. So, a certain amount of animal protein is the actual mischief maker when it comes to longevity. This means certain carbs (those without lectins, or with lectins with which your microbes have been familiar for millennia) are not as problematic as the Atkins and Paleo folks have taught you, as long as you minimize certain animal proteins.

And hastening the aging process is not the only result of eating excessive amounts of protein. Remember, eating simple sugars increases production of insulin, the fat storage hormone, just as eating fat boosts the level of leptin, the hormone that signals your brain when you are full. But you may not know that when you consume sugars along with certain proteins more prevalent in animals than plants, they stimulate cells' ultimate aging receptor, which senses energy availability. We will discuss this aging receptor in chapter 9.

Energy—think food—is usually available cyclically, based on the circadian rhythms of seasons and daylight. If energy is plentiful, then it is time to grow and make things, meaning babies. When energy is scarce, it is time to batten down the hatches, get rid of hangers-on, and wait things out. During scarce times we use the fat we stored; meanwhile, our mitochondria switch from sugar (glucose) burning to fat burning, in what is called metabolic flexibility. Most of my patients with multiple diseases have lost all metabolic flexibility. This means that a diet high in both sugars and protein encourages weight gain and makes a person more susceptible to disease—and therefore could and indeed does reduce life span, but also health span and life enhancement.

Here's another paradox for you: Your genes want you to reproduce and replace yourself. Once that happens, your genes couldn't care less how long you live—okay, you do need enough time to get your offspring to the point where they are able to survive on their own—and then they do everything they can to get out of the way. That middle-age spread is a perfect example of what I am taking about. We are supposed to die off once we replace ourselves. But if we want to live as long and as healthy a life as possible, we need to eat differently.

A Paleo Diet That Endures

LET'S RETURN TO my previous conundrum, the Kitavans, a small tribe of farmers who inhabit an equally small island in Papua New Guinea. According to Swedish physician Staffan Lindeberg, who has been studying the tribe's diet for decades, the Kitavans obtain 60 percent of their calories from carbohydrates, 30 percent from fat (most of it saturated fat), and only 10 percent from protein. Most of the islanders smoke, they are not very active, but they live well into their nineties without medical care. Their diet seems to contradict most of the conventional assumptions about what constitutes a healthy diet, and yet the tribe seems untouched by most of the diseases of modern man.

Lindeberg's study, in which he matched 220 Kitavans with as many Swedish subjects of the same age and gender, provided provocative results.[7] Kitavan men age twenty and older had a lower body mass index (BMI), lower blood pressure, and lower total LDL ("bad") cholesterol than those of comparable Swedish men. Both groups displayed similar HDL ("good") cholesterol readings. Kitavan women over the age of sixty had lower levels of APoB (apolipopoprotein B), a marker for LDL cholesterol associated with heart and vascular disease, than their Swedish counterparts. Furthermore, Kitavans never experience strokes or heart attacks.

When Is a Carb Not a Carb?

SO HOW DO the Kitavans stay slim and avoid heart attacks, despite eating mostly carbohydrates and a large amount of primarily saturated fats, both of which are considered a recipe for obesity (and heart disease, in the case of the fats) in the West? The answer lies in the fact that the carbohydrates the Kitavans consume are primarily resistant starches, which give you a free (well, almost free) pass when it comes to their caloric content. If that sounds too good to be true, welcome to the world of resistant starches. This subset of starches behaves differently in your GI tract than do corn, rice, wheat, and other typical starches or simple sugars. Instead of being quickly converted to glucose (blood sugar), which is burned for energy or stored as fat, yams, taro, plantains, and other resistant starches simply pass through your small intestine intact. These foods are resistant to the enzymes that break complex starches—hence their name.

That means you don't absorb the calories as sugar, which would prompt an insulin surge—but what is even better is that these starches are just what the doctor ordered for your gut microbes, which happily devour resistant starches and grow, meanwhile converting them to short-chain fatty acids such as acetate, propionate, and butyrate (the colon's preferred fuel, as well as a perfect fuel for neurons). Resistant starches also increase the proportion of "good" bacteria in your gut, just as a prebiotic does, not only enhancing digestion and nutrient absorption but also fostering the growth of bugs that nurture the mucous layer of your gut.[8] More mucus means fewer lectins getting through to rip open the tight junctions and start the whole lectin-induced cycle of weight gain and misery.[9]

In addition to not raising blood sugar or insulin levels, resistant starch assists in controlling your weight by:

- Reducing calorie count when substituted for wheat flour and other quickly metabolized carbohydrates.[10]
- Making you feel full longer and therefore consume less food.[11]
- Boosting fat burning and reducing fat storage after a meal.[12]

You need not live on an island and eat taro day in and day out to get the benefits of resistant starch. In Part II, I'll introduce you to more sources of the microbe-friendly food and explain how to prepare them to maximize their benefits.

How Leaves Become a High-Fat Diet!

A gorilla is a classic herbivore, subsisting primarily on leaves. (Yes, they do occasionally inadvertently scarf down an insect or three on the leaves.) Surprisingly, a gorilla eats sixteen pounds of "fat-free" leaves a day, but 60 to 70 percent of the calories the animal absorbs after digestion is in the form of fats! How can that be? Well, the gut microbes, good little guest workers that they are, break down the cell walls of plants and ferment the energy into usable fuel, principally the fats we just discussed, which the animal can absorb. As a result, the gorilla "eats" an extremely high-fat diet! Just like the Kitavans!

Other Long-Lived Thin Peoples

I SHOULD MENTION that with the rise of globalization, traditional diets are increasingly giving way to the SAD, or perhaps more appropriately, what is now the typical Western diet. But the Kitavans don't have a lock on longevity and good health. Okinawans, Cretans, and Sardinians are known for their longevity. Although their diets differ, both also consume foods that feed gut bacteria. If you carefully examine the diets of long-lived societies, including the Seventh-day Adventists of Loma Linda, California, where I was a professor for years, a remarkable pattern emerges from seemingly disparate diets. The Okinowans and the Kitavans eat a diet very high in resistant starches, from a purple sweet potato and taro root, respectively; the Cretans and Sardinians eat a very high-fat (olive oil) diet, while the Adventists eat a diet composed of 60 percent fat, despite being vegetarians.

What could possibly be the common thread? It's the minimal intake of animal protein. Most of these long-lived cultures get most of their calories from sources other than protein. And even the high "carb" eaters, like the Kitavans and the Okinowans, turn their resistant starches into usable fat, courtesy of their gut bugs. We'll revisit these long-lived societies in Part II.

Blame Pizza and Chicken for Fat Kids

IT'S OBVIOUS THAT the American diet has changed dramatically in the last century. In that same time, and particularly in the last fifty years, we (and our children) have become significantly heavier. For her 2009 doctoral dissertation in the urban studies and public affairs program at the University of Akron, Lisaann Schelli Gittner explored the connection between the changes in the American diet and the rise in childhood obesity.[13] Her thesis, entitled *From Farm to Fat Kids,* explored one of the unintended consequences of government agricultural policies, which significantly changed the food supply. This created a niche for inexpensive processed and refined foods, and their increasing use correlated with the growing incidence of obese kids. Beginning in the 1960s, the intensive planting of crops such as corn, wheat, sugar beets, canola (rapeseed), and soybeans made for a very different supply of plant food than was available around 1900. This shift in crops led to a change in diet from grass-fed meats and their fats (butter and lard), chickens that ate bugs, lots of root vegetables, and very limited amounts of fruit to one high in polyunsaturated fats, sugar, massive amounts of fruit products like apple juice, and other processed foods, and one low in vegetables. The increase in BMI of children over these years mirrored these changing patterns in food consumption.

But despite all this, only two foods correlated perfectly with rising obesity rates in kids. Not surprisingly, they were pizza and chicken. In the 1970s, kids started eating lots of both these foods. Just check out the lunch menu in any public school. The more pizza and chicken kids consumed per year, the higher their average BMI. Although Gittner's focus was public affairs, not lectins, both of these foods are lectin bombs. The typical pizza contains at least three ingredients full of them: wheat, cheese full of casein A-1 and insulinlike growth factor, and tomato sauce. How about the chicken? Unlike its forebears, which foraged in the barnyard for grubs and insects, today's typical hen spends its brief life eating soy and corn, and laced with the estrogenlike compounds arsenic and phthalates. Dip this chicken in wheat flour breading mix and deep-fry it in peanut or soybean oil and you have a perfect lectin and estrogen bomb. Eat these two foods on a regular basis and your lectin load grows—and with it, your weight almost certainly will as well.

You now have a thorough understanding of how we got into this intertwined health crisis, thanks to subtle changes in your foods, personal care products, lighting, and a host of new drugs, and why your excess weight and health problems really aren't your fault. Now it's time to take back your body and your life. As I tell my patients, your body is the only home you will ever live in. If you spend the same effort on this home that you spend on your house or apartment or car, the dividends will last a long, vibrant lifetime. Let's move on to Part II, where I'll supply you with the tools and guidance you'll need to achieve a healthy weight, along with vibrant health.

Introducing the Plant Paradox Program

Revamp Your Habits

Okay, this is what you have been waiting for. Now that you know the science behind the Plant Paradox Program and what it has done for countless others, it's time to jump in and take control of your health by finding out what it can do for *you*. But before you get started, I want you to commit to memory the four rules that govern the program, along with the following statement, which is the most important thing I have to say in all of Part II: *Every time you waver, every time you rationalize something about what you plan to eat, every time you hear a little voice in your head saying, "But this is healthy food," stop and return immediately to Rule Number 1* (below).

Let me tell you what I have learned from every patient I have cared for over the past sixteen years as director of the Center for Restorative Medicine, which informs Rule Number 1: what you stop eating is more important than what you start eating. My patient Tony, whose vitiligo was cured after he started the program, is a perfect example. When the pigment in his skin returned, I could have said that his skin miraculously normalized because my dietary program was extremely anti-inflammatory, high in antioxidants, low in simple carbs, high in olive oil, and blah, blah, blah. The creators of all diets make these kinds of proclamations. But quite frankly, most of this rationale about why a dietary program works is wrong. Why? Because it wasn't what I told Tony to eat that made the big difference in his health; rather, it was what I told him *not* to eat that cured him.

Follow the Rules

THESE FOUR SIMPLE rules will enable you to experience success on the Plant Paradox Program.

RULE NUMBER 1: What You *Stop* Eating Has Far More Impact on Your Health Than What You *Start* Eating

As far as I know, Professor John Soothill of Great Ormond Street in London, my old hospital, was the first person to state this rule. If you get no further than this rule, and if you actually follow the Plant Paradox food lists, I can virtually guarantee that you will achieve remarkably good and sustainable health. Now, I'm not suggesting that you simply stop eating, although the ability of a simple water fast to cure any number of diseases is staggering.[1] But this rule does confirm Hippocrates's dictum that "all disease begins in the gut." If you stop damaging your gut, you'll be healthier overall. Your gut holobiome accounts for 90 percent of the cells that make you "you" and contains 99 percent of all the genetic material that makes you "you"—so what goes on in your gut, unlike Las Vegas, doesn't stay in your gut. Which brings us to my second rule.

RULE NUMBER 2: Pay Attention to the Care and Feeding of Your Gut Bugs, and They Will Handle the Care and Feeding of You. After All, You Are Their Home.

Another way of expressing this rule is: Give your gut bugs what they want, and nobody gets hurt. That sounds pretty easy, except for one thing. Part I should have convinced you by now that most of us have a virtual wasteland inside our gut. Years of using antibiotics, antacids, and NSAIDs, plus the high-fat, high-sugar Western diet, have decimated the once-dense "rain forest" of our gut. A "food desert" is an area where quality food is unavailable, even if people want to eat it. Imagine your gut as a vast, almost uninhabitable food desert, where only the bad bugs can survive and actually thrive on the stuff you throw down to them. Remember Audrey II, the carnivorous plant in *Little Shop of Horrors*, who was always screaming, "Feed me, Seymour. Feed me!"? Similarly, the bad bugs are demanding more sugar, refined carbs, and saturated fat—in other words, junk food. That's exactly what the bad bugs love to dine on, which takes us back to Rule Number 1. Stop feeding the gang members what they thrive on, and they will leave town. It is as simple as that.

SUCCESS STORY

Every Little Bit Counts

Twenty-three-year-old Lydia B. had a persistent cough and sore throat, which her well-meaning doctor was treating with round after round of broad-spectrum antibiotics. She developed a rash, which her doctor called an "antibiotic drug rash." When it failed to clear up, he sent her to a rheumatologist, who diagnosed her with lupus and started her on high doses of steroids. The rash resolved, but by then acne, weight gain, and mood swings—all the result of steroid use—had made this formerly vivacious young woman obese and miserable. Her story was classic: her gut buddies had been carpet-bombed, the gang members had moved in, and her own immune system had begun to mistakenly attack her.

When I came on board, our job was to initiate an all-out effort to stop the incoming attacks from lectins, restore the gut wall, and rebuild the gut buddies. We started to rapidly taper her off steroids and instituted the Plant Paradox Program. Within three months, Lydia was completely off steroids, the acne had cleared, the rashes on her face and arms had disappeared, and the excess weight was falling off. Her depression has also lifted. All was well.

Then, one morning a few months later, Lydia came running into the office in a panic. By chance, I was sitting at the front desk, filling out a form, and looked up to see this lovely woman covered from head to toe with huge red blotches, the classic *erythema multiforme*, a symptom of an autoimmune reaction in lupus. She sheepishly admitted that she had had a piece of sourdough bread the night before, and woke up with this gift. Luckily, a little Benadryl and quercetin tided her over, but it was a lesson she'll never forget.

RULE NUMBER 3: Fruit Might as Well Be Candy

Forget any idea that fruit is a health food. As you've learned, eating fruit in season allowed our ancestors to fatten up for the winter, but now fruit is ubiquitous 365 days a year. The next time you ask for a fruit salad as a "healthy" breakfast, I suggest that instead you order a bowl of Skittles candy. Go ahead—it's the same poisonous stuff. The corollary to Rule Number 3 is this: If it has seeds, it's a fruit! That means that a zucchini, a tomato, a bell pepper, an eggplant, and a pickle are all fruits! And when you eat them, they deliver the same chemical message to your genes and your brain as a more obvious fruit, such as an apple, does: Store fat for the winter. Moreover (and this will surprise most of you), eating the fructose in fruit causes your kidneys to swell and suffer injury, which can destroy them.[2]

Just to be clear, there *are* three fruits that you can have, so long as you eat them when they are still green: bananas, mangoes, and papayas. Unripe tropical fruit has not yet increased its sugar (fructose) content. Instead, it is made up of resistant starches, the things your good gut bugs love to dine on, but we mere humans don't have the enzymes to digest. Green papaya and mango are great sliced in a salad. Green banana flour comes in handy for making grain-free pancakes and baked goods. Our dear friend the avocado is the only acceptable ripe fruit because it contains nary a trace of sugar and is composed of good fat and soluble fiber, which help you lose weight and absorb fat-soluble vitamins and antioxidants.

I covered the next concept several times in Part I, but it is so important that it deserves to be my fourth and final rule.

RULE NUMBER 4: You Are What the Thing You Are Eating, Ate

If you prefer, think of this as a piece of parental advice: When you sleep with someone, you are sleeping with everyone that person ever slept with! If you eat meat, poultry, farm-raised fish, eggs, and dairy products, you are largely an ear of corn and a pile of soybeans, because that is what almost all industrially raised food animals are regularly fed.

The Elephant *Not* in the Room

WHY HAVE I not mentioned how many calories you can consume a day? The old rule, that a calorie in equals a calorie out, assumes that *you* are absorbing all those calories. It doesn't factor in the fact that on the Plant Paradox Program, your gut buddies have an amazing ability to consume a lot of the calories that you ingest. They use those calories to grow lots of little clones, either making the calories unavailable to you or changing them into life-promoting special fats that power you. On this program, you will make sure that your gut buddies get their fair share, which means you can actually eat far more food than you used to eat and still lose weight. I kid you not. In fact, as my friend Dr. Terry Wahls likes to say, you'll see evidence of this with the large bowel movement "snakes" coiled in your toilet!

We'll get into specifics about what you will and will not be eating below and then again in greater detail in the following chapters. Your food choices will expand as you heal your gut and your tolerance for certain lectin-containing foods grows as you advance through the three phases of the Plant Paradox Program. But unlike most "diet plans," there will be no calorie counting or carb counting. All you have to watch is your intake of animal protein.

Feasting on Corn

CORN IS OMNIPRESENT in the standard American diet, especially in processed foods. Fast food restaurants rely on corn oil, cornstarch, cornmeal, corn syrup, and a host of other ingredients extracted from corn. When scientists examined approximately 480 burgers from a gamut of fast food restaurants, they found that almost all of them, a whopping 93 percent, contained a "signature" C-4 carbon that indicates that the meat that comprised the burger came from corn (meaning the animal's diet was corn-heavy).[3] If that drives you to order a chicken sandwich next time you grab a bite at a fast food restaurant, hear this: The meat in chicken sandwiches were similarly made from corn. In fact, all the chicken served in the fast food places in the study originated from one source, Tyson, which feeds chickens corn—and only corn. There is no escaping corn in such chain restaurants.

If 93 percent of the ground beef in a burger originated with corn, the next logical question may be "How much of me originated with corn?" Do you want to hear the good news first? It's less than 93 percent. Now for the bad news: Scientists at the University of California–Berkeley carbon-tested strands of hair from typical Americans and found that 69 percent was from corn.[4] (Even health guru Sanjay Gupta's hair analysis found the exact same percentage of carbon from corn.[5]) And here's the shocker: When the same carbon test was performed on strands of hair from typical Europeans, the corn content was a mere 5 percent.

Unfortunately, there's even worse news. Most field corn (the type fed to livestock) grown in the United States is a genetically modified version called Bt corn. A gene for a potent lectin from the snowdrop plant is inserted into this corn to improve its insect resistance. And once that lectin makes it into corn and is fed to cows, chickens, and pigs, and then you eat those animals or drink cow's milk, it makes its way into you! This is a lectin to which everyone reacts, and it's even found in the breast milk of American mothers.

Another sobering point: Genetically modified corn produces

osteopenia and osteoporosis in chickens.[6] (And you thought only postmenopausal women developed these two bone-deterioration diseases.) One reason chickens are crammed together in their pens is that their leg bones are so brittle from their diet that they fracture when the birds try to walk. So, ladies, the next time you take your osteoporosis medication in the morning and have a boneless chicken breast for lunch or dinner, ask yourself a variation of that age-old question: Which came first, the chicken or the osteoporosis? Actually, the correct answer is corn. Again, you are eating the stuff that these animals ate.[7]

Because our livestock have been routinely given antibiotics, they have become hosts to multiple forms of antibiotic-resistant bacteria. Almost weekly, we hear another report of a meat or chicken recall because of an outbreak of deadly diarrhea.

Wait—I'm not done yet. It turns out that chicken (eggs and flesh), pork, beef, and cow's milk are contaminated with aflatoxins, toxic by-products of molds and fungi that grow on corn, wheat, and soybeans. These compounds are toxic to animals and humans, and their consumption has been linked to genetic changes and cancer.[8] Cereal grains and soybeans (the type fed to poultry) are particularly subject to aflatoxin contamination.[9] While the U.S. Department of Agriculture sets standards for the amount of fungal toxins that are allowed in corn, grains, and soybeans fed to our chickens, turkeys, cows, and pigs, there is no control over or requirement about the maximum amount of these toxins that are allowed in the finished products—the meats that we eat and the milk that we drink. And, quite frankly, it's a staggeringly high amount. It seems the USDA is more concerned about food animals consuming these toxins than humans eating those same toxins in animals. Think about that the next time you order a serving of Chicken McNuggets. You might be getting a double whammy of aflatoxins from the chicken as well as the breading. Add a glass of milk and you up your chances of toxification.

She'd Rather Switch than Fight Multiple Sclerosis

Marcia D., a beautiful twenty-nine-year-old, was referred to me with chronic progressive multiple sclerosis (MS), despite taking heavy immunosuppressant meds and following a gluten-free, mostly vegetarian diet. Persistent brain fog and progressive numbness of her left hand made getting to and from work difficult, so she had to work from home. She had noted some improvement after going gluten-free, but some of her favorite gluten-free foods—like corn chips, potatoes, and tomatoes— seemed to worsen her symptoms. As usual, her blood work showed the typical pattern of lectin sensitivity and exposure to foods that contain them. Out those foods went, and within three months, Marcia was back at work and off the immuno-suppressant drugs, and the brain fog and numbness were gone.

That was five years ago. Her recent blood work reflects the banishment of lectins from her diet, although I do get the occasional phone call for help. I remember one panicked call well. She had awakened one morning with her left fingers going numb and her brain foggy. "What were you doing last night?" I asked. "I was with some friends and had a slice of gluten-free pizza," she replied. Now, gluten-free pizza is a fabulous lectin bomb, usually with a crust made of oat, corn, or rice flour, plus tomato sauce and cheese made from cows with the casein A-1 mutation. You get the idea. I asked Marcia what she expected by eating that pizza? Her answer was that she was thirty-three years old and had to have a life! "Fine," I replied. "Do that and enjoy your life from a wheelchair. It's always your choice." She has never wavered since that morning.

The Buddy System

BACK TO RULE Number 2, which applies to the good bugs, your gut buddies. Friendly bacteria are like neighbors who are invested in the neighborhood (your body). Your objective is to protect and encourage their growth, but typically their needs and wants have been pushed aside in favor of the bad bugs. As a result, the good bugs are hiding in their homes, afraid to come out. But if you starve the bad guys and throw the good guys a lifeline, the good guys will reemerge to support the neighborhood. What's more, those good bacteria will start asking you for more of what they need to succeed. I've been amused and pleased through the years when dyed-in-the-wool "meat and potatoes" people come back to see me after a couple months on the program and tell me that they now crave salads full of green things. In fact, when they go a couple of days without one, they are ready to kill to get to the salad bar! They are completely shocked by their own behavior, which is now controlled by a new set of microbes, their true gut buddies, giving out new sets of instructions. These good bacteria are saying loud and clear to their hosts, "Please help take care of our home."

The most important gift your gut buddies can give you is to direct your appetite and manage your cravings. This frees you from the constant battle to control your desires, along with the chore of calorie counting and the effort to demonize those wonderful-looking junk foods. Give your gut buddies what they want and they will return the favor.[10] Soon, the bad bugs responsible for those cravings will have left the building.

Those unremitting cravings that often torture people on high-protein, high-fat, low-carbohydrate diets do not occur when the source of protein is fish and there are plenty of resistant carbs from greens and tubers. But the fats in high-protein diets tend to come from the lard in beef and saturated fats in other farm animals. The LPSs in your gut hop on these saturated fats to sneak through the wall of your gut; then they are directly transported to the hunger center in your brain, the hypothalamus. There, the resulting inflammation in your brain sparks your hunger.

This absence of constant hunger is one way in which the Plant Paradox Program differs significantly from Paleo and some ketogenic diets, both of which include plenty of animal fats. The Plant Paradox Program contains only appropriate animal fats—and let me remind you that there are vegetarian and vegan versions of the program for those who eat no meat, fish, or poultry and for those who also don't touch dairy or eggs. People who insist that we need to eat animal protein will soon learn what any gorilla knows: there is a huge amount of muscle-building protein in leaves. Not convinced? Just look at a horse. He didn't get those sleek muscles from munching on burgers.

An Overview of the Plant Paradox Program

THE REVOLUTIONARY APPROACH of the Plant Paradox Program will help you achieve both optimal health and the ability to manage your weight by feeding you and your good gut bugs what you both need. We'll get into the specifics of the three phases that constitute the Plant Paradox Program in the following three chapters. Meanwhile, here are the basics:

- **PHASE 1:** This three-day cleanse begins the process of repairing your gut, fortifying the good microbes, and banishing most of the bad microbes. At the end of the three days, your gut organisms will have changed, and therefore, your gut has changed. But you must move directly from Phase 1 to Phase 2 to prevent the almost immediate return of the bad guys.
- **PHASE 2:** Here is where the Plant Paradox Program really kicks in. All I ask is that you give me two weeks, and in return I'll give you back your life. After two weeks, you will feel and see the change—it is that powerful. And after six weeks, you'll have engrained these new eating habits. During this time, I'm going to ask you to eliminate or reduce certain foods and eat more of others. Here's an overview:
  - Initially, you'll eliminate major lectins (grains and legumes, including corn and soybeans, which also contain estrogenlike substances), GMO foods, crops treated with Roundup, and many saturated fats. This includes whole-grain products, which hypersensitize the immune system. But fear not, vegetarians and vegans, I have a solution for you below.
  - Eliminate all sugars and artificial sweeteners.
  - Minimize intake of most omega-6 fats, which prompt the body's attack mode, encouraging fat storage and hunger.
  - Eliminate industrial farm—raised poultry (including so-called free-range poultry) and livestock (along with their dairy products) and all farm-raised fish, which are fed antibiotics, corn, and beans full of omega-6s and laced with Roundup.

- You may have a small serving of nuts, guacamole, or simply half a Hass avocado as a snack.[11] You will find that over
  time, if you are eating the right foods, you no longer feel
  the need for snacks. The wrong foods, on the other hand,
  simply make you hungrier.
- Avoid using all endocrine-disrupting products.
- Instead, you'll consume the following:
  - All leafy greens and certain vegetables, and a sub-
    stantial amount of tubers and other foods that contain
    resistant starch. Initially, you will give fruit the boot.
    Later, you can reintroduce it only in its real season, and
    only as "candy."
  - Consume more omega-3 fats, particularly those found
    in fish oil, perilla oil, flaxseed oil, and other approved
    oils, such as avocado, walnut, olive, or macadamia nut,
    as well as medium-chain triglycerides (MCTs), all of
    which allow speedy repair of the gut barrier.
  - Consume no more than 8 ounces of animal protein a day
    (remember, fish and shellfish are animals), primarily as
    wild-caught fish and shellfish, which are high in ome-
    ga-3 fatty acids and have no artery-destroying Neu5Gc,
    as well as eggs from pastured or omega-3-fed chickens.
  - Only 4 ounces of your daily protein should come from
    grass-fed or pasture-raised meat, which have more
    omega-3 and fewer omega-6 oils than animals fed
    grains and soy, but still do contain lots of Neu5Gc.
  - Consume dairy products only from certain breeds of
    cows or from sheep, goats, and water buffalo, which
    make casein A-2. However, in general, with the ex-
    ception of ghee, limit all dairy products, owing to the
    presence of Neu5Gc.

- **PHASE 3** (optional): Reduce intake of all animal protein, including fish, to a total of 2 to 4 ounces a day and fast intermittently.
- The Keto Plant Paradox Intensive Care Program, introduced in chapter 10, is designed for those of you with diabetes, cancer, or kidney failure, or who have been diagnosed with neurologic diseases such as dementia, Parkinson's, Alzheimer's, or ALS. If that describes you, do the Three-Day Kick-Start Cleanse, then go directly to chapter 10 and dive in. I'll provide instructions to determine when, if ever, you may segue to Phase 2.

Glad Tidings for Vegetarians and Vegans

MY PRACTICE INCLUDES a large number of vegetarians and vegans who have asked for my help over the years. Unfortunately, most of them were what I call "pasta-grain-bean-atarians." Asking them to give up their usual sources of plant protein, regardless of the fact that these foods were making them sick, has been a struggle for them and for me. Fortunately, by working with my vegetarian and vegan "canaries," I have found ways around the problem. Here's the first piece of good news: A pressure cooker will destroy the lectins in beans and other legumes, which are a fantastic source of nonvegetable protein, as well as in vegetables in the nightshade and squash families (actually fruits). Better yet, pressure-cooked beans, shorn of their offending lectins, serve as a smorgasbord for your gut buddies, and can improve longevity and enhance memory. More good news: Most natural foods stores and Whole Foods stock brands of beans and other legumes in cans that are not lined with BPA. Westbrae Natural and Eden Foods are two such brands. (Eden Foods pressure-cooks the beans in the can.) Thus vegetarians and vegans can consume small amounts of properly prepared legumes and certain other lectin-containing foods in Phase 2 of the Plant Paradox Program.

Unfortunately, the lectins in wheat, rye, barley, and oats—yes, the gluten-containing grains—cannot be destroyed, so these foods remain off-limits. But using a pressure cooker does destroy the lectins in other grains and pseudo-grains, making them safe for consumption. (See "Not Grandma's Pressure Cooker," below.) In fact, because the lectins are destroyed, their role in weight gain is also reduced. But please do not introduce these foods until Phase 3, if at all. Remember, humans have no need for these grains.

Let me embrace my vegan and vegetarian colleagues and friends once more, along with anyone else who wants to reduce his or her intake of animal protein. All that stands between you and true health are the lectins in beans and certain grains that can be destroyed in a few minutes on your countertop.

Not Grandma's Pressure Cooker

You may be disinclined to purchase a pressure cooker, fearing that it could be dangerous. Almost everyone who grew up in the 1950s has heard about a pressure cooker exploding and creating a terrible mess, and perhaps even burning the cook. Pressure cookers from that era had just one mechanical regulator, which could allow pressure to build up with disastrous effects. Today's appliances are a whole different story, thanks to a metal interlocking lid designed to withstand enormous pressure, an airtight gasket, and a relief valve to allow the device to maintain a constant pressure. They are also surprisingly affordable. Look for an automatic one, such as the Cuisinart or Instant Pot brands, which shut off when the cooking cycle is complete. For a hassle-free, lectin-free lifestyle, a good pressure cooker can't be beat.

What Is the Right Amount of Protein?

Consuming sufficient protein is essential to power your body and build muscle. And the protein you consume must provide the essential amino acids that supply the building blocks of protein you cannot make yourself. However, most Americans consume far more protein, particularly animal protein, than they need. Government subsidies of corn, other grains, and soybeans that are fed to industrial-farmed animals, poultry, and even fish mean that animal protein has become ridiculously inexpensive. No matter how cheap, no one needs to eat a pound of sirloin at a sitting. As we've discussed, overconsuming and then having to metabolize large amounts of protein into sugar is associated with higher blood sugar levels, obesity, and a shorter life span.[12] Moreover, certain amino acids in animal protein—methionine, leucine, and isoleucine—seem to be real culprits for promoting rapid aging and cancer growth.[13]

So how much protein do you *actually* need? Most protein recommendations are based not on your weight but on your lean body mass, which requires a number of complex calculations to ascertain. But to make it really easy, both Dr. Valter Longo of the Longevity Institute at the University of Southern California and I agree that people require *only 0.37 grams of protein per kilogram of body weight.*[14] Since 1 kilogram equals 2.2 pounds, a 150-pound man needs about 25 grams of protein daily and a 125-pound woman about 21 grams. You can calculate this for yourself by dividing your weight in pounds by 2.2 to get your weight in kilograms, and then multiplying that number by 0.37 to get your required daily grams of protein. To give you a general sense, you'll get 20 grams of protein from one scoop of protein powder, about two and a half whole eggs, a Quest bar, 2 to 3 ounces of fish or chicken, a 3-ounce can of tuna, a 3.75-ounce can of sardines, or 4 ounces of canned crabmeat. To best judge your intake of animal protein, just remember the rule "Eat one and you're done," meaning a single 3-ounce serving a day.

And please, do not fall into the "protein-combining" trap, which means that you must eat all essential amino acids at every meal. This is total nonsense from an evolutionary standpoint. Your ancestors didn't examine their food choices each meal to make sure that they were getting the right combination of proteins. Your body recycles essential amino acids; you don't need a fresh batch of each and every essential amino acid from protein on a daily basis.

To complicate matters, the calculations above do not take into account that every day we recycle about 20 grams of our own protein that has sloughed from our intestines and mucus. In other words, both mucus and your gut lining cells contain protein, and when mucus is produced or your gut lining cells die and are replaced, we digest these proteins in our gut. Your digestive system is very economical! If you want to be a real protein-calculating purist, you could eliminate another half of the already low protein recommendation because you are recycling your own protein daily. As you can see, our protein needs are shockingly small.

In actual practice, this means that if you had two medium eggs at breakfast (about 15 grams of protein), a big salad topped with an ounce of soft goat cheese (about 5 grams) for lunch, a couple of tablespoons of pistachios (about 3 grams) for a snack, and 3 ounces of salmon with dinner (22 grams), you'd be far exceeding your protein needs—and I am not even counting the protein in the vegetables you are eating. Yes, there is protein in vegetables. Half a cup of steamed cauliflower supplies 1 gram of protein; a medium baked sweet potato, 2 grams; and an artichoke, about 4 grams. Protein adds up quickly, and as you'll see, I'm going to be lenient about the amount of protein you can have initially on the Plant Paradox Program. But by Phase 3, for very good reasons, you are going to try to significantly restrict both your overall protein intake and the amount of animal protein.

Forget Your Excuses and Get Inspired

IN PART I, I talked about supposedly healthy foods that do not live up to their name. As a plant paradox newbie, you may have still some lingering doubts about the wisdom of cutting out whole grains, organic chicken, cow's milk yogurt, edamame, tofu, and other foods that are marketed as "healthy." You'll need to get over that hurdle to succeed on the Plant Paradox Program. On the one hand, the program is very simple—what other diet has only four rules?—but, admittedly, it does require some mental and physical realignment if you have been eating the typical overproteinized American diet, or even if you have been dutifully consuming what you think is healthy food. Ditto if you have been eating a variety of vegetables without understanding the significant differences between, say, a potato and a yam. Below are some of the most common excuses, as exemplified by the experiences of some of my patients who have become plant paradox advocates after changing their way of eating and experiencing dramatic changes in their health—and often their weight. When you read of their dramatic recoveries, you will probably decide that you, too, are willing to make some relatively small changes in order to have major changes in your health, weight, and overall sense of well-being.

Don't let any of these excuses keep you from moving forward with the program.

EXCUSE #1: You Are Already Slim, Fit, and Active

If so, you may feel there is no need to change your way of eating. What follows is the story of an outwardly fit man who did not know that he had a serious health problem, with increased risk for even more serious problems. Fortunately, when he found out, he decided to do something about it. Resigning himself to accept the inevitable was never an option.

EXCUSE #1 SUCCESS STORY

An Extreme Athlete Betters All His Numbers

Simon V. came to see me on the advice of a friend. He was forty years old, cycled 150 to 200 miles a week, was slim and muscular, and from all appearances was in great shape. Initially, he was interested in improving his athletic performance, but a test revealed that he was not going to enjoy a healthy life span. His oxidized LDL ("bad") cholesterol level, an indicator of how sticky your cholesterol is, was extremely high, and he had low HDL ("good") cholesterol. He also carried what's commonly called the Alzheimer's gene, known as ApoE4 (30 percent of us carry that gene). Fortunately, I am the world's expert on the dietary approach for people with ApoE4. After adopting the Plant Paradox Program, Simon reduced his body fat to a remarkably low

8 percent and lost eight pounds. His oxidized LDL went from 107 to 47, which is within the normal range, and his HDL is now up to 62, also in the normal range. Not only did Simon improve his chances for living a long, healthy life, he also bettered his athletic performance. He can now sustain a heart rate of 180 beats per minute for thirty minutes, and his resting heart rate dropped an additional eight points.

EXCUSE #2: You Are Worried That the Program Requires a Deep Understanding of Human Metabolism and Nutritional Concepts

The good news is that I have several patients who have Down syndrome or are otherwise intellectually challenged, who have had great results. I also have a number of patients who don't speak English who have seen positive outcomes. Although it is important to read this entire book to understand why the Plant Paradox Program works, its success often comes down to knowing and abiding by the two lists of food to either eat or avoid.

EXCUSE #2 SUCCESS STORY

Ensuring a Healthy Future

Molly S. has Down syndrome, along with a host of health problems. At forty-seven, she a had fatty liver, high cholesterol, and prediabetes, and was in kidney failure. She was also obese. Her mother was worried about Molly's long-term future, considering her cluster of medical issues, and they both came to see me.

Molly's mother was particularly concerned that at the special school Molly attended, the students were fed cookies and ice cream and other problematic snacks. Once Molly's mother understood the Plant Paradox Program herself, she implemented it right along with Molly, explaining to her daughter how to follow it and preparing food for her to take to school. Molly followed the program to the letter, and within six months had lost thirty pounds. Her kidney function has returned to normal, and all her numbers for cholesterol, liver function, and blood pressure also normalized. Molly learned that the foods being pushed on her at her school were making her ill. Now she tries to help her classmates avoid them, too.

EXCUSE #3: You're Too Old to Make Significant Changes in Your Eating and Other Habits (or You Think Your Loved Ones Are)

A lot of the patients I see in my Palm Springs clinic are retirees. I am constantly inspired by the willingness of elderly or extremely ill people to make changes that will better their lives. Here is just one such inspiring story that drives home the point that I see every day. It is never too late to improve your health. You replace about 90 percent of your old cells with new ones every three months, regardless of your age. Giving those new cells high-quality building materials to work with via the foods you eat and what you feed your bugs will absolutely make a new you!

It's Never Too Late to Make Better Choices!

I first met Rebecca L. ten years ago, when she was eighty-five. As the sole caregiver for her mentally disabled sixty-year-old daughter, she told me at our first office visit, "You've got to help me. I can't die." At that time, Rebecca had severe coronary artery disease, congestive heart failure, diabetes, and heartburn. Her arthritis and obesity made it difficult for her to walk. Well, by following the Plant Paradox Program, she lost seventy pounds and has kept it off. All of her health problems are a distant memory, so she is no longer taking any medications. At ninety-five, this striking redhead now has a live-in boyfriend who is only eighty-five!

With this inspiration under your (soon to be smaller) belt, I trust you are champing at the bit to get going. But if you still have some lingering doubts, consider these facts.

- Great apes eat fruit to gain weight for the winter. What makes you different? Nothing.
- Farmers use grains, corn, and beans to fatten livestock for slaughter. What makes you different? Nothing.
- Horses are fed oats to fatten them for the winter when forage is hard to come by. What makes you different? Nothing.

Every time you think the "rules" don't apply to you, you have to answer the same question: What makes you think that you are any different? I think you know the answer.

Unless you *don't* want to slim down and *don't* want to improve your overall health, let's move on to the cleanse phase of the Plant Paradox Program.

Phase 1

Kick-Start with a Three-Day Cleanse

Welcome to Phase 1 of the Plant Paradox Program, the Three-Day Kick-Start Cleanse. As you now know, bacteria and other single-cell organisms can control you in many ways, including creating an insatiable appetite and making you crave the wrong foods. These invaders have taken over, "partying" in your gut, while you suffer the consequences. It is time to drive them out.

Just as a gardener or farmer prepares the soil before planting, you need to prepare the environment in your gut before you sow the seeds of wellness. Think of the French word *"terroir,"* which refers to the combination of soil, climate, and region that produces a distinctive wine, as a metaphor for the individual environment in your gut. Based on my experience studying tens of thousands of patients, I can assure you that if your gut is damaged, you can eat all sorts of good-for-you foods but you simply won't benefit from them. That's where this three-day cleanse—or modified fast, if you prefer to think of it that way—comes in; it begins the process of restoring your gut.

Well-designed studies have shown that a three-day cleanse completely changes the types of bacteria that inhabit your gut—yet within a day of reverting to your old habits, all the good guys leave and the bad guys move back in.[1] But here's an important point: While everyone has been focusing on the bugs that live in your colon, recent research suggests that the *real* war is happening in your small intestine.[2] Doctors and scientists have been focused on testing patients' stools because we haven't had the tools to reach the small intestine, but that's where the action begins. Only the Plant Paradox Program focuses on your entire gut and the buddies that live everywhere in and on you.

Because it is so important to keep those gut buddies around, you will move directly into Phase 2 after three days on the cleanse. Despite the solid research on how a three-day cleanse changes gut flora cited above, these three days are optional. Feel free to start in Phase 2 if you prefer, but understand that it will take a bit longer to achieve results.

PHASE 1 Strategies

PREPARE YOUR GUT for "planting" a new crop by weeding out the bad things and preparing the "soil" for the good things. In just three days, this modified fast or cleanse doesn't just repair your gut, it also repels invaders—the gut busters—by starving many of the gut bacteria that make us sick and fat and stimulate an immune response. The complete cleanse is composed of three components, and while I recommend you follow all three protocols, you will still see results even if you just follow the three-day food plan.

COMPONENT 1: On and Off the Menu

During this short cleanse, you will eat no dairy, grains or pseudo-grains, fruit, sugar, seeds, eggs, soy, nightshade plants, roots, or

tubers. Also off the menu are corn, soy, canola, or other inflammatory oils, along with any form of beef or other farm animal meat.
Instead, you *will* eat delectable dishes made with vegetables and
small amounts of fish or pastured chicken. We also provide vegetarian and vegan options for recipes that include fish or chicken.
This three-day protocol is based on the Kick-Start Cleanse, which
my good friend Irina Skoeries designed for the Plant Paradox Program. The founder of Catalyst Cuisine, Irina developed the recipes
for this phase, some of which also recur in the Phase 2 meal plan.
Meal plans for Phase 1 appear on pages 289–290 and include vegan
and vegetarian versions. Recipes start on page 315 and similarly
provide vegan and vegetarian variations. Using the principles I
teach, Irina cured herself of rheumatoid arthritis, which had crip-
pled her. By removing all the proscribed foods, you, too, will ex-
tinguish the flames of inflammation, allowing your body to begin
the process of healing.

The ingredients for the cleanse recipes can be found at most
well-stocked supermarkets. Irina also now has a successful
healthy meal delivery service, available throughout the continen-
tal United States, which ships meals in an insulated container. You
can order the three-day cleanse from her and save yourself some
work. (For more information, visit www.catalystcuisine.com.) Or
you can modify her recipes or use your own, as long as you follow
these guidelines:

Vegetables
- Welcome to the wonderful world of vegetables, with particular
  emphasis on the cabbage family, including bok choy, broccoli,
  Brussels sprouts, any color and type of cabbage, cauliflower, kale,
  and mustard greens. Greens include endive, all kinds of lettuce, spinach, Swiss chard, and watercress. Also on the menu are

artichokes, asparagus, celery, fennel, and radishes, along with such fresh herbs as mint, parsley, basil, and cilantro, plus garlic and all kinds of onions, including leeks and chives. Don't forget the ocean vegetables kelp and seaweed, including sheets of nori.

- You can eat as much as you want of these vegetables, either cooked or raw. If you have irritable bowel syndrome (IBS), SIBO, diarrhea, or another gut issue, limit the raw veggies and cook the rest thoroughly.

Protein

- Consume no more than 8 ounces of wild-caught fish (such as salmon, shellfish, or mollusks) or pastured chicken a day in two 4-ounce portions (about the size of a deck of cards). Certain Quorn products, tempeh (without grains), and hemp tofu are also acceptable.

Fats and Oils

- You can and should have a whole Hass avocado each day. Olives of any kind are also permitted.
- Use only avocado oil, coconut oil, macadamia nut oil, sesame seed oil, walnut oil, extra-virgin olive oil, hemp seed oil, and flaxseed oil. MCT oil (sometimes called liquid coconut oil), perilla oil, and Thrive algae oil, which we will discuss later, are also good choices but may be difficult to find in stores. They are all available online.

Snacks

- Have one or two small snacks of Romaine Lettuce Boats Filled with Guacamole (page 320), or simply half an avocado splashed with lemon juice, or ¼ cup of Dr. G.'s New and Improved World-Famous Nut Mix (page 333), or any combination of the approved nuts.

Condiments and Seasonings
- Use fresh lemon juice, vinegar, mustard, freshly cracked black pepper and sea salt, and your favorite herbs and spices.
- Avoid any commercially prepared salad dressings or sauces.

Beverages
- Have a Green Smoothie (page 315) each morning.
- Drink 8 cups a day of tap or filtered water, or San Pellegrino or other Italian sparkling mineral water (or Acqua Panna, a still mineral water).
- Also drink plenty of green, black, or herbal tea, or regular or decaffeinated coffee.
- If you wish, sweeten your tea or coffee with stevia extract (preferably SweetLeaf, which also contains inulin) or Just Like Sugar (inulin).

And Don't Forget
- Get at least eight hours of sleep.
- Exercise in moderation, preferably outdoors.

Only the Best

THE SOURCE AND quality of the foods you use to make your meals and snacks are critical. Preferably:

- All vegetables should be 100 percent organic.
- Vegetables can be fresh or frozen. If fresh, they should be in season and grown locally with sustainable farming practices, if at all possible.
- All fish and shellfish should be wild caught.
- All chicken should be pastured.

But as I always say, just do the best you can. Following these guidelines ensures that the foods you'll be eating provide the maximum amount of nutrients and the least amount of disruptors and lectins. I realize that occasionally, if the organic version is unavailable, you may have to use conventional produce, but it's important to understand that the purer the ingredients, the better the results of the cleanse.

To ensure that you are not creating inflammation when cooking or dressing foods, you'll be using only certain oils. Phase 1 recipes (see pages 315–324) use avocado oil for sautéing, but you can also cook with most of the oils listed above. Extra-virgin olive oil should never be exposed to high heat, but low heat is fine. Hemp seed and flaxseed oils should not be heated at all, so confine their use to dressing salads and other vegetables.

See "Make the Cleanse Easy" on page 314 for time-saving tips.

COMPONENT 2: Prepare the "Soil" and Remove the "Weeds"

My oldest patient, Michelle Q., whom I profiled in my first book, is now 105 years old! She still walks into my office in her two-inch-high heels, dressed to the nines, with her hair and makeup impeccable. When she became my patient fifteen years ago, I asked her why she had come to see me. She answered that I was the only doctor who talked just like the late, great nutritionist Gaylord Hauser, who changed her life when she was in her twenties. Thanks to Michelle, I have read everything that Hauser ever wrote, and over the years I have incorporated much of what he taught into my practice. I have tested his dictums on myself, as well as on my patients, and not surprisingly, the sophisticated blood tests that I use have confirmed most of his teachings.

Hauser's first rule was to start with as clean a slate within your gut as possible. His herbal laxative was designed to do just that, by preparing your gut for "planting" a new crop by weeding out the bad things and preparing the "soil" for good things. While not critical, Hauser's recommendation to clean the gut with an herbal laxative called Swiss Kriss or the equivalent has been good advice for nearly a century, and it will absolutely kick-start the great results of the Plant Paradox Program.

You can find Swiss Kriss in any pharmacy or order it online. The active ingredient is the laxative herb senna, or sennosides—each tablet contains 8.5 mg. Other gang-member-destroying ingredients include anise seed, calendula flower, caraway seed, hibiscus, peach leaves, peppermint oil, and strawberry leaves, along with some binding agents. An adult dose is two tablets, taken at bedtime. If you do not want to do this or are concerned about the potential discomfort it might cause, let me stress that using this laxative is absolutely optional. If you do opt to use it, take it the night before you begin the cleanse, along with a glass of water. (If you prefer the flake form of the product, take half a teaspoon.) There is no need to repeat it on the following days. It is a good idea to start this part of the Three-Day Kick-Start Cleanse when you are planning to be at home the next morning.

COMPONENT 3: Supplemental Assistance

Ideally, you shouldn't just stop with preparing the soil and killing the "weeds." I have been very impressed with the ability of several natural supplements to kill bad gut bacteria, molds, and fungi. None of these are absolutely essential; however, if you suffer from IBS, leaky gut, or any autoimmune condition, please consider adding these to your initial regimen. I'll provide doses in the supplement section (pages 273–285). The suggested supplements include:

- Oregon grape root extract or its active ingredient berberine
- Grapefruit seed extract (not to be confused with another great supplement, grape seed extract)
- Mushrooms or mushroom extracts
- Spices such as black pepper, cloves, cinnamon, and wormwood to kill parasites, fungi, and other bad gut flora

Reap the Rewards

LET ME REMIND you that by following a fast or cleanse, even in a mere three days you can change the balance of microbes in your system to more friendly species. That's the good news. But if you just do a cleanse or fast and then return to your old way of eating, any improvement in your gut flora will be short-lived and the bad guys will return with a vengeance. On the other hand, if you immediately transition to a gut buddy–promoting diet, namely Phase 2 of the Plant Paradox Program, beginning the day after you complete the cleanse, you will be on your way to solidifying the gains you've achieved.

At the end of the three days, you will:

- Absolutely change the balance of your gut bacteria for the better.
- Almost certainly lose three or four excess pounds, which will be primarily water weight.
- Dramatically reduce inflammation.
- Have an improved sense of well-being thanks to reduced inflammation.

- Solidify the gains (and losses) you've achieved by moving immediately on to Phase 2.

Tips for Success

DURING THESE THREE days, you will eat delicious food; however, your body will likely miss all the addictive (and inflammation-promoting) foods to which it is accustomed. You might experience some hunger and perhaps some energy depletion. If you find that you need to eat more than the suggested meals on the Phase 1 meal plan, select items from the list of acceptable vegetables, but do not have more than the two servings of guacamole or avocado or any additional fish or chicken. And before turning to more food, try drinking a couple of cups of tap or filtered water.

You may well hate me for those seventy-two hours! But by Day 4, when you move to Phase 2, you will love the fact that your energy has returned in spades and your jeans are noticeably looser.

Before we move to Phase 2, and at the risk of sounding like a broken record, it is absolutely crucial that you segue immediately from Phase 1 to Phase 2. To keep your gut buddies working for the home team, begin Phase 2 on the morning of Day 4. Turn the page to get up to speed on this next phase.

Phase 2

Repair and Restore

If your boat is sinking and water is gushing into the hull, instead of bailing faster or using a bigger bucket, both of which are an exercise in futility, you need to plug the holes. Likewise, if you have a health problem, slowing its progress, as modern medicine suggests, is not a solution; instead, you need to stop the problem in its tracks. Only then can your body start to heal itself. Believe me, your body has the ability to restore itself to perfect health, once you eliminate the foods and other forces that prevent it from healing.

Now that you've initiated the weeding phase of the Plant Paradox Program, it's time to begin the six-week (minimum) repair process. The first step is to stop eating the foods full of lectins that are continually blowing holes in the walls of your gut. If you did the three-day cleanse, you have already begun to eliminate such foods. Once more, let me emphasize the point embodied in Rule Number 1 (see chapter 6, page 168)—contrary to everything you've been led to believe, it's the things you *don't* eat that will dramatically change your health. Once you have that principle firmly established in your mind and practice it on a daily basis, you can move on to Rule Number 2, which says that eating certain foods and taking certain supplements nourish the good bacteria—aka "gut buddies"—and their friends, which have begun to come out of hiding during the three days of Phase 1. Simultaneously, you'll continue to starve the bad bacteria by eliminating the foods they thrive on, along with other disruptive products that hinder healing.

Make no mistake. For the first two weeks, this will be a challenge, because you will be removing a huge number of so-called healthy foods, which are actually making you sick. You might even suffer some withdrawal symptoms, such as low energy, headaches, grouchiness, and muscle cramps. If so, understand that it merely confirms the old adage: the definition of an addict is someone who uses or eats something that he or knows is killing him, but does so nonetheless. All I ask is that you give me two weeks during which you will hate me, and then see how much you like me after that. But remember, although you will see the changes in two weeks, it takes at least six weeks to cement new habits. Stay the course for six weeks and you will find that it becomes virtually automatic.

The short food lists I promised you follow. For the next two weeks, you should eat foods only from the Say "Yes Please" list, and you should not eat any foods from the Just Say "No" list. The Phase 2 recipes (pages 315–363) include many of these "Yes Please" foods. Phase 2 meal plans appear on pages 290–294, again including vegan and vegetarian variations. (Depending on how you respond to the first two weeks, you may be able to slowly and incrementally start reintroducing some lectin-containing foods on that list, but I strongly advise you to not add such foods for the full six weeks.) I suggest you copy this list and carry it with you wherever you go. Take it to the supermarket and restaurants. Keep a copy at your workplace. Refer to it often. Soon, following it will become second nature.

For those of you impatient folks who just couldn't wait to start the Plant Paradox Program and jumped here without reading

Part I, the list is followed by a quick summary of why I am telling
you to do these "crazy" things. I sincerely hope that as you begin to
see the results of following the program, you will take the time to
read the earlier chapters. It will help you understand why the Plant
Paradox Program works and why it is a lifetime approach to eating,
not a quickie diet to follow and then revert to your old habits.

THE SAY "YES PLEASE" LIST OF ACCEPTABLE FOODS

Oils
Algae oil (Thrive
  culinary brand)
Olive oil
Coconut oil
Macadamia oil
MCT oil
Avocado oil
Perilla oil
Walnut oil
Red palm oil
Rice bran oil
Sesame oil
Flavored cod liver oil

Sweeteners
Stevia (SweetLeaf is my
  favorite)
Just Like Sugar (made
  from chicory root
  [inulin])
Inulin
Yacón
Monk fruit
Luo han guo (the
  Nutresse brand is
  good)
Erythritol (Swerve
  is my favorite as
  it also contains
  oligosaccharides)
Xylitol

Nuts and Seeds
(½ cup/day)
Macadamia nuts

Walnuts
Pistachios
Pecans
Coconut (not coconut
  water)
Coconut milk
  (unsweetened dairy
  substitute)
Coconut milk/cream
  (unsweetened, full-fat
  canned)
Hazelnuts
Chestnuts
Brazil nuts (in limited
  amounts)
Pine nuts (in limited
  amounts)
Flaxseeds
Hemp seeds
Hemp protein powder
Psyllium

Olives
All

Dark Chocolate
72% or greater (1 oz./day)

Vinegars
All (without added
  sugar)

Herbs and Seasonings
All except chili pepper
  flakes
Miso

Energy Bars
Quest bars: Lemon
  Cream Pie, Banana
  Nut, Strawberry
  Cheesecake,
  Cinnamon Roll, and
  Double Chocolate
  Chunk only
B-Up bars (sometimes
  found as Yup bars):
  Chocolate Mint,
  Chocolate Chip
  Cookie Dough, and
  Sugar Cookie only
Human Food Bar
  (humanfoodbar.com)
Adapt Bar: Coconut
  and Chocolate
  (adaptyourlife.com)

Flours
Coconut
Almond
Hazelnut
Sesame (and seeds)
Chestnut
Cassava
Green banana
Sweet potato
Tiger nut
Grape seed
Arrowroot

Ice Cream
Coconut Milk Dairy-
  Free Frozen Dessert

THE SAY "YES PLEASE" LIST OF ACCEPTABLE FOODS, *CONTINUED*

(the So Delicious blue label, which contains only 1 gram of sugar)
LaLoo's goat's milk ice cream

"Foodles" (my name for acceptable noodles)
Cappelo's fettuccine and other pastas
Pasta Slim
Shirataki noodles
Kelp noodles
Miracle Noodles and kanten pasta
Miracle Rice
Korean sweet potato noodles

Dairy Products (1 oz. cheese or 4 oz. yogurt/day)
Real Parmesan (Parmigiano-Reggiano)
French/Italian butter
Buffalo butter (available at Trader Joe's)
Ghee
Goat yogurt (plain)
Goat milk as creamer
Goat cheese
Butter
Goat and sheep kefir
Sheep cheese and yogurt (plain)
Coconut yogurt
French/Italian cheese
Switzerland cheese
Buffalo mozzarella (Italy)
Whey protein powder
Casein A-2 milk (as creamer only)
Organic heavy cream
Organic sour cream

Organic cream cheese

Wine (6 oz./day)
Red

Spirits (1 oz./day)

Fish (any wild-caught—4 oz./day)
Whitefish
Freshwater bass
Alaskan halibut
Canned tuna
Alaskan salmon
Hawaiian fish
Shrimp
Crab
Lobster
Scallops
Calamari/squid
Clams
Oysters
Mussels
Sardines
Anchovies

Fruits (limit all but avocado)
Avocados
Blueberries
Raspberries
Blackberries
Strawberries
Cherries
Crispy pears (Anjou, Bosc, Comice)
Pomegranates
Kiwis
Apples
Citrus (no juices)
Nectarines
Peaches
Plums
Apricots
Figs
Dates

Vegetables

Cruciferous Vegetables
Broccoli
Brussels sprouts
Cauliflower
Bok choy
Napa cabbage
Chinese cabbage
Swiss chard
Arugula
Watercress
Collards
Kohlrabi
Kale
Green and red cabbage
Radicchio
Raw sauerkraut
Kimchi

Other Vegetables
Nopales cactus
Celery
Onions
Leeks
Chives
Scallions
Chicory
Carrots (raw)
Carrot greens
Artichokes
Beets (raw)
Radishes
Daikon radish
Jerusalem artichokes/ sunchokes
Hearts of palm
Cilantro
Okra
Asparagus
Garlic
Mushrooms

Leafy Greens
Romaine

Red and green leaf
   lettuce
Mesclun (baby greens)
Spinach
Endive
Dandelion greens
Butter lettuce
Fennel
Escarole
Mustard greens
Mizuna
Parsley
Basil
Mint
Purslane
Perilla
Algae
Seaweed
Sea vegetables

Resistant Starches
Tortillas (Siete brand—
   only those made with
   cassava and coconut
   flour or almond flour)
Bread and bagels made
   by Barely Bread
Julian Bakery Paleo
   Wraps (made with
   coconut flour) and
   Paleo Coconut Flakes
   Cereal

(In Moderation)
Green plantains
Green bananas
Baobab fruit
Cassava (tapioca)
Sweet potatoes or yams
Rutabaga
Parsnips
Yucca
Celery root (celeriac)
Glucomannan (konjac
   root)
Persimmon
Jicama
Taro root
Turnips
Tiger nuts
Green mango
Millet
Sorghum
Green papaya

Pastured Poultry (not
free-range—4 oz./day)
Chicken
Turkey
Ostrich
Pastured or omega-3
   eggs (up to 4 daily)
Duck
Goose

Pheasant
Grouse
Dove
Quail

Meat (grass-fed and
grass-finished—4 oz./
day)
Bison
Wild game
Venison
Boar
Elk
Pork (humanely raised)
Lamb
Beef
Prosciutto

Plant-Based "Meats"
Quorn: Chik'n Tenders,
   Grounds, Chik'n
   Cutlets, Turk'y Roast,
   Bacon-Style Slices
Hemp tofu
Hilary's Root
   Veggie Burger
   (hilaryseatwell.com)
Tempeh (grain-free
   only)

THE JUST SAY "NO" LIST OF LECTIN-CONTAINING FOODS

**Refined, Starchy
Foods**
Pasta
Rice
Potatoes
Potato chips
Milk
Bread
Tortillas
Pastry
Flour
Crackers
Cookies

Cereal
Sugar
Agave
Sweet One or Sunett
   (Acesulfame K)
Splenda (Sucralose)
NutraSweet
   (Aspartame)
Sweet'n Low (Saccharin)
Diet drinks
Maltodextrin

Vegetables
Peas
Sugar snap peas
Legumes*
Green beans
Chickpeas* (including as
   hummus)
Soy
Tofu
Edamame
Soy protein
Textured vegetable
   protein (TVP)

THE JUST SAY "NO" LIST OF LECTIN-CONTAINING FOODS, *CONTINUED*

Pea protein
All beans, including
   sprouts
All lentils*
*Vegans and vegetarians
can have these legumes
in Phase 2, but only if they
are properly prepared in
a pressure cooker.

Nuts and Seeds
Pumpkin
Sunflower
Chia
Peanuts
Cashews

Fruits (some called
vegetables)
Cucumbers
Zucchini
Pumpkins
Squashes (any kind)
Melons (any kind)
Eggplant
Tomatoes
Bell peppers
Chili peppers
Goji berries

**Non–Southern
European Cow's
Milk Products** (these
contain casein A-1)
Yogurt (including Greek
   yogurt)
Ice cream
Frozen yogurt
Cheese
Ricotta
Cottage cheese

**KefirGrains, Sprouted
Grains, Pseudo-
Grains, and Grasses**
Wheat (pressure
   cooking does not
   remove lectins from
   any form of wheat)
Einkorn wheat
Kamut
Oats (cannot pressure
   cook)
Quinoa
Rye (cannot pressure
   cook)
Bulgur
White rice

Brown rice
Wild rice
Barley (cannot pressure
   cook)
Buckwheat
Kashi
Spelt
Corn
Corn products
Cornstarch
Corn syrup
Popcorn
Wheatgrass
Barley grass

Oils
Soy
Grape seed
Corn
Peanut
Cottonseed
Safflower
Sunflower
"Partially hydrogenated"
Vegetable
Canola

No Means No

THE JUST SAY "NO" list is so named because *no* human being ever ate
any of the foods on it until at least ten thousand years ago, when man
began to cultivate grains and other crops. Until that point, grains,
pseudo-grains, and beans were not part of our forebears' diet. As
a result, our ancestors and their gut buddies never encountered or
dealt with the lectins from these seeds. In terms of evolution, getting to know and develop an immunological tolerance to a new lec-

tin within a ten-thousand-year span is like speed dating—it simply cannot be done. These modern seeds are totally different from the plants and other foods that form the basis of the Plant Paradox Program. In contrast, the ancient foods you will be eating have been the sources of vibrant human nutrition for millions of years. Perhaps just as important, the lectins and polyphenols in these beneficial plants and their leaves have been prevalent in the human diet for so long that your immune system and your gut buddies have developed an intimate and symbiotic relationship with them.

Yes, you read that right. Not all lectins are problematic; however, it does take time, lots of time, for our kind to handle them and the messages they convey. Because this messaging has been constant and consistent over millions of years, these plants foster human health. (While I am on the subject, let me again make it crystal clear that you are not going to eliminate *all* lectins from your diet. However, you can control which ones you consume and how much.)

So, again, I ask you: Do you want to trust a plant that mankind has dealt with and with which it has developed a mutual admiration for over millions of years, or one that humans first encountered just a few thousand years ago?[1] If you are hesitant to answer, let me have Dirty Harry answer for you: "You just got to ask yourself one question, 'do I feel lucky?' Well, do ya, punk?" After treating tens of thousands of patients, I can assure you that the folks who thought that they would get lucky by eating whatever they wanted are the same folks who believe that the house wants you to win at a casino.

White Is Right

AS WE DISCUSSED in earlier chapters, all cultures have tried to deal with the lectins that were making its members ill. For ten thousand years, mankind has been trying to make bread white. The vast majority of the nasty lectins, especially wheat germ agglutinin (WGA), are in the bran, which makes the bread brown. Most cultures have been successful in getting rid of the bran—think of French baguettes or Italian white pasta. Italians would never countenance whole-grain pasta! (Meanwhile, brown bread was relegated to the poor.) The same lesson applies to rice, the dietary staple of four billion people. Over the eight thousand years rice has been cultivated, why has every effort been made to remove the hull to create white rice? Well, the hull contains the lectins, and these smart folks have figured out how to eliminate them. However, recently all that changed with the fateful advice to eat "whole-grain goodness." Let's reiterate what we learned in Part I: "Whole-grain goodness" is a modern disaster—and in fact something that your ancestors desperately and successfully tried to eliminate or lessen ever since grains entered the diet. Whole-grain baguettes, croissants, pasta, sushi rice, and soba noodles? Absolute nonsense first, and poison second.

The King of Lectins

AS WE LEARNED, beans, peas, soybeans, lentils, and other members of the legume family (often referred to as the so-called pulses) are another relatively recent agricultural addition to the human diet. An individual bean may be small, but with the highest lectin content of any food group, beans can have a big impact. Five raw black beans or kidney beans will clot your bloodstream within five minutes. Ricin, the lectin found in the castor bean, a plant native to Africa but now thriving in Southern California, is the most potent lectin known. A couple of molecules of ricin will kill a human within minutes, making it a favorite espionage tool. Remember, plants don't like you, and they (and their babies) are armed and dangerous!

Want some examples of bean chemical warfare? Massive outbreaks of "food poisoning" have occurred in schools and hospitals when, as part of a "healthy eating days" program, cafeterias unwittingly served undercooked beans.[2] According to the Centers for Disease Control, 20 percent of the food poisoning cases in the United States are the result of lectins in undercooked beans.[3] Does this sound like a health food? Eating canned beans can also raise your blood pressure, thanks to both the BPA in the lining of most cans and the lectin content.[4] Best to give canned beans a wide berth. Ditto for tofu and edamame (green soybeans), along with any other unfermented soy products. They are most definitely not the health foods they are made out to be. Remember, these are foods that we use to fatten animals for slaughter. What makes you any different?

Despite these serious concerns about legumes, pressure cooking is a great way to destroy the lectins and retain the nutrition in lentils, kidney beans, and the rest of this large and varied plant family. (See page 180 and "Not Grandma's Pressure Cooker," page 181.)

The Dairy Dilemma

ANOTHER OF OUR culture's food icons, placed high on the healthy foods honor roll, is milk, which has no place in a health-conscious diet—or at least cow's milk doesn't. Let me remind you that if you think you are lactose-intolerant, or if milk stimulates mucus production, you are actually reacting to the lectinlike casein A-1 protein (see chapter 2 for a complete explanation of the casein A-1 mutation and its effect on cows around the world). Fortunately, goats and sheep are not affected by this mutation, making their milk and dairy products acceptable on the Plant Paradox Program, with the word of warning that they all have Neu5Gc, the sugar molecule associated with cancer and heart disease.

New World Lectins

WE HAVE DISCUSSED how Christopher Columbus's "discovery" of the Americas led to the introduction of New World plants to Europe, Africa, and the Far East. As a side note, my Paleo friends just don't seem to understand that no European, African, or Asian had ever been exposed to these plants (and their lectins) before Columbus sailed the ocean blue. Therefore, why they have any place on the Paleo diet is perplexing. The same folks who rail against the evils of grains—and I'm with them on that—love American plants, including the nightshade[5] and squash families, along with peanuts and cashews, and sunflower, chia, and pumpkin seeds. Contemplate this: The lectins in the nightshade family include solanine, a neurotoxin.[6] Again, all New World plants have troublesome lectins that most of mankind has eaten for no more than five hundred years. Even Native Americans came from Asia, so these plants are "new" to all of us.

According to my friend and colleague Loren Cordain, Ph.D., author of *The Paleo Diet*, the first book on the subject, studies that were conducted to see whether humans could absorb the omega-3 fats in chia seeds proved that indeed they could. There was only one hitch: The researchers had hoped to prove that these omega-3 fats would reduce inflammation. But in fact, inflammation markers in the subjects who ate chia seeds went up slightly, rather than decreased, as had been expected.[7] You may be getting some omega-3 fatty acids from chia seeds but their lectin content outweighs any benefit.

The Most Popular Nut Is Not a Nut

The peanut, which originated in the Americas, is a legume, not a nut. As such, it is loaded with killer lectins. Did you know that 94 percent of humans carry a preformed antibody to the peanut lectin?[8] Get this: The lectin in peanut oil produces atherosclerosis in experimental animals, including even our primate cousins the rhesus monkey—but when that lectin is removed from the oil, atherosclerosis does not develop.[9] And here's a stunner: When peanuts are fed to humans and their resulting bowel movements are fed to rats, precancerous lesions appear in the rat colons.[10] All these dangerous effects are the result of consuming the peanut lectin. Think about that the next time you are out at the ballpark!

The Irritating Cashew Nut

Despite its name, like the peanut, the cashew nut is not a nut. Originally found in the Amazon rain forests, it, too, is a bean, which hangs separately from the fruit. Thanks to its potent lectins, Amazonians always threw the "nut" away and ate only the fruit. The shell around the nut is such an irritant that cashew workers must wear protective gloves. There are numerous reports in the dermatological medical literature of outbreaks of rashes after consuming cashew nut butter or the nuts themselves.[11] Cashews are actually in the same botanical family as poison ivy. Keep that in mind before you munch on some cashews. And in my clinical experience, cashews dramatically increase inflammation, particularly in my patients with rheumatoid arthritis.

The Cashew Connection

Here's an example of what can happen when just a single problematic food sneaks back into your diet. Patrice L. was an extremely thin woman who had battled rheumatoid arthritis since her teenage years and had the joint deformities to show for it. At age fifty-nine, she was afraid of the effect that long-term steroids and immunosuppressants were having on her, especially with her advancing osteoporosis. We started the Plant Paradox Program and within three months, she was off steroids and all other medications and all her inflammation markers had normalized. Once she felt good, we started our routine three-month blood test and follow-up program. On her second-year visit, a typical marker that I follow for lectin ingestion (TNF-alpha) was mildly elevated for the first time since her markers had normalized. I asked if she was cheating on the program at all, and Patrice was aghast! "No. Never. Why would I?" she replied. So, we went down the "bad food" list. True to her word, she was avoiding all the usual suspects like the plague. Then we got to cashews. She said she had completely forgotten that they were on the avoid list and had recently been on a cashew kick! In fact, there was a bag in her car that she had been munching on the way to her appointment. One month later, a recheck showed her inflammation was gone—along with the cashews.

American Bad Guys

TWO OF THE worst lectin additions to our diet are the American grain known as corn (maize) and the pseudo-grain quinoa. We have talked at length about the dangers of corn, but did you know that the French banned corn as unfit for human consumption in 1900 and allowed its use only to fatten pigs? This was prompted by an outbreak of congenital mental retardation (cretinism) in northern Italians, who had adopted corn as their main grain. As you now know, corn is not a natural food for cows either.[12]

The American pseudo-grain quinoa is just as troubling. The Incas had three detoxification processes to remove the lectins in quinoa. First, they soaked it, then they let it rot (fermented it), and finally they cooked it. If you've used quinoa, you'll know that the first two of those instructions are not on the package directions. Need I add that most folks who go gluten-free regard quinoa as a great substitute for the grains they have foresworn? In fact, the lectins in this pseodo-grain quinoa only further mess with their gut wall.

SUCCESS STORY

Mother Knows Best!

Alicia M., a forty-year-old Peruvian, relocated to Los Angeles from Lima a year ago but continued to eat her traditional diet, which included quinoa as her staple starch. However, since her move, her bowels and overall health had become a mess. Bloating, sleep troubles, IBS, and brain fog welcomed her to America. Yet she continued her native diet (and shunned American fast food poisons)—until she sought my help.

When we got to quinoa on the Just Say "No" list, Patrice was shocked! She had eaten it all her life without any problem. When I started to explain that the Incas had three steps to eliminate the lectins in quinoa before they ate it, her eyes flew open wide. "Oh my gosh!" she exclaimed. "My mother always said you could not eat quinoa without first pressure cooking it. I thought that was just an old wives' tale, so I have been eating it without pressure cooking it since coming to America. And you are not going to believe this, but my mother visited two weeks ago and bought me a pressure cooker! She was right, but I thought that she was just being old-fashioned."

Six weeks later, I got the call that I was expecting. "You and Mom were right," Patrice told me. "I'm back to normal, and I love my pressure cooker!"

Dealing with Deadly Nightshades

YOU'LL RECALL THAT the nightshade family includes eggplants, potatoes, peppers, goji berries, and tomatoes. Would it surprise you to know that Italians refused to eat tomatoes for two centuries after their native son Columbus brought them home? To this day, Italians peel and deseed tomatoes before making tomato sauce because the peels and seeds contain the lectins. The clever Italians also hybridized the Roma tomato to maximize the ratio of pulp to skin and seeds. Cooks then blanch the tomato in boiling water, pull off the skin, cut the fruit in half, squeeze out the seeds, and presto—pulp minus the skin and seeds. And by the way, tomato sauce and pizza were invented just a little over 120 years ago, making them very new foods in evolutionary terms.

The same approach applies to cooked Italian red peppers. When you open a glass jar of them, do you see any peels and seeds? No. They have been removed, which is not necessarily the case in most American products. The Indians of the American southwest always roast, peel, and deseed their peppers, again to rid them of lectins. Likewise, you won't see peels and seeds in a can of green chilies. Once more, the lectins have been removed. And why are Tabasco and other hot sauces fermented? Because using bacteria to break down the lectins is a time-honored method of lessening the lectin load, just as the Incas did with their quinoa. There is substantial evidence that fermentation significantly reduces lectin content. For example, fermentation in sourdough kills gluten.[13] And fermentation eliminates 98 percent of the lectins in lentils.[14] If you are willing to invest the time, you can banish lectins with the age-old technique of fermentation—although a pressure cooker can do the job in a fraction of the time. Just remember that this won't work with gluten-containing grains.

While we are on the subject of methods used to minimize the impact of lectins, let me overturn a few more myths. Soaking dried grains does not remove gluten or WGA. And sprouting legumes does not make them any easier to digest. In fact, it actually increases lectin content.[15] Feeding sprouted beans or grains to lab animals has been shown to cause cancer.[16] However, as we will discuss further in the next chapter, removing the skins and seeds from tomatoes and peppers and peeling and deseeding squash does reduce the lectin load. Speaking of squash . . .

The Squash Family

WITH THE EXCEPTION of the cucumber, which was first described in India three thousand years ago, but only made its way to Africa and Europe with Columbian trade, the squash family hails from the Americas. As such, its members have lectins that have been foreign to humans for most of their evolution. It bears repeating that any "vegetable" with seeds, such as pumpkin or zucchini, is a fruit, which will have grown only during the summer. And sugars in these summer fruits that we call vegetables signal your central operating system that winter is coming. This means there are two reasons to avoid the squash family: the lectin content and the store-fat-for-winter message they convey to your body.

SUCCESS STORY

The Attack of the Tomatoes

When fifty-year-old Renate Z. sought my help, she was taking three medications and using two rescue inhalers to manage her severe asthma, which was accompanied by severe arthritis, hypertension, and high cholesterol. Within a month of starting the Plant Paradox Program, she had stopped all her medications, including her blood pressure pills, and tossed her inhalers. She also lost thirty pounds over the next six months. When I saw her ten months into the program, she mentioned that about a month earlier she was hungry one night and went to the refrigerator, where her husband had left a container of grape tomatoes in plain view. Renate hadn't had tomatoes in nine months and said to herself, "What the heck. I'll have just three." Fifteen minutes later, she suffered a massive asthma attack! Because she had thrown out her inhalers and medications, she had to call 911. The night in the hospital made her a firm believer in the ability of plants to harm their predator using chemical warfare. She hasn't wavered since.

You Are What *They* Ate

YES, I HAVE said this a few times already, but it is so important that it bears repeating (again). If you feed grains or beans to fish, chicken, cows, pigs, or lambs, they become walking, clucking, and swimming ears of corn or bushels of soybeans. This transformation has occurred only in the last fifty years, coincident with our epidemic of health problems. Some of the most dangerous plant lectins now lurk in the meat of our favorite animal foods. This is but one reason to moderate protein intake. My research and that of others have confirmed that we are overproteinized as a society. From childhood, we are programmed to become protein-aholics. And eating modern animal protein is a major cause of our obesity crisis.[17] As you will soon learn, the single factor that stands out in long-lived societies is the very small amount of protein, and particularly animal protein, that its members consume during their long life span. Limiting animal protein—and let me remind you that a fish is an animal as well—extends health span and life span.

Good Fats, Bad Fats

THE OILS LISTED in the Just Say "No" list on pages 203–204 are all chemically derived from lectin-bearing seeds or beans, meaning they should be avoided as much as possible. I used to include canola oil, made from rapeseed, on my acceptable foods list; however, almost all canola oil now comes from GMO seeds, so I have removed it. For now, and for at least two weeks, I also want you to limit your intake of all long-chain saturated fats, such as coconut oil and animal fats, along with most other mono- and polyunsaturated long-chain fats, such as olive oil, avocado oil, and MCT oil. Also limit your consumption of cheese, sour cream, heavy cream, and cream cheese (even from grass-fed animals), all of which contain saturated fats.

Instead of using olive or coconut oil in this period, I recommend perilla oil. It has the highest content of rosemarinic acid (from rosemary), which improves cognition and memory.[18] You may not have heard of it, but it is the primary cooking oil in Korea, Japan, and China. You can find it at Asian markets, natural foods stores, and Whole Foods, as well as from online sources. Perilla oil also has the highest content of alpha linolenic acid,[19] a form of omega-3 fat used in the Lyon (France) Heart Diet, which has been shown to be more effective at preventing heart disease than the low-fat American Heart Association diet.[20] The Lyon Heart Diet established the gold standard for heart-healthy diets in 1994. Another good alternative is MCT oil (MCT stands for medium-chain triglycerides), which is 100 percent composed of ketones. It is sometimes called liquid coconut oil because it remains liquid even at cold temperatures. The body burns MCT ketones for fuel easily without turning them into body fat. Unlike regular coconut oil, it contains none of the long-chain fatty acids on which those nasty lipopolysaccharides (LPSs) can ride. Other good choices include macadamia nut oil, walnut oil, avocado oil, Thrive algae oil, and ghee. (Ghee is clarified butter, meaning that the milk solids—protein—have been removed and with them the offending lectinlike casein.) You can also use citrus-flavored cod liver oil on salad or to dress cooked vegetables.

Along with perilla oil, which does the best job, all of the oils and fats on the Say "Yes Please" list block LPSs from breaching the gut barrier. Unlike other polyunsaturated fats, long-chain fish oil omega-3s also block the entry of LPSs past your gut wall.[21] I've mentioned before that LPSs ride into your body from your gut on saturated fats. But these fats can't get through without special transport molecules called chylomicrons. The LPSs stow away on chylomicrons, which are formed to carry the long-chain saturated fats, and hitch a ride to get through the gut wall. And the last thing you want are LPSs invading your body right now. Sadly, even my best friend, olive oil, should be limited for the first two weeks of this phase of the Plant Paradox Program, as it, too, is carried by chylomicrons.

A word of advice to any Paleo and ketogenic followers who believe that saturated fats are good for you: A recent study shows that saturated fats such as lard increase hunger and appetite by delivering LPSs to the brain's hunger center;[22] by contrast, fish oil does exactly the opposite, actually sending signals to the brain that help you moderate your food intake![23] Is it any wonder that so many Paleo recipes are for desserts? One popular Paleo blogger's site is called "All Day I Dream About Food." That's the last thing that will happen as the Plant Paradox Program kicks in.

The Program: Phase 2

NOW THAT YOU have the food list and some accompanying information, and assuming you have done the three-day cleanse (or chosen not to), it is time to put the rest of the program into action. You will follow Phase 2 for six weeks. Why so long? Although you can begin to repair your gut and drive out most of the gang members in a few days with the Phase 1 cleanse, some of them are still lurking, plotting to take over the neighborhood again. During Phase 2, you can't let your guard down as you follow the list of acceptable foods. I've found that people typically need at least six weeks to change ingrained habits. Let's be clear, habits and addictions are hard to break, as anyone who has detoxed or cleansed at a rehab center or spa for a couple of weeks knows all too well. Yes, you will start to feel great in a couple of weeks, but please, don't be fooled. The bad bugs are still there, marginalized to be sure, but just waiting for a chance to regain their advantage. Please, show them no mercy for a full six weeks. After what they've done to you, you need to punish them unmercifully, and starve them out of your life.

Continue to Plug the Holes

What will you be avoiding or omitting to allow your body to heal?

- As indicated on the Just Say "No" list, eliminate most high lectin–containing foods, including vegetables in the nightshade family and vegetables with seeds—the exception being avocados—as well as grains, pasta, bread, cereal, crackers, etc.
- Omit all out-of-season fruit (except those with resistant starches, the not-yet-ripe fruits on the Say "Yes Please" list, and avocados). Preferably, give all other fruit the boot! Modern fruit is as bad as candy.
- Avoid long-chain saturated fats, as well as limiting olive oil and coconut oil, for the first two weeks to block LPSs from breaching the gut wall.
- Consume no more than 4 ounces of all animal protein twice a day (for 8 ounces total). For instance, if you have two eggs for breakfast, wait until dinner for the next 4-ounce portion of animal protein.
- Who Neu? Consider eating less beef, pork, and lamb to reduce your Neu5Gc intake (see pages 156–158). This applies to grass-fed animals as well.
- Consume only pasture-raised chicken, duck, and turkey.
- Try to make wild fish and shellfish a significant portion of your protein intake, but avoid any farm-raised fish (do not be fooled

by claims that it is organic), particularly salmon, tilapia, cat-fish, or shrimp.

- Avoid fish high on the food chain such as swordfish, grouper, tilefish, and sushi-grade tuna, which accumulate more mercury and other heavy metals.
- Vegetarians and vegans should omit tofu and other unfermented soy products.

Continue to Feed the Gut Buddies

What *will* you be eating to feed the residents of the condo that is you?

- Maximize your resistant starch intake to allow your friendly gut bugs to produce short-chain fatty acids and ketones (the fats you can use directly as fuel) that you can absorb from your gut (see page 160). These starches include plantains, taro root, shi-rataki noodles, and other nongrain "pastas," parsnips, turnips, jicama, celery root, and Jerusalem artichokes (sunchokes), as well as unripe fruits such as green bananas, mangoes, and pa-payas.
- Eat lots of fructooligosaccharides (FOS), a form of indigestible (for you) sugar in the form of inulin and its cousin yacón, on which your gut bugs thrive. These compounds are found in veg-etables such as radicchio, Belgian endive, Jerusalem artichokes (sunchokes), okra, artichokes, onions, and garlic. They are also available as powders and in sweeteners such as SweetLeaf and Just Like Sugar. (See "Your Gut Buddies Get to Eat Sugar," page 221.)
- Eat raw or cooked mushrooms, which provide more unique FOS to pamper your gut buddies.

- Consume as many leafy green vegetables and vegetables in the cabbage family (crucifers) as possible. (See "The Crucifer Paradox," page 221.)
- Increase gram-positive bacteria and their friends (the "gut buddies") by consuming polyphenol compounds in pulp from all acceptable fruits. Put your juicer back to work by "reverse juicing." Juice your fruits, toss the juice (which is where the "candy" lurks), and add the pulp to a smoothie, or blend it with plain goat, sheep, or coconut yogurt and toss into any salad dressing.
- Consume lemon juice and vinegars, including balsamic vinegar from Modena, Italy, which also contains polyphenols.
- In addition to cooking with the acceptable oils, take a fish oil capsule before each meal. Or mix flavored cod liver oil—I love Carlson's lemon or orange flavors—with an acceptable oil to dress salads or cooked veggies. Vegans and vegetarians can use an algal DHA capsule instead.
- Nuts—particularly pistachios, walnuts, macadamias, and pecans, which are full of polyphenols—promote the growth of "gut buddies." Nut consumption is also associated with reduced risk of overall mortality.[24] You can have ¼ cup of Dr. G.'s New and Improved World-Famous Nut Mix (page 333) twice daily.
- Consume figs (which are technically flowers, not fruit), and use dates or dried figs as a sweetener in limited amounts. Both are full of the FOS that boost the growth of good gut bugs and overall health. Add figs and dates to salads or toss a couple of dates into a smoothie.

I realize that this is a lot to absorb, but let me remind you to do the best you can do with what you have and where you are. See the Say "Yes Please" list for more specifics. If you are unfamiliar with any of these foods, see pages 201–203 and 302–311 for sources and further explanation.

The Crucifer Paradox

Although you should eat as many vegetables in the cabbage family (crucifers) as possible, if you have been told or suspect that you have IBS or "leaky gut," remember my advice to over-cook all crucifers initially. When eaten raw or in large quantities, these vegetables often cause stomach upset and diarrhea. If you are new to them, increase your intake gradually. Crucifers, including sauerkraut, activate specialized white blood cells in the intestinal lining, and those cells contain receptors that calm the immune system gone awry. Compounds in cruciferous veggies thus alert the border patrol on your gut wall to calm down and not to shoot anything that moves. These receptors are called the Ah receptors. When activated, your immune cells say, "Ah." Now you know why Mom made you eat your broccoli!

Your Gut Buddies Get to Eat Sugar

Your gut buddies require indigestible (for you) sugars for proper growth and function, particularly the guys that guard and feed the cells that line your gut. These indigestible sugars are called prebiotics, not to be confused with probiotics, which are the friendly bacteria that are the seeds for your new rain forest. Unless you feed probiotics what they need to grow, meaning prebiotics, they will perish. Fructooligosaccharides (FOS) are a special form of prebiotic, which feed the gut buddies that live near your gut wall, stimulating the mucus production that protects you from lectins and LPSs. Want more good news? Many prebiotics contain polyphenols. According to research at the Cleveland Clinic, the polyphenols in fruit pulp also paralyze certain enzymes in gut bugs, preventing them from converting the animal proteins carnitine and choline into an artery-damaging compound called TMAO.[25]

Bid Adieu to Gut Busters

As well as making the dietary changes above, stop taking antibiotics if at all possible. Note, however, that you should always check with your health-care provider before doing so. In addition:

- Eliminate all stomach-acid-blocking drugs. Instead, use antacids such as Rolaids or Tums as necessary. You will be shocked at how quickly your heartburn will disappear when following this program. You can also take betaine or marshmallow root and chew DGL. (For more information, go to www.DrGundry.com.)
- Eliminate NSAIDs and replace with Tylenol, or preferably 5-loxin (boswellia extract). There are several good products that contain boswellia such as Now D-Flame and MRM Joint Synergy. (Again, for more information, go to www.DrGundry.com.)

Additional Important Supplements

I have already advised you to take a fish oil supplement before each meal, but let me get a bit more specific. In terms of dosage, take the capsule with the highest number of milligrams of DHA you can afford—you'll need about 1000 mg per day. In addition to protecting the lining of your gut, fish oil consumption is associated with a bigger hippocampus and overall larger brain size, making it an important tool in avoiding dementia and other neurological problems associated with aging.[26]

I cannot emphasize enough that the vast majority of people are profoundly vitamin D deficient. In my opinion, vitamin D is the single most important missing ingredient necessary to restore your gut health and therefore your overall health. It is essential to stimulate the growth of enterocyte stem cells, which repair the gut wall that has been damaged by lectins on a daily basis.[27] In my fifteen years of experience as a practitioner of restorative medicine, pushing vitamin D blood levels up to 70 to 100 ng/ml per day is necessary for most people, and may require upward of 40,000 IUs a day to achieve. I have absolutely no qualms keeping my patients' levels of vitamin D greater than 100 ml, which is where I keep mine. However, unless a health-care professional is checking your levels, limit yourself to 5000 to 10,000 IUs initially.

In addition:
- Restore gut flora with targeted probiotics *Bacillus coagulans* (BC30), available at any drugstore under the trade name Schiff Digestive Advantage, or other probiotics such as *L. reuteri* and *saccharomyces boulardii*, and stomach mucus enhancers like DGL (deglycyrrhizinated licorice root), slippery elm, and marshmallow root.
- Repel invaders by rebuilding stomach acid with betaine and grapefruit seed extract.
- Repair the gut wall with vitamin D and fish oil, as discussed above, as well as with L-glutamine (a protein that feeds gut cells), butyric acid from ghee, polyphenols like grape seed extract and pycnogenol, and anthocyanins, the polyphenols in

dark berries like blackberries. All are available over the counter.

· Reactivate and calm white blood cells in the intestinal lining with the supplements indole-3-carbinol and DIM, or simply increase your intake of cruciferous veggies.

· For recommended doses and a schedule, go to www.DrGundry .com.

SUCCESS STORY

Taming the Relish

Jane Y., a fifty-year-old nurse who lives in the Pacific Northwest, had been troubled by intractable migraines for most of her life. She had run the gamut of treatment options without success. Jane sought me out after hearing of my successes with other migraine sufferers, including myself—I know from personal experience how awful migraines can be. She immediately started the Plant Paradox Program and within days her migraines abated. She was delighted, but after a few months she visited to discuss a dilemma. One of Jane's passions is canning (and eating) a zucchini and tomato relish she makes with the vegetables in her garden. With both fruits now off limits and canning time fast approaching, she was in a quandary. I suggested that we do a lectin challenge: she should can half of her relish using her traditional canning method, and the other half using a pressure cooker. Jane returned home delighted, and a few weeks later she called me. Not surprising, within a few minutes of eating her regular canned relish, wham, a migraine struck. But the next day, when she gingerly tasted her pressure-cooked relish, nothing happened. She ate some more, and, again, nothing. Jane was back in business with her relish! Thanks to her lectin sensitivity, she has gone on to become one of my most cherished lectin testers. Despite her best efforts with pressure cooking wheat, oats, rye, and barley for an hour (that is a long time in a pressure cooker), she still gets migraines from these grains.

Putting It All Together

MY PATIENTS HAVE been remarkably successful in constructing a diet that they can live with, literally and figuratively, just by following the two food lists and the above rules. Having said that, a few tips are in order.

• **BREAKFAST** may seem daunting initially, but it is actually pretty easy. My wife, Penny, and I have a Green Smoothie (page 315) nearly every day, unless I am doing intermittent fasting, which is discussed in the next chapter. Bars from the approved list—certain Quest bars, certain Yup bars, the Human Food Bar, and the Adapt Bar—also all work well. The first two contain 20 grams of animal protein apiece, so the protein content adds up quickly. But by far, my patients' favorite breakfasts are my muffins, either the cinnamon and flaxseed (pages 327–328) or the coconut and almond flour (pages 325–326) variety. Ready in just a couple of minutes in the microwave, they can be easily transported to work or school. Try the Perfect Plantain Pancakes (pages 330–331) on the weekend. Finally, two pastured or omega-3 eggs or ¼ cup of Dr. G.'s New and Improved World-Famous Nut Mix (page 333) are filling, meaning you can probably skip a morning snack. Got to have yogurt? I prefer plain (unflavored and unsweetened) coconut milk yogurt, but if that is unavailable, plain goat or sheep milk yogurt will do fine. Both are casein A-2, which is good, although they do contain Neu5Gc.

- **SNACKS**. You can have a morning and afternoon snack in this phase, at least initially. The advent of single-serving organic guacamole—it contains no peppers—by Wholly Guacamole, available at most Costco stores, has made portable guacamole my go-to snack, if I need one. Buy sliced jicama at Trader Joe's or Whole Foods to serve as dipping "chips," or bake up a batch of Paradox Crackers (page 332). Alternatively, carry cut-up pieces of romaine lettuce or Napa or Belgian endive in a mason jar or stainless steel container. Or reach for ¼ cup of my nut mix. Just don't overdo it on the nut front, since they are notoriously difficult to stop eating.

- **LUNCH ON THE RUN**. This is the meal my patients find the least challenging to adapt to their new lifestyle. A salad always hits the spot! Carry it with you premade, or purchase it at most grocery stores or a salad bar. Keep in mind that most prepared salad dressings, even the better ones, are made with toxic oils—and often corn syrup. Carry a portion of balsamic or another vinegar mixed with extra-virgin olive oil in a small shaker bottle instead. In a restaurant, ask for dressing on the side, or simply order olive oil and vinegar. No olive oil? Vinegar and/or lemon juice will do just fine.

- **DINNER**. This is where you get to have fun and feed your gut buddies what they like. That means that animal protein plays a supporting role in your meals, not the central one with which most of us grew up. Consider the palm of your hand (don't include the fingers) as the size of your protein portion for the night. I would prefer that you choose wild, nonthreatened smaller fish or wild shellfish. A reliable guide is available at the Monterey Aquarium (www.seafoodwatch.org). Always consider incorporating the protein into a salad—think of a Caesar salad topped with grilled or boiled shrimp—or tossed with shirataki noodles, kelp noodles, Miracle Noodles, Cappello's fettuccine, or another acceptable form of "pasta." A spiralizer is a great tool for turning root vegetables into "noodles." My wife and I share a large mixing bowl of salad every night, regardless of what else we are eating—and several nights a week, it is all we have for dinner! Let me assure you, we are never hungry. Vegetarians can use the approved types of Quorn, a mushroomlike product with a meaty texture; hemp "tofu," available at Whole Foods; or tempeh without grains, found in most grocery stores or health food stores. Hilary's Root Veggie Burger is a delicious product I discovered recently, but avoid the lectin bombs in other veggie burgers at all costs. See the recipes starting on page 315 for more suggestions.

Get Out of the Dinner Rut

I ALWAYS TRY to encourage my patients to rotate vegetable choices with seasonal availability, but I realize that studies show that most people rotate between five and six go-to vegetables. Why not try to buck that trend? After all, each vegetable has a unique set of phytonutrients. Changing them frequently delights your gut buddies. And mixing things up helps avoid mealtime monotony.

Thanks to misguided nutritional advice, dinner is often associated with having a starch. But that advice rarely if ever includes a certain category of starches that you and I should cherish, the resistant starches, aka soluble fibers. These are tightly bound chains of sugar molecules that are nearly impossible for your digestive enzymes to break down to be absorbed—which is why they are called resistant. These unabsorbed sugars arrive deep in your intestines, where your gut buddies are just waiting for their favorite meal! The gut bacteria convert these sugars into short-chain saturated fats that power you and your intestinal cells. And the best news is that the gang members can't use these sugars for fuel, so they are starved out. Enjoy that sweet potato, or some turnips, parsnips, or rutabagas, among an array of other choices on the Say "Yes Please" list. Your gut buddies will thank you.

After about six weeks, most people really start hitting their groove. If you are one of them, it is time to join me at the next stage of your health journey. However, if you are not ready, you can stay in this phase longer.

In fact, there is really no need to move on. Some of my patients have taken a year to regrow the rain forest in their gut. You may take even longer. Everybody is different. You may even choose to spend the rest of your healthy life in this phase. There are plenty of healthy options available to you, and there's no need to compare yourself to other people—this is not a race.

That being said, if your

- weight returns to normal,
- aches and pains alleviate or vanish,
- brain fog clears,
- persistent gut issues and any autoimmune symptoms abate,

then it is probably time to meet me in the next chapter.

Phase 3

Reap the Rewards

Phase 3 is akin to the harvest, when you enjoy the sustained benefits of the symbiotic relationship between what you consider yourself and your holobiome: vitality, weight management, and longevity blessed with good health. Think of it this way: Your goal is to die young at a very old age.

Once their "inner you," the gut, is happily stabilized, most of my patients who initially came to me to lose weight notice that this desired result is part and parcel of their overall improved health. In other words, if you are doing everything right, you will return to your appropriate weight, whether you were underweight or overweight when you started the Plant Paradox Program. My autoimmune and arthritis patients revel in their pain-free and energized new lives. In fact, all my patients who attain success with the program embrace the fact that it is a lifestyle, not simply a diet.

You'll achieve two things in this lifestyle phase. First, you will ascertain whether your gut has indeed healed, and that your gut buddies are happy and empowered to keep you in continued good health. Second, you can test whether you can reintroduce certain lectins—but only if those gut bugs are happy and only after the minimum of six weeks spent in Phase 2. Don't feel you have to rush to test your tolerance for lectins just because forty-two days have elapsed. If you prefer, continue to follow the meal plans for Phase 2, including vegan and vegetarian variations, which start on page 290. If you are in no hurry to try adding back some formerly problematic lectin foods, on page 295 you will find meal plans for a Phase 3 Five-Day Modified Vegan Fast you can follow on a monthly basis if you wish.

Patience Will Be Rewarded

HOW LONG BEYOND the six weeks before you can try to reintroduce some lectins? When you achieve the goal of ongoing good health depends, of course, on the particular condition or set of conditions you had when you started the Plant Paradox Program. Thanks to the sophisticated blood tests I run on my patients every three months, I can spot when a patient's rain forest has been restored and the gang members and their LPSs have vacated the premises. However, my patients can also usually sense themselves when this occurs. So, I'm going to let you decide when it is time (if ever) to try reintroducing small amounts of lectin-containing foods into your gut.

How do you make that decision?

- Have your bowel movements become normal? One test that many of my successful patients report is that they no longer need toilet paper. You are reading that correctly. Think about it. Do you see your dog using toilet paper? There's no need with perfectly formed poops. Your great ape cousins don't need TP either. If everything is as it should be, there is no sense of urgency as a result of loose or poorly formed stools to push out lectins or bad bugs. It's a fascinating test to tell that things are returning to normal. Need I remind you that all illness starts in the gut?

- Have your joints stopped hurting?
- Has your brain fog cleared?
- Has your skin cleared, is your face glowing, and has any acne disappeared?
- Is your energy level over the top?
- Do you sleep without restlessness or awakening several times a night?
- If you were overweight, are you now wearing a smaller size? Or, if you were underweight at the start, are you filling out your clothes more?

If the answer to any of these questions is no, please don't get antsy and make the mistake of trying to leave Phase 2 prematurely. You're not ready yet.

Similarly, if you have been diagnosed with an autoimmune condition, or even suspect that you have one, or if you had your tonsils removed, are hypothyroid, have arthritis or heart disease, have chronic sinus issues, or you see yourself in any of the accounts of my "canaries," those folks who are supersensitive to lectins, I urge you not to waver in your avoidance of the foods on the Just Say "No" list. All too often, I have witnessed the reversal of good fortune as the result of small and seemingly harmless missteps. Don't be in too much of a hurry to experiment with your tolerance for foods you have given up for the last month and a half.

Fortunately, most of you are not "canaries"! And in this phase, I want to teach you some techniques to ensure that you have a lifestyle you can live with, literally and physically. I'm also going to illuminate the tricks shared by most long-lived societies, along with the cutting-edge research that confirms the principles that you'll put into practice. Despite what you may have heard about the so-called blue zones (see "What Are the Blue Zones?" page 239), most of these cultures have striking similarities that escape cursory inspection. The common misconception is that these cultures *appear* to have very different dietary practices—the staple foods differ among them—but, in fact, they all share a unifying dietary practice, which I have already mentioned. This universal practice is the restricted consumption of animal protein, which I believe is the key to a vibrant health span.

As a native of Nebraska, which dubs itself the Beef State, along with its official designation as the Cornhusker State—what do you think those cows eat?—it saddens me to admonish you about this fact. But the truth is that animal protein intake is low in all these long-lived societies. Animal and (now) human studies validate that long life is associated with eating minimal amounts of meat, poultry, and even fish.[1]

Finally, I am going to show you that perhaps you can have your cake and eat it, too—no, not that kind of cake—by employing the practice commonly referred to as intermittent fasting. This involves periodically prolonging the periods of time between meals, or just restricting protein consumption and overall calories intake a certain number of days each month or each week. I am going to take you through this step by step.

SUCCESS STORY

The Food Chain Up Close and Personal

Patrick M., a forty-five-year-old executive from the midwest with chronic fatigue syndrome, arthritis, and hypertension, sought my help after he had visited some of the finest spas and health centers in Switzerland, all to no avail. Within six weeks of going on the Plant Paradox Program, all his symptoms cleared and he was able to stop his blood pressure medications. He also felt alert and his arthritis abated, allowing him to resume his active travel schedule. When we spoke by telephone six months into the program, Patrick noted that he was doing well except when he dined out on the road. Despite eating his safe fall-back foods of chicken or shrimp, his symptoms returned. He speculated that it might be because flour, and the gluten it supposedly contained, had been used in cooking these foods. What he hadn't grasped was that the chicken or shrimp served in a restaurant had probably been fed corn and soybeans, meaning that he was eating what the thing he was eating ate. Within a month of stopping these "safe foods," Patrick reported that he was no longer experiencing any fatigue or pain. The trigger wasn't hidden gluten; rather, it was the shrimp and chicken, which might as well have been corn and soybeans.

The Program: Phase 3

UNLIKE THE FIRST two phases, which have a suggested duration, this is really a lifestyle. Staying on this phase indefinitely will greatly enhance your chances of living to a ripe old age without being plagued with an array of health issues. You will continue to eat much the way you have been eating, and depending upon your tolerance for lectins, you can make some dietary changes.

- Continue to eat foods on the Say "Yes Please" list (pages 201–203), consuming primarily locally grown foods that have been picked when ripe (meaning in-season produce).
- Once your gut is repaired, consume more ketogenic fats. These

are medium-chain saturated fatty acids such as MCT oil or coconut oil that kick-start fat burning, rather than being stored as fat.

- Continue to avoid the Just Say "No" foods (pages 203–204). However, if you wish to and can do so, gradually reintroduce small amounts of immature (no seeds or only tiny seeds) lectin-bearing foods such as cucumbers, zucchini, and Japanese eggplant to test your tolerance. Try one at a time for a week before trying another food.
- Later, if you can handle these foods, try to introduce heirloom tomatoes and peppers that have been seeded and had the skins removed. Give each a week to see how you do, before introducing another.
- Next, try to introduce pressure-cooked legumes in small amounts. Again, do this one week at a time. Hey, there's no rush—you've got the rest of your life, after all.
- Finally, after you've reintroduced the lectin-containing foods and are doing well, you might be able to introduce Indian white basmati rice *in extreme moderation* or other grains and pseudo-grains that have been pressure cooked—with the exception of barley, rye, oats, and wheat, all of which contain gluten. We'll discuss pressure cooking later in this chapter.
- Eat less food overall and have less frequent meals. As you'll learn in chapter 10, this will give your gut, brain, and mitochondria the chance to rest between doing the work of digestion and energy production, as well as minimize the time that LPSs are loose in your body.
- Progressively reduce your animal protein to no more than 2 ounces per day; instead, derive the vast majority of protein from leaves, certain vegetables, mushrooms, nuts, and hemp.
- Continue to take the supplements recommended in Phase 2.
- Periodically, try to fast and restrict your caloric intake, partic-

ularly in the form of animal protein. I'll present some specifics on how to do this later in the chapter.

· Restore daily and seasonal rhythms with exposure to daylight, ideally for an hour each day, at or near midday. Also get eight hours of sleep a night and regular exercise.

· Avoid blue light as much as possible in the evenings and use one or more of the blocking strategies discussed in "Blue Light Trojan Horses" (page 129).

A Nut Allergy "Cured"!

When Amelia W. asked me for help, she was fifty-one years old and had diabetes, high blood pressure, and high cholesterol. She also said she had such a severe allergy to all nuts that she carried an EpiPen of epinephrine (adrenaline) in case she had an attack after accidentally eating nuts in a restaurant. I explained to her that her immune system was so activated by lectins and LPSs that it was shooting at any foreign protein regardless of whether it was friend or foe. She shrugged her shoulders, nodded, and said, "Sure, just help me lose weight." She started the Plant Paradox Program. Six months later, she was down thirty pounds, and her diabetes, hypertension, and cholesterol problems were only a memory. However, it was her recent experience at a restaurant that caught my attention.

Amelia and a girlfriend had a Caesar salad at a hip place in Los Angeles. During the meal, she noticed that her eyes were itchy and watering a bit, but she tossed it off as the result of a lot of dust in the air. When she awoke the next morning, her eyes were still a bit puffy. She thought nothing more about it until her girlfriend called in horror two days later to say that she had discovered that the restaurant used walnuts in the creamy Caesar dressing! But instead of calling her attorney, my patient bought a bag of pistachios and another of macadamia nuts. She started with tiny bites and waited. Nothing happened! More nuts, bigger bites, but still nothing happened. Then a handful of nuts, but still no reaction. She now was eating nuts with abandon! She wanted me to know that she was cured. In fact, though, she wasn't cured of anything. Her immune system had been reeducated by her gut buddies to chill out, and those nuts were her gut buddies' friends—and now her friends as well.

Testing the Waters

BEANS AND OTHER LEGUMES: Even my nonvegetarian and nonvegan patients miss their beans, and as I noted in chapter 6, you can try to reintroduce legumes as long as you cook them in a modern one-touch pressure cooker. Simply follow the cooking directions that come with your machine. Beans are a great source of resistant starches, the sugars that your gut bugs can use, as long as you remove those nasty lectins. When compared with animal protein, bean protein is associated with greater longevity, at least in a head-to-head comparison between beans and beef.[2] Interestingly, when compared with red meats, eating fish or chicken did not appear to reduce longevity.

THE SAFEST GRAIN: Of the four billion people who use rice as their staple grain, most opt for white rice. Rice eaters traditionally have little or no heart disease, a fact that I attribute to the lack of wheat germ agglutinin (WGA) from wheat in their diet. In my opinion, if you are going to add a grain back into your diet, the safest option is white basmati rice from India—not the American strain. Indian white basmati rice has the most resistant starch of any variety. You can make the starch even more resistant by refrigerating rice after cooking, and then reheating before using it, or making a cold rice salad. That said, if you have diabetes, prediabetes, or cancer, or if weight loss is your goal, stay away from even this relatively benign grain. And do remember sorghum and millet are the only grains that contain no lectins, meaning they are safe from the get-go.

Only in America

NIGHTSHADES: The Italians and French learned two centuries ago to peel and seed tomatoes before eating them or even when cooking with them. Tomatoes, peppers, eggplant, and other members of the nightshade family are the next group of lectin-containing foods to try to reintroduce—in limited quantities, of course, and always peeled and deseeded. Americans have been slower to adopt these techniques to defang the nightshade family. To easily peel tomatoes, immerse them in boiling water for about 30 seconds. Or pierce tomatoes on a long fork and rotate them over the flame of your gas burner. Do the same with peppers until they blacken and then place in a paper bag to cool. The skin will easily peel off.

SQUASH: As with tomatoes, peel skin and eliminate the seeds before eating squash. Alternatively, eat baby summer squash. Do not spiralize mature squash unless you peel and deseed them first. Peel and remove the seeds of winter squash before cooking as well. Regardless, always keep in mind that these are fruits, not vegetables, and long ago our forebears ate them only to gain weight for the winter.

A word of warning: The fructose in these fruits, even though we call them vegetables, is often enough to initiate weight regain, as a number of my well-meaning patients have experienced. If your scale is heading in the wrong direction after reintroducing these fruits, simply reverse course. Cease and desist eating any food that stimulates weight gain or makes it difficult to control your appetite. The same advice applies to pressure-cooked grains or beans. Remember, there is no human need for these foods. A two-by-three-inch muscle in your mouth—that's right, it's called your tongue!—should not rule (or ruin) your health.

A Pound of Flesh, No Way!

I HAVE MENTIONED the dangers of excessive intake of animal protein earlier, but now it is time to really start the culling process. Two recent human studies have hammered the final nail in the animal protein coffin, a fact already established in animal studies.[3] Both studies conclude that meat consumption contributes to the current epidemic of obesity as much as, if not more than, our staggeringly high consumption of sugar does. Yes, you read that correctly. Eating meat makes you as fat as eating sugar does! Luckily, no such strong association was found with fish or shellfish consumption. I recommend these two as the best choices for nonvegans and non-vegetarians. Moreover, red meat contains Neu5Gc, the sugar molecule linked to both cancer and heart disease. Think about that the next time you Paleo folks reach for that grass-fed steak, hot dog, or slab of bacon. Instead, enjoy some wild salmon or shrimp.

The combination of meat and the bread or buns on which it is served at fast food restaurants creates the perfect storm in a way you would never expect. The simple sugars in the fries, chips, bun, or bread enter your bloodstream as sugar almost immediately. In fact, a single slice of whole wheat bread raises your blood sugar higher and faster than four tablespoons of straight sugar. The meat that you ate is more slowly digested, entering your bloodstream slightly later. Unfortunately, your cells are full of the sugar from the bun or fries you ate so there is no need for more calories. Little did you know, when this occurs, that protein converts to sugar, which immediately turns into fat.

What Are the Blue Zones?

Journalist Dan Buettner teamed up with *National Geographic* to visit and research parts of the world where people live the longest, reaching the century mark at ten times the overall rate achieved in the United States. After publishing an article about his findings in the magazine, Buettner went on to write the best-selling book *The Blue Zones*. And the winners are: the Italian island of Sardinia; Okinawa, Japan; Loma Linda, California (yes, where I once was a professor); the Nicoya Peninsula of Costa Rica; and the Greek island of Ikaria. The key is that all these different dietary styles share one thing and one thing only: they dramatically limit animal protein. Stay tuned as we are going to do a deep dive into this subject shortly.

A Look at the Mediterranean Diet

SHARP-EYED READERS WILL notice that two of the blue zones are found on islands in the Mediterranean, so perhaps you are thinking you should just eat the Mediterranean diet and not have to give up grains. I know—I love bread, too! It is positively addictive. Sadly, I have to inform you that meta-analysis shows that cereal grains are actually a *negative* component of this diet,[4] which is countered by vegetables rich in polyphenols, as well as the olive oil and red wine consumed in the region. In fact, because the lectins in grain bind to joint cartilage, Italians overall have significantly high rates of arthritis;[5] Sardinians have a high proportion of autoimmune diseases; and my Adventist friends from Loma Linda keep their orthopedic surgery department very busy. Remember, your goal is longevity with vibrant health, not just limping along for another year on the planet.

SUCCESS STORY

When Bread Is Not Bread

Susan R. emigrated from Hungary to Los Angeles seeking a movie career. But shortly after arriving, the twenty-seven-year-old began experiencing severe stomach pain, cramps, and bloody diarrhea. When a workup revealed Crohn's disease, her doctor recommended she start immune-suppressing drugs. Shocked that this was her fate at such an early age, she visited me at the urging of an actor friend. Laboratory tests showed classic lectin intolerance and massive inflammation. Susan started the Plant Paradox Program and within two weeks, the abdominal pain began to subside and her bowel movements became normal. She continued to thrive and returned to her active life. About a year later, she returned to Hungary, where, at the urging of her family, she dined on local breads and yogurt, both of which had been forbidden on my program. To her delight, she suffered absolutely no gastric distress. Back in Los Angeles, convinced that she was cured, she began eating local yogurt and breads. Within days, all her previous problems returned with a vengeance. A quick visit with me confirmed that her immune system was reactivated. How could that be?

When she was in her homeland, Susan was eating bread that had been made with yeast and sourdough cultures, and with wheat that hadn't been sprayed with Roundup. The yeast and sourdough starters ate the lectins in the wheat. And the milk used to make the yogurt came from casein A-2 cows that had not been feed corn or soybeans with a Roundup chaser. With nothing to disturb her gut buddies, she was fine. But when Susan returned and ate American yogurt and bread, what she was eating was totally unlike what she had eaten in Hungary. The bread wasn't simply bread and the yogurt wasn't simply yogurt because you are not just what you eat, but also how what you are eating was prepared and raised.

Susan's story has a happy ending. In this country, she avoids our lethal foods, but when she is in Hungary, she eats the same foods (which, of course, are not the same at all), and they nourish her and her gut buddies.

The Protein Connection

STILL DON'T BELIEVE that moderating animal protein intake is the answer to a long, healthy life? As Simon and Garfunkel sang, "A man hears what he wants to hear and disregards the rest." Let's take a look at the science. With the exception of one rhesus monkey study conducted at the National Institute on Aging (NIA),[6] calorie restriction has been shown to extend life span in all animals (including a

University of Wisconsin study of rhesus monkeys.)[7] While calorie-restricted monkeys had a better health span than did their conventionally fed companions in both studies, monkeys in both groups died at the same age only in the NIA study. The University of Wisconsin, using the same breed, reached the opposite conclusion, that indeed calorie restriction increased life span. Who was right? When Wisconsin researchers looked at the data of the NIA study, they found and reported that all the NIA animals were calorie-restricted, and the proteins used in the two studies might be the real explanation of differences, since the University of Wisconsin monkeys ate less protein and more carbs. (Astute readers will note that this mimics the habits of the people in blue zones.) Researchers at St. Louis University, who have followed members of the CR Society International for years—these folks restrict their calories, eating about 20 to 30 percent fewer calories than normal—decided to put the animal protein hypothesis to yet another test.

Despite eating a lot fewer calories, the CR folks had IGF-1 levels (see "Want to Live to Be 100?" pages 243–244) that were about the same as those of people eating a normal diet. No wonder those rhesus monkeys of the NIA study didn't live longer than their more rotund study mates. The researchers then recruited vegans and measured their IGF-1 levels, only to find them much lower than those of the calorie-restricted group. For the ultimate test, several CR members were asked to cut their animal protein consumption without changing their total calorie intake. Lo and behold, down went their IGF-1 scores to parallel those of the vegans.[8] This means that if you want to be in the game—meaning the game of life—for the long haul, cut down on animal protein or cut it out entirely. I recommend no more than 2 ounces a day. Want more than that at a sitting? No problem, just go animal-protein-free for a day or so and your protein bank account will even out.

Want to Live to Be 100?

For years I have routinely measured my patients' levels of insulinlike growth factor 1 (IGF-1), an easily measured marker for aging.[9] Both animal and human studies show that the lower your IGF-1, the longer you live, and the less chance for developing cancer. The two factors in animal and human studies, including my own studies, that correlate to lowered IGF-1 are consuming less sugar and consuming less animal protein—specifically, certain amino acids. These amino acids, particularly methionine, leucine, and isoleucine, which are far more prevalent in animal protein than plant-based proteins, activate the cellular sensor of energy availability, mTOR, or just TOR, for "target of rapamycin." (Rapamycin is a transplant drug that was being testing during my early days at Loma Linda University. Any transplant drug has to undergo years of animal testing for both safety and long-term side effects.) Imagine the researchers' surprise when animals treated with rapamycin had an extended, not a shorter, life span,[10] since most transplant drugs shorten life span! The search for the cause of this phenomenon revealed that the main driver of longevity is a receptor for energy availability on all cells. Researchers, who usually don't lack fancy names to call things, called the receptor the "mammalian target of rapamycin" or mTor. We now know that the equivalent sensor exists in all living things, even worms, so it is simply called TOR.

TOR senses energy availability. If it senses lots of energy—think food and summer—it is time to grow and TOR stimulates cellular growth by activating IGF-1. If TOR senses little energy—think winter, drought, or starvation—it is time to batten down the hatches, cut back all nonessential functions, and kick any cell not pulling its own weight off the island; in that process, therefore, IGF-1 is lowered. While TOR cannot be measured—it is a receptor or sensor—its downstream messenger, IGF-1, tells cells to either grow or go into hibernation and wait for better times. By measuring IGF-1 (and lowering it with our food choices, such as less animal protein), we can manage our rate of aging. Scary, but true. My ninety- and hundred-year-olds all have very low IGF-1 and so should you.

How Low Can You Go?

WHERE'S THE BOTTOM in terms of protein consumption? My former colleague Dr. Gary Fraser at Loma Linda University probably has the answer. In his studies of the long-lived Seventh-day Adventists and a meta-analysis of six other studies, he has clearly shown that vegan Adventists live the longest, followed by vegetarian Adventists who limit dairy fats.[11] Vegetarian Adventists who do consume dairy come next, and the Adventists who occasionally eat chicken or fish bring up the rear in terms of longevity. What does this mean for you? It means that eating animal protein is not necessary for good health and that completely avoiding animal protein produced the greatest longevity among an already extremely long-lived people. If you are still thinking you can't do without lots of burgers, chops, and steaks, consider this: The risk of developing Alzheimer's correlates directly with the amount of meat consumed.[12] Now just imagine what could happen with a lectin-limited all-plant diet!

As impressive as these studies are, they must be balanced against the other masters of longevity in the blue zones, for whom small amounts of animal protein, particularly seafood, are an integral part of their diet. Dan Buettner, the author of *The Blue Zones*, hadn't heard of the very old residents of the mainland Italian town of Acciaroli, located south of Naples. This village has the largest percentage of centenarians recorded—30 percent of the town's residents are more than one hundred years old—who attribute their remarkable health to eating anchovies with rosemary every day, and washing it down with generous amounts of wine. Having said that, my own studies confirm the connection between the intake of animal protein and sugar (even fruit sugar) and IGF-1 levels. My advice is to embrace appropriate plants as your preferred protein source, maybe throw in some small fish and rosemary, and look forward to a long and healthy life.

Fasting and Ketones

Fasting is perfectly natural. Ignore "experts" who claim fasting is dangerous. Humans once fasted regularly, not because it was trendy or they wanted to cleanse their gut, but rather for a more basic reason: food was not always available. A study performed in 1972 is instructive. Researchers put twenty-three obese subjects on a sixty-day starvation diet. First they were injected with insulin, which removes sugar from the bloodstream. Immediately all got severe symptoms of hypoglycemia (low blood sugar), with sweats, low blood pressure, and fainting. At the end of the sixty days, they were all once more injected with insulin; this time, even though their blood sugar levels were extremely low, they were completely alert and bright. Blood drawn from veins exiting their brains proved that their brains were burning ketones for energy instead of glucose, and therefore did not require glucose.[13] This is proof that humans can adapt to use ketones as a primary fuel when we are without sources of sugar from carbs and protein.[14] Keep in mind that almost all the great religious traditions have some form of fasting as part of their spiritual practice. Mormons who practice a weekly one-day fast live significantly longer than their nonfasting, although also very healthy, Mormon brethren.[15]

An Alternative to Animal Protein Restriction

NOT READY TO forgo animal protein completely? Okay, I hear you. What if I told you that there was another way out? Valter Longo of the Longevity Institute at the University of Southern California has shown that a monthly five-day modified vegan fast of approximately 900 calories gives the same results in terms of IGF-1 and other markers of aging, as does an entire month of a traditional calorie-restricted diet.[16] Therefore, if you limit calories and avoid animal protein for just five days each month, you get the same benefits as though you joined the CR Society International for the whole month, but without the effort. It is akin to doing specific exercises for one or two days a week and achieving the same physical fitness results as exercising every day (actually, that's true, too, as research shows[17]).

So, how about it? This next month, just follow the vegan version of the Three-Day Kick-Start Cleanse from Phase 1, which contains about 900 calories (pages 289–290), for five days instead of three, and watch what happens. You'll find meal plans for this Five-Day Modified Vegan Fast on page 295. My wife and I love this addition to our lifestyle! You can repeat two days from the Phase 1 cleanse, or make any changes that keep your daily calorie intake in that range.

Then follow the Phase 3 Plant Paradox guidelines for the rest of the month—most people can occasionally depart from this for a few days while traveling or on a special occasion—and you've got a program that you can probably live with for a very long, healthy time.

Another Alternative

IF THAT IS too extreme for you, then try intermittent fasting (IF). The initial IF programs centered on the idea that twice a week you would drastically cut calories to 500 to 600 a day, and then eat normally for the rest of the week. To get an idea of what that looks like, it could be three approved protein bars a day, or six or eight pastured or omega-3 eggs, or five bags of Romaine lettuce with approximately three tablespoons of olive oil plus vinegar (guess which I choose!). In my clinic, I usually advise patients to fast on Monday and Thursday. On Monday you are coming off the weekend, so cutting back makes easy good sense. After two days off the fast, you cut back again on Thursday so you have the whole weekend to relax again. By the way, my patients usually lose about a pound a week using this technique.

A Third Option

STILL NOT CONVINCED? My colleague and friend Dr. Dale Bredesen, a leading dementia researcher at UCLA and the Buck Institute for Research on Aging, and I agree that the longer you go between meals, the more metabolic flexibility you develop in your mitochondria, the tiny power stations in your cells, especially in the neurons of your brain. How long? Every day, try going for 16 hours without eating. In practical terms, this means if you finish dinner at 6:00 p.m., you'll have brunch the next day at 10:00 a.m. Or finish dinner at 8:00 p.m., and a noon lunch will be your first meal the next day. Remember, the meaning of breakfast is "break fast." The farther you extend this time period, the better.[18] I am not just now jumping on this bandwagon. If you read my first book, you may recall that from January through May of each year, I fast for 22 out of 24 hours each day during the week, eating all my calories between 6:00 and 8:00 p.m. and drinking generous amounts of green tea and mint tea, as well as a cup of coffee in the morning. I have continued this practice for the last ten years, so I know not only that it is doable, but that it is also sustainable. After all, you are reading this book to find out how to make your life sustainable, aren't you?

An Intensive Care Approach

SOME OF THE patients who arrive at my center are on their last gasp, often with physical issues such as severe diabetes, cancer, or kidney failure, or with newly diagnosed dementia or Parkinson's or other neurological diseases. Such dire cases need intensive care because the energy-producing organelles of their cells, their mitochondria, are in shock. And these folks need to go immediately to Dr. Gundry's "intensive care unit." If that describes you, or you have a loved one with one or more of these conditions, I've designed a modification of the Plant Paradox Program to deal with these seemingly different conditions. The adaptation is called the Keto Plant Paradox Intensive Care Program, and it's detailed in the next chapter. I'll give you a hint: Such conditions actually all have a common cause. And I'll give you one guess, dear reader, what that might be.

The Keto Plant Paradox
Intensive Care Program

A great number of my patients find me after all else has failed. Others turn up when they are suddenly confronted with a diagnosis of diabetes, cancer, Parkinson's disease, Alzheimer's disease or another form of dementia, or another life-threatening condition. It should come as no surprise that I believe that the underlying mechanism that unleashes all these outcomes is the breakdown of the intestinal barrier by lectins, in cahoots with the Seven Deadly Disruptors. As a result, those lectins and the LPSs (the lipopolysaccharides I've dubbed little pieces of shit) gain admittance to the body. In terms of dementia and Parkinson's, specialized white blood cells called glial cells protect neurons (nerve cells) like bodyguards or handlers. When they detect lectins or LPSs nearby, they crowd around the neurons that they are pledged to protect, kind of like circling the wagons in the old western movies or pulling up the drawbridges from the moat surrounding the castle. Sadly, these glial cells protect the nerve so well that even simple nourishment can't get to the nerve cell and the nerves die. Moreover, lectins and LPSs on the loose set in motion a fundamental metabolic derangement in how mitochondria, the energy-producing factories in all cells, process sugars and fats. Read on to see how this happens.

The Mighty Mitochondria

AS A CHILD of the 1950s and 1960s, I can't help but think of mitochondria as Mighty Mouse and millions of his clones—that's because they really do come to save the day, every day. Hundreds of millions of years ago, the precursors of all living cells engulfed bacteria that became our mitochondria. These mitochondria developed a symbiotic relationship with their host cells and stayed on to produce the energy-generating molecule called ATP that all cells need to function. Mitochondria—or Mighty Mice, if you will—actually have their own DNA, which divide at the same time their host cells divide. Mitochondria shoulder the workload of handling the calories you consume, using sugars and fats to produce ATP in an assembly line called the Krebs cycle. Like any workers, mitochondria can do only so much work in a day and need a little downtime now and then to catch their breath.

Until recently, the circadian clock worked well for Mighty Mice. During the day, they worked nonstop, turning all the sugar and protein (which itself turns to sugar) you ate into ATP. Then at night, your mitochondria slowed down, cut back, and maybe even caught a few z's while the boss slept. The mitochondria's metabolic duties do not grind to a halt at night, but they do shift to a slow burn in the absence of sugar and protein intake, relying instead on a special form of fat called ketones. As I explained in chapter 9, ketones are normally generated from fat cells when sugar supplies are low. Compare this system to a hybrid car, which runs on gas and gets a battery recharge from the engine while running. It stores this electrical energy to draw on once the gas is gone or the engine is off. Likewise, at night, when you are not eating, mitochondria draw on your "battery" power in the form of ketones to create ATP.

We've discussed the impact of circadian rhythms on your me-

tabolism earlier. In the summer, when food is plentiful, the mitochondria probably have to put in some overtime, and perhaps they
even occasionally refuse entry to the delivery vans bringing in
sugar and protein and dumping some fat in a landfill (your belly).
Not that long ago, that would not have normally been a problem.
Why? Because come winter, Mighty Mouse and his look-alikes
could slow down since the boss was taking time off and not eating
much, so fat could be used to make ATP in lieu of sugar. Sending
some fat in ketones to mitochondria during periods of food scar-
city is just what the doctor ordered: It takes only half the effort to
turn ketones into ATP than it does with sugar, which makes the
workers happy and conserves the body's stores of energy in times
of need!

A Mitochondrial Mix-up

BUT WHAT HAPPENS when Mighty Mouse and team are chronically
overworked trying to handle that huge number of calories you eat,
day in, day out, 24/7, 365 days a year? Stressed out and underap-
preciated, they start calling in sick and refuse to shoulder that extra workload. The power grid (ATP production by mitochondria) is
strained and rolling blackouts start to dim the lights. The trucks
that deliver sugar have now nowhere to go and instead dump more
of their cargo (fat) into the landfill. When your mitochondria
are under this kind of strain, your energy sputters to a stop. Your
brain—think of it as upper-level management—has no idea what is
going on down on the factory floor and angrily keeps telling the
workers (mitochondria) to produce or find more sugar to turn into
energy—on the double. That's because your brain is starving to
death from an energy deficit. Now think of your immune system

as cops. Because there is no energy to pay them, they cut back on patrols. With the lights down low and the cops nowhere in sight, the criminal element—in the form of cancer cells, for example— moves in, happy to use all that sugar that's lying around, free for the taking. This scenario doesn't sound like any comic book I've ever read, but it does have the awful ring of familiarity. Happily, however, it is not a hopeless situation.

By now, you probably have a pretty good idea of why this sad state of affairs occurred. Be patient with me while I explain how my plan will extricate you. It requires a quick lesson in enzymes. When you eat sugar or protein—remember protein is the "new sugar" and is converted to sugar[1]—your pancreas squirts out insulin to usher sugar into the mitochondrial factories. However, if the factories are running at full tilt, insulin and its sugar cargo are turned away at the receiving dock. Instead, insulin instructs an enzyme called lipoprotein lipase to make fat cells turn sugar into more fat to store for later use. If you continue to eat sugar or protein—or if you have been eating lectins, which also block the loading docks—your poor pancreas keeps making more and more insulin to ferry all that cargo around and get it converted to fat. This is called insulin resistance, but in reality, Mighty Mouse and team have gone on a work slowdown, or even on strike, to protest the unfair working conditions.

At their core, all the various diseases cited at the opening of the chapter involve a metabolic derangement, a mismatch between energy consumed and the ability of your workers (Mighty Mouse) to handle it, caused by the overconsumption of energy (food), primarily in the form of sugars and protein. Toss in saturated fats that transport LPSs into you, and lectins that release more LPSs, and it's no wonder the workers are on strike!

❧

ALS Stopped in Its Tracks

I met Art S. four years ago, when he drove his motorized wheelchair into my exam room. At sixty-five, he was in the final stages of ALS, better known as Lou Gehrig's disease, the condition recently made famous by the Ice Bucket Challenge. Art was completely paralyzed except for two fingers on his right hand with which he operated the wheelchair controls. Bright and alert, with a loving wife and kids, he had been told that he would need a tracheostomy and a ventilator in order to continue to live. By wheeling himself in to see me, Art chose another path. Four years later, as a practitioner and evangelist of my Keto Plant Paradox Program, he still steers his wheelchair through Costco, still uses his two fingers, and still breathes on his own without a tracheostomy or ventilator. If you know anything about the progression of ALS, you know that what you just read is supposed to be impossible. In fact, it's not impossible, as Art will gladly tell anyone who will listen to his still strong voice.

The Ketone Conundrum

SO WHY NOT just cut way back on sugar and protein and take the workload off your mitochondria by simply burning all that stored fat as fuel? Unfortunately, it's not that easy. If you ever did the Atkins diet, you'll remember that Dr. Atkins wanted everyone to get into ketosis, which he believed would burn stored body fat. But, alas, your mitochondria cannot process fat directly from your fat cells. Instead, an enzyme called hormone-sensitive lipase has to turn your stored fat into a usable form of fat called a ketone.

Your body works in elegant ways. Insulin is the single hormone to which this enzyme is sensitive. So, if your insulin level is high, your brain assumes that you must be chowing down for the coming winter, converting everything you eat into fat to tide you over when pickings are slim. And it assumes that the last thing you want to do right then is convert that fat into ketones. So, insulin keeps hormone-sensitive lipase from working.

On the other hand, if it's winter and you're not eating much, hormone-sensitive lipase is unblocked because there is no insulin being produced—and away you go, making ketones to send to Mighty Mouse et al. Once upon a time, this ketone backup fuel kept humans alive during times when food was in short supply. But we no longer have to scrounge for food in the winter. If you eat 365 days a year as though it is endless summer, your insulin level stays high, the workers are on strike, and you can't access all that stored fat because high insulin is blocking hormone-sensitive lipase. Think water, water everywhere, and not a drop to drink!

And this is exactly the scenario that halts a lot of followers of low-carb, high-protein diets, such as Atkins, South Beach, Protein Power, and Paleo. Even cutting out sugar does not diminish insulin levels, because of all that protein. Again, the excess protein morphs into sugar and results in insulin release, which blocks the action of the hormone-sensitive lipase, preventing fat from converting to ketones. The side effects of this blockage typically manifest as headaches, low energy, aches, and the so-called Atkins or low-carb flu. To be clear, you have to cut out not only sugars but also proteins to stop this process. Really? Both? Fat chance of that happening, you say. In fact, you are right. Fat will give you a chance!

❧

Eating Fat Is the Key to Unlocking Fat Storage

SO HOW DO we fix this? As you probably suspected, given the title of this chapter, it involves ketones. Contrary to those low-carb, high-protein diets, you have to dramatically drop *both* sources of insulin-raising calories—sugar and protein—to get insulin levels to drop and to reduce the workload on your poor mitochondria. But how do you get ketones into those tiny powerhouses when your body can't make them? Thankfully, there's a way around this roadblock, without the suffering involved with the "low-carb flu." Like the old expression, if you can't beat them, join them. As you learned earlier, most of us eating the standard American diet have so much insulin currently blocking ketone production that producing our own ketones from our fat is really difficult. But plants have given us a break, another paradox. Luckily, you can eat or drink ketones that plants have already made for you. Several plant fats are composed of ketones, and paradoxically, despite being fats from plants, they can help you out of this mess.

Medium-chain triglycerides (found in MCT oil) are 100 percent composed of ketones, which can plug directly into the Krebs cycle without any help from insulin. Solid coconut oil (meaning it is solid below about 70 degrees) contains about 65 percent MCTs, making it another source of ketones. Another source of MCTs is red palm oil, also known as palm fruit oil, which is made of about 50 percent ketones. Butyrate, named for the ketone in butter, is the short-chain fatty acid in butter, goat butter, and ghee (clarified butter), and it's yet another small source of ketones. This gives us a lot of choices right off the bat.

But let me remind you: Protein is every bit as much your enemy as are sugar and carbohydrates. (Talk about paradoxes!) That is why many well-meaning ketogenic dieters will never get into and maintain ketosis—they make the mistake of taking their good MCT fats while still eating a generous dollop of animal protein in the form of bacon, spareribs, beef, sausages, cold cuts, and other fatty meats, as well as high-fat cheeses. Please understand that you can swallow ketones all day but, as long as you keep eating animal proteins (which keep your insulin levels high), you will never get to the point of breaking down your own fat into ketones, which promotes weight loss. Moreover, for those of you who have cancer, let me remind you that cancer cells love animal products. See pages 157–158 for a refresher course on Neu5Gc and cancer.

The Cancer Connection—and More

LET'S TAKE A moment to thank Nobel Prize–winning German physician Otto Warburg, who in the 1930s discovered the Achilles' heel of all cancer cell metabolism. Unlike in normal cells, the mitochondria in cancer cells are unable to use ketones to generate ATP. Nor do they choose to combine sugar with oxygen to generate ATP, the way normal cells act. Instead, cancer cell mitochondria rely on the extremely inefficient system of sugar fermentation also used by yeasts and bacteria. This means that the average cancer cell needs up to eighteen times more sugar to grow and divide than do normal cells![2] That's not all. Cancer cells prefer to ferment sugar in the form of fructose rather than glucose, so there's another reason to give fruit the boot (and you will do that almost completely with this plan).[3] If you or someone you love has cancer, we are going to starve those guys out of existence.

❧

Diabetes and Cancer Have Disappeared

Melinda Y., a new seventy-seven-year-old patient, had diabetes, which was in itself serious, but her bigger problem was the large squamous cell cancers on both her legs. The tumors were too large for surgery and chemotherapy is notoriously ineffective for lesions this large. She had heard in online chat rooms that all would not be lost if she followed what I had suggested for other cancer patients. She flew into Palm Springs for a visit. I immediately placed her on the Keto Plant Paradox Intensive Care Program. Within six months, not only did her diabetes disappear, but her cancers also completely resolved. It's an amazing but true story about the power of this program!

While we are starving cancer cells, every other cell in your body, including your brain, can also use ketones to power Mighty Mouse and his clones. As a cardiac surgeon, I know that heart cells much prefer ketones to glucose for everyday energy use or when under intense performance challenges, such as running a marathon.

If you are experiencing memory loss, Parkinson's, or neuropathy, exciting research suggests that the exhausted Mighty Mice in your nerve cells can come back to life if they are fed ketones instead of sugar.[4]

Slim, but Still Diabetic

As a fifty-five-year-old dentist, Ralph K. was a health-care provider, but his own health was poor, through no fault of his own.

Although he was slim, his type 1 diabetes made him dependent on insulin and had caused diabetic heart disease. He had already suffered a heart attack and had had stents implanted. Despite taking high doses of statin drugs, his cholesterol numbers were terrible. Ralph's prognosis was not good when he was referred to me. However, all that changed once he adopted the Keto Plant Paradox Intensive Care Program. His diabetes markers are now normal, his insulin requirements have fallen dramatically, he is off statins, and all his cholesterol numbers have been in the normal range for three years.

Diabetes and Kidney Failure Are Curable

IF YOU HAVE diabetes, let me reiterate that ketones do *not* need insulin to be delivered to your mitochondria. They get a free pass! Unlike everything you have almost certainly been told by your diabetic educator, fat is your friend. Say it with gusto: "Fat is my friend!" Another important thing you should understand is that protein, carbs, and fruit are your enemies and fat and ketones are your friends.[5] In contrast to the teachings of nutritionists who deal with the condition, diabetes is just a metabolic derangement brought about by too much protein, sugar, and fruit overworking your poor mitochondria. Diabetes is completely curable, a fact I see every single day.

Speaking of fruit, fructose is one of the leading causes of kidney failure, one that you and your doctor, even your nephrologist, are almost certainly unaware of. Fructose is such a toxin that 60 percent of it is shunted toward the liver, where it is converted to the form of fat called triglycerides (which causes heart disease) and to uric acid, which raises blood pressure, causes gout, and directly damages your kidneys' filtration system.[6] Thirty percent of fructose that you consume doesn't go to your liver but heads right to your kidneys, where it causes a more direct insult to their filtering system.[7] Remember, fruit is candy, toxic candy. As we've learned, fruit was good for one thing long ago and that was to fatten you for winter. We could tolerate its toxicity for a few months in exchange for fat, because during the other nine months, we could recover from the onslaught to our kidneys. But now your kidneys receive 365 days of direct insult with no break in sight. To be clear, with the Keto Plant Paradox Intensive Care Program, you will immediately eliminate the vast majority of toxins that are killing your kidneys—namely, lectins, fruits, and excessive amounts of animal protein.

SUCCESS STORY

Kidney Failure Averted

When I met him at the age of eighty-one, Jerome M. was HIV-positive and in end-stage kidney failure as a result of an autoimmune disease called glomerulonephritis. This disease causes inflammation of the filtering system in the kidneys, known as glomeruli, which remove waste and excess fluid. He was taking high doses of the steroid prednisone and was scheduled for dialysis. Jerome agreed to go on the ketogenic version of the Plant Paradox Program. After ten months, he was able to stop the prednisone. In that time, his creatinine level dropped from 1.7 to 1.1 (1.0 is normal), and his cystatin C level, a high-tech kidney function test, dropped from 1.84 to 1.04 (normal is 0.97). His GFR (glomerular filtration rate) also improved, going from 40 to 65, which is in the safe zone. He has now been off the prednisone for two years and never did need dialysis.

Spare the Kidneys

The best example of ketosis in action is a pregnant hibernating bear. She enters her den pregnant but doesn't eat or drink for five months. During that time, she gestates her young, gives birth, suckles her cubs, and emerges from the den skinny but with all her muscle mass intact. If she didn't spare her muscles, she couldn't hunt for food for her cubs. But the most amazing feat of all is that she doesn't urinate for five months. How does she do all this? She lives on the ketones from the fat that she stored for the winter. Now, kidneys have really only two jobs to do: get rid of water that you drink or consume in foods, and filter out protein waste by-products. Like diesel fuel, protein burns dirty; ketones, on the other hand, burn clean, like natural gas. Mama Bear burns ketones and drinks nothing, so her kidneys have nothing to do, and therefore she has nothing to urinate.

The kidney-sparing effect of the Keto Plant Paradox Intensive Care Program never ceases to amaze me. I even kept my elderly Yorkshire terrier alive after she was sent home from the vet, who said that she would be dead within the month with kidney failure and to simply keep her comfortable. Boy, did I keep her comfortable! She went on the raw pancetta diet—dogs are carnivores, after all. By eating only the profoundly fatty Italian bacon, perfect for carnivores, but less so for humans, her edema and ascites (water in the abdomen) disappeared, and she rejoined our other three dogs and me on our morning jog. She lived two more years, dying at a normal ripe old age.

No Need for Dialysis

At sixty-one, Guadalupe O. was obese, severely insulin-resistant, and in diabetic renal failure. She was scheduled for shunt placement and dialysis. Her daughter, who is a manicurist at the salon that cuts my hair—a shout-out to Tracy!—had heard about what I was doing in my clinic, so she brought her mother, who speaks no English, to see me. Guadalupe's diabetes was out of control, with an HbA1C of 12 (normal is less than 5.6) and her kidney function was nearing a GFR of 10 (safe is greater than 90). No wonder she was about to be put on dialysis. The poisons in her blood were at enormous levels. She immediately started the Keto Plant Paradox Intensive Care Program. That was three years ago and Maria remains off dialysis to this day. Her HbA1c has dropped to as low as 5.8, but usually runs around 6.0 without insulin shots. She has dropped about thirty pounds, but her traditional diet of corn tortillas and beans and fruit prove to be a powerful attraction at times. Whenever we see her weight increase or her renal function start to worsen, her daughter helps her get back on track. No one should be on dialysis at her age.

The Keto Plant Paradox Intensive Care Program in Practice

AS YOU CAN see, these very outwardly different health conditions all stem from a single and correctable cause of mitochondrial dysfunction. If you have such a condition, instead of the basic Plant

Paradox Program, I strongly advise you to follow this variation, which further significantly reduces animal proteins and completely forbids fruits and seeded veggies (which are fruits).

THE KETO PLANT PARADOX INTENSIVE CARE PROGRAM LIST OF ACCEPTABLE FOODS

Oils
Algae oil (Thrive culinary brand)
Olive oil
Coconut oil
Macadamia oil
MCT oil
Avocado oil
Perilla oil
Walnut oil
Red palm oil
Rice bran oil
Sesame oil
Flavored cod liver oil

Sweeteners
Stevia (SweetLeaf is my favorite)
Just Like Sugar (made from chicory root [inulin])
Inulin
Yacón
Monk fruit
Luo han guo (the Nutresse brand is good)
Erythritol (Swerve is my favorite as it also contains oligosaccharides)
Xylitol

Nuts and Seeds
(½ cup/day)
Macadamia nuts
Walnuts
Pistachios
Pecans
Coconut (not coconut water)
Coconut milk (unsweetened dairy substitute)
Coconut cream (unsweetened canned)
Hazelnuts
Chestnuts
Flaxseeds
Hemp seeds
Hemp protein powder
Psyllium
Pine nuts (in limited amounts)
Brazil nuts (in limited amounts)

Olives
All

Dark Chocolate
90% or greater (1 oz./day)

Vinegars
All (without added sugar)

Herbs and Seasonings
All except chili pepper flakes
Miso

"Fat Bomb Keto" Bars
Adapt Bar: Coconut and Chocolate

Flours
Coconut
Almond
Hazelnut
Sesame (and seeds)
Chestnut
Cassava
Green banana
Sweet potato
Tiger nut
Grape seed
Arrowroot

Ice Cream
Coconut
Milk Dairy-Free Frozen Dessert (the So Delicious blue label, which contains only 1 gram of sugar)

"Foodles" (my name for acceptable noodles)
Capello's fettuccine and its other pastas
Pasta Slim
Shirataki noodles
Kelp noodles
Miracle Noodles and kanten pasta
Miracle Rice

Dairy Products (1 oz. cheese or 4 oz. yogurt/day)
French/Italian butter
Buffalo butter (available at Trader Joe's)
Ghee
Goat butter
Goat cheese
Butter
Ghee
Goat Brie
Goat and sheep kefir
Sheep cheese (plain)
Coconut yogurt
High-fat French/Italian cheeses such as triple-cream Brie)
High-fat Switzerland cheese
Buffalo mozzarella (Italy)
Organic heavy cream
Organic sour cream
Organic cream cheese

Wine (6 oz./day)
Red

Spirits (½ oz./day)

Fish (any wild-caught—2 to 4 oz./day)
Whitefish
Freshwater bass
Alaskan halibut
Canned tuna
Alaskan salmon (canned, fresh, smoked)
Hawaiian fish
Shrimp
Crab
Lobster
Scallops
Calamari/squid
Clams
Oysters
Mussels
Sardines
Anchovies

Fruit
Avocado

Vegetables

Cruciferous Vegetables
Broccoli
Brussels sprouts
Cauliflower
Bok choy
Napa cabbage
Chinese cabbage
Swiss chard
Arugula
Watercress
Collards
Kale
Green and red cabbage
Radicchio
Raw sauerkraut
Kimchi

Other Vegetables
Nopales cactus
Celery
Onions
Leeks
Chives
Scallions
Chicory
Carrots (raw)
Carrot greens
Artichokes
Beets (raw)
Radishes
Daikon radish
Jerusalem artichokes/sunchokes
Hearts of palm
Cilantro
Okra
Asparagus
Garlic

Leafy Greens
Romaine
Red and green leaf lettuce
Kohlrabi
Mesclun (baby greens)
Spinach
Endive
Dandelion greens
Butter lettuce
Fennel
Escarole
Mustard greens
Mizuna
Parsley
Basil
Mint
Purslane
Perilla
Algae
Seaweed
Sea vegetables
Mushrooms

Resistant Starches (in moderation)
Siete brand tortillas made with cassava and coconut flour or almond flour
Bread and bagels made by Barely Bread
Julian Bakery Paleo Wraps (made with coconut flour) and Paleo Coconut Flakes Cereal
Green plantains
Green bananas
Baobab fruit
Cassava (tapioca)
Sweet potatoes or yams
Rutabaga
Parsnips
Yucca
Celery root (celeriac)
Glucomannan (konjac root)

THE KETO PLANT PARADOX INTENSIVE CARE PROGRAM LIST OF ACCEPTABLE FOODS, *CONTINUED*

Persimmon
Jicama
Taro root
Turnips
Tiger nuts
Green mango
Millet
Sorghum
Green papaya

Pastured Poultry (not free-range—2 to 4 oz./day)
Chicken
Turkey
Ostrich

Pastured or omega-3 eggs (up to 4 yolks daily but only 1 white)
Duck
Goose
Pheasant
Dove
Grouse
Quail

Meat (grass-fed—2 to 4 oz./day)
Bison
Wild game
Venison
Boar

Elk
Pork (humanely raised)
Lamb
Beef
Prosciutto

Plant-Based "Meats"
Quorn: Chik'n Tenders, Grounds, Chik'n Cutlets, Turk'y Roast, and Bacon Style Slices
Hemp tofu
Hilary's Veggie Burger (hilaryeatwell.com)
Tempeh (grain-free only)

THE KETO PLANT PARADOX INTENSIVE CARE PROGRAM'S JUST SAY "NO" LIST OF LECTIN-CONTAINING FOODS

Refined, Starchy Foods
Pasta
Rice
Potatoes
Potato chips
Milk
Bread
Tortillas (except for the two Siete products above)
Pastry
Flours made from grains and pseudo-grains
Cookies
Crackers
Cereal
Sugar
Agave
Splenda (sucralose)
SweetOne or Sunett (acesulfame K)

NutraSweet (aspartame)
Splenda (sucralose)
Sweet'n Low (saccharin)
Diet drinks
Maltodextrin

Vegetables
Peas
Sugar snap peas
Legumes
Green beans
Chickpeas (including as hummus)
Soy
Tofu
Edamame
Soy protein
Textured vegetable protein (TVP)
All beans, including sprouts
All lentils

Nuts and Seeds
Pumpkin
Sunflower
Chia
Peanuts
Cashews

Fruits (some we call vegetables)
All fruits, including berries
Cucumbers
Zucchini
Pumpkins
Squashes (any kind)
Melons (any kind)
Eggplant
Tomatoes
Bell peppers
Chili peppers
Goji berries

Non–Southern European Cow's Milk Products (these contain casein A-1)
Yogurt
Greek yogurt
Ice cream
Frozen yogurts
Cheese
Ricotta
Cottage cheese
Kefir
Casein protein powders

Grain-or Soybean-Fed Fish, Shellfish, Poultry, Beef, Lamb, and Pork

Sprouted Grains, Pseudo-Grains, and Grasses

Whole Grains
Wheat (pressure cooking does not remove lectins from any form of wheat)
Einkorn wheat
Kamut
Oats (cannot pressure cook)
Quinoa
Rye (cannot pressure cook)
Bulgur
Brown rice
White rice
Wild rice
Barley (cannot pressure cook)

Buckwheat
Kashi
Spelt
Corn
Corn products
Cornstarch
Corn syrup
Popcorn
Wheatgrass
Barley grass

Oils
Soy
Grape seed
Corn
Peanut
Cottonseed
Safflower
Sunflower
"Partially hydrogenated"
Vegetable
Canola

What You'll Eat

THE SAY "YES PLEASE" list for the Keto Plant Paradox Intensive Care Program eliminates almost all fruits, except those that are listed as resistant starches. All other fruits move to the Just Say "No" list. This is the main change, and everything else remains nearly the same as the basic program. Consume absolutely no fruit except for avocados, green bananas and plantains, green mangos, and green papayas. (Okay, nitpickers, okra is fine, too. It is technically a fruit, but that mucusy stuff that many people hate binds lectins like a magnet.) As far as fats go, initially concentrate on medium-chain fatty acids or the short-chain fatty acids in butter or ghee, but a word of warning: Too much coconut oil or MCT oil in too short a time can give you diarrhea.

As a starting point, aim for about 3 tablespoons spread out across the day and work your way up to what your system can tolerate. Meal plans for the Keto Plant Paradox Intensive Care Program appear on pages 297–300. All Phase 1 and Phase 2 recipes are appropriate for this ketogenic program.

A Few More Specifics

- Macadamias become the preferred nut, with other nuts taking a supporting role.
- The sugar-free coconut milk frozen dessert remains, but the goat ice cream is now a no-no.
- You can still treat yourself to extra dark chocolate, but be sure it contains at least 90 percent cacao. Lindt makes such a bar, which is widely available.
- Animal protein sources drop to no more than 4 ounces—the size of a deck of cards—a day, preferably in the form of wild fish, shellfish, and mollusks.
- If you have cancer, try eliminating animal proteins altogether. They contain a greater concentration of the amino acids that cancer cells use than do plant sources of protein. The leaves, tubers, and root vegetables you are eating provide all the protein[8] you need but your cancer calls cannot use.
- Egg yolks are virtually pure fat, and one your brain needs to function properly. Try a three-yolk, one-whole-egg omelet cooked in coconut oil or ghee, and filled with sliced avocado, mushrooms, and onions. Sprinkle with turmeric, and splash it with more ghee or macadamia, perilla, or olive oil before serving.
- Vegans can have half a Hass avocado with a dollop of coconut oil. Hemp seeds are a good source of fat and plant protein. Walnuts have the highest plant protein content of the nut choices.[9]

- Greens, other acceptable vegetables, and resistant starches take on the role of being fat-delivery devices. I often tell my Keto Plant Paradox patients that the only purpose of food is to get fat into their mouths. For example, broccoli enables you to consume perilla oil, MCT oil, ghee, or any of the other approved oils. One of my favorite dishes is to simmer cauliflower in canned coconut cream, available at Trader Joe's, with curry powder and eat it with a spoon. Drench, and I do mean drench, your salads with olive oil, perilla oil, macadamia nut oil, or better yet, mix olive oil or these other oils with MCT oil in a one-to-one ratio. MCTs are flavorless, making them a perfect addition to smoothies.

Boost Fat Burning

INTERMITTENT FASTING OR stretching out the length between meals is especially effective early in the Keto Plant Paradox Program, since taking the load off your stressed-out mitochondria is one of your principal goals. But unlike people on the conventional Plant Paradox Program, you folks don't yet have the metabolic flexibility to access and use all that fat you have stored between meals. Instead, when you are not eating you should supplement every few hours with a tablespoon of MCT oil or coconut oil; otherwise, you may experience brain fog, feel weak, or get dizzy. Artisana, Kelapo, Carrington Farms, and Spectrum all offer single-serving packets of coconut oil, which makes it easy to get your shots if you are on the go. Another good alternative is to have an Adapt bar. After a month or two, try eliminating one dose of coconut oil. If you feel fine, start to stretch out the time between meals.

A Diet for Life

HOW LONG SHOULD you follow the Keto Plant Paradox Intensive Care Program? The answer varies, depending on the condition that prompted its use. If you have cancer or neurological or memory issues, stay on it for the rest of your (longer and better) life. If you have been addressing issues of obesity, diabetes, or kidney failure and have succeeded in achieving improved health, the good news is that after two or three months, you may be able to switch to the regular Plant Paradox Program. Start with Phase 2, addressed in chapter 9. On the other hand, if you go off the rails when you switch to this more liberal version of the program, return to the Keto program ASAP.

A few words of parting: As I've said before, none of the phases of the Plant Paradox Program or this variation should be considered a race to the finish. The object is not to get through the program as quickly as possible. Rather than a competition, regard the program as a path to a lifestyle you can live with, a lifestyle that is life- and health-affirming. Always do what you can do, with what you've got, wherever you are. If you fall off the wagon for a day or two, simply climb back on. Once you have experienced the health enhancements the Plant Paradox Program (in either form) offers, why would you do anything else?

I will leave you with two particularly inspiring patient stories. May they encourage you to try the Keto Plant Paradox Intensive Care Program if you are facing a critical health issue.

He Beat Cancer Twice

A single parent with three lovely children, Earl F. is fifty-three and HIV-positive. He first came to see me ten years ago, but I did not see him again for four years, when he reappeared, looking sheepish. He had just been diagnosed by biopsy with prostate cancer, with a Gleason Score of $3 + 3 = 6$, which indicates the relative aggressiveness of the cancer and therefore its severity. He had also gained twenty pounds in the interval. Could I help him beat the cancer? Earl went on the Keto Plant Paradox Intensive Care Program, eating generous amounts of flaxseeds, and supplementing with the Brassica tea patented by Johns Hopkins. Two months later, a much slimmer Earl's repeat biopsies showed no prostate cancer. He thanked me, and like before, disappeared, canceling his scheduled appointments.

Three years later, he suddenly surfaced again, looking sheepish and with a large healing incision on his scalp. He had recently undergone extensive neurosurgery to remove part of a huge glioblastoma multiforme, one of the most feared forms of brain cancer. Unfortunately, the tumor's location was such that not all of it could be removed. Earl was receiving both chemo and radiation therapy, but his research had convinced him that things looked bleak. Could I help again? Luckily, he was an old hand at the Keto Plant Paradox Program, and we dove right in. We upped his vitamin D levels, to above 110 ng/ml, and added additional cancer-arresting supplements. Once we saw that he was making progress with the diet and his lab results, Earl scheduled his next appointment.

But as before, he disappeared. Then, two and a half years after his surgery, he walked back into the office bearing CT scans,

MRIs, and PET scans of his brain, all of which showed no tumor and only scar tissue. He also brought a picture of his three kids to show me how they were growing, and announced that they all were going to hike around Europe for the summer. The Keto Plant Paradox Program had returned their dad to them—twice. I sure hope those kids make Dad eat a lot of olive oil over there!

Dementia Slowed

George P. was eighty-five when his son moved his wife and him to Palm Springs from their home in Florida, after George was diagnosed with moderate to severe Alzheimer's disease. The relocation had not gone well. When a person with dementia is removed from his familiar surroundings, the dementia almost always worsens, as was the case with George, and he began wandering at night. The family was living on a tight budget, so a twenty-four-hour care or a memory care facility was not in the cards. After his son brought George to see me, testing revealed the presence of the ApoE4 genotype, commonly called the Alzheimer's gene. He also had high insulin levels and sugar levels, typical of people with George's condition. His poor brain was starving for sugar.

The entire family went on the Keto Plant Paradox Intensive Care Program and I added some brain-enhancing supplements for George. Within a couple of months, he stopped wandering at night. A few more months and he was engaging his son and wife in conversations and jokes, just as he had years earlier. I saw George every three months like clockwork for his new blood work, often drawing his blood myself to have more time to assess his status. About a year after his first appointment, I walked into my exam room to draw George's blood. On this day, his son and wife, who were always with him, were nowhere in sight. "Where's your family?" I asked. "Home," he replied. "Well, did someone drive you here?" I asked. "No," he replied, "I drove myself." The shocked look on my face must have surprised him. Getting up from his chair, he put his hand on my shoulder and said, "Look, I've been coming here every few months for over a year now. Don't you think I'd remember the way by now?" If I ever needed reassurance of my faith in the power of food, his question said it all.

Plant Paradox Supplement Recommendations

About twenty years ago, I used to tell my patients that supplements made expensive urine. That was before I started measuring the effects of vitamins, minerals, and plant compounds such as polyphenols, flavonoids, and other phytonutrients in my patients' biomarkers of inflammation. I also perform actual measurements of each patient's vascular flexibility, using an Endopat device, an FDA-approved system that measures the ability of blood vessels in the arm to respond positively with increased blood flow following a brief period of blood flow restriction. I can now reliably tell when patients have changed their supplement regimen or even changed brands, based upon these tests.[1]

Let me tell you why nutrient supplementation is a critical component of the Plant Paradox Program. I can choose no better source to convince you of that than the United States federal government. Here is the actual wording in U. S. Senate Document 74–264: **"The alarming fact is that foods—fruits, vegetables and grains—now being raised on millions of acres of land that no longer contains enough of certain needed nutrients, are starving us—no matter how much we eat of them."**[2]

When I lecture on this subject to health-care professionals, I always ask them to guess the date of this document's release, so I'll do

274 The Plant Paradox

the same with you. A hint: this is not new information. How about it? Was the report issued in 2000? 1990? 1960? Not even close. It was written in 1936! Eighty-one years ago. Even then, scientists knew that our soil had been depleted of vitamins, minerals, and its own microbiome. And that was in the days before the use of petrochemical fertilizers, pesticides, biocides, and Roundup. The mind boggles at what our soil contains now (and what it doesn't contain). And we know for a fact that it's worse, as detailed in a 2003 report comparing the mineral content of vegetables and fruits from 1940 to 1991.[3]

Why is this so important to you and your health? The reason my program is called the Plant Paradox Program is that plants are both our bane and our salvation. Our ancient hunter-gatherer ancestors consumed more than 250 different plants annually on a rotating, seasonal basis. Those plants' roots delved deep into six feet of organic loam soil, teeming with bacteria and fungi to create an amazing *terroir* of minerals and phytochemicals within the plants' tubers, leaves, flowers, and fruits. The meat and fat from the animals that our forebears killed and ate also contained these phytochemicals, because the animals they ate also ate those plants.

Let's say that you eat an organic diet, you eat seasonally, you frequent your farmers' market, and you consume wild seafood, pastured chicken and eggs, and grass-fed meats and cheeses from A-2 cows, as well as from sheep and goats. These are all great habits. Isn't that enough? Well, if you think that by doing so, you can get all the phytonutrients that our ancestors ingested from 250 different plant species, perhaps you would be interested in buying the Brooklyn Bridge! As the lab tests on many of my patients who are faithful organic eaters show, getting all of the nutrients you need simply cannot be done without supplements.

What are the supplements in which most people are deficient, and how do you replace them?

Vitamin D$_3$

AS I MENTIONED previously, the biggest shock to me is that most Americans have very low levels of vitamin D$_3$.[4] About 80 percent of the Californians in my practice were vitamin D deficient when they first enrolled, including 100 percent of my autoimmune and lectin-intolerant patients. I have been shocked by how much supplementation some of my autoimmune patients need to get their vitamin D blood levels up to what I consider normal, which is 70 to 105 ng/ml for serum 25-hydroxyvitamin D, the active form of vitamin D in your body. Because I measure vitamin D levels every three months, I can be aggressive with replacement, but if you are just beginning this program, please add just 5000 IUs of vitamin D$_3$ daily. For autoimmune disease, start with 10,000 a day. In the last seventeen years, I have yet to see a case of vitamin D toxicity. In fact, I doubt that it exists.

The B Vitamins, Especially Methylfolate and Methylcobalamin

MANY OF THE B vitamins are produced by gut bacteria, so if your gut rain forest has been decimated, it is likely that you are deficient in both methylfolate (the active form of folic acid) and methylcobalamin (the active form of vitamin B$_{12}$, sometimes called methyl B$_{12}$). Moreover, more than half of the world's population has one or more mutations of the methylenetetrahydrofolate reductase (MTHFR) genes, which limits their ability to make the active forms of both vitamins. Many people, including myself, call the MTHFR mutation the Mother F'er gene thanks to how the acronym looks— but if you were to say it out loud on network television, you would be bleeped. Visit MTHFR discussion websites and you will hear people blaming a long list of health problems on this gene. The good news is that by swallowing a methylfolate 1000 mcg tablet each day and putting a 1000 to 5000 mcg methyl B_{12} under your tongue, you can bypass the genetic mutation. Since you have about a 50 percent chance of carrying one or more of these single or double mutations, I think it is worth taking the active forms of methylfolate and methyl B_{12} just in case. Although they will not hurt you, if you are one of the few with one or both of the double mutations, you may notice increased excitability or conversely depression. Visit my website (www.DrGundry.com) for more information on how to proceed should this happen.

Why should you take these B vitamin supplements? Simply put, they contribute a methyl group to an amino acid called homocysteine in your bloodstream and convert it to a harmless substance. An elevated homocysteine level is correlated with damage to the inner lining of your blood vessels that is on a par with elevated cholesterol levels. The B vitamin supplements almost always lower these levels to within normal range.

The G6

YEARS AGO, WHEN *Dr. Gundry's Diet Evolution* was first published, I was asked to name the six most important classes of supplements that I felt everyone should have in their armamentarium for great health. We termed this the G6, in reference to the meeting of heads of state (now expanded to the G7) to determine the future course of the world (and in reference to the first letter of my last name). Here is my G6 list:

Polyphenols

Perhaps the most important class of compounds missing from your diet is the plant phytochemicals called polyphenols. Plants design these compounds to resist insects and protect against sunburn (yes, fruit gets sunburned), so polyphenols provide you with a host of beneficial effects when metabolized by your gut bacteria. These benefits include blocking the formation of the atherosclerosis-causing trimethylamine N-oxide (TMAO) from the animal proteins carnitine and choline, and, as I mentioned above, actively dilating your blood vessels. These compounds are so important that I formulated my own blend called Vital Reds, available at www.GundryMD.com. The product combines thirty-four different polyphenols, as well as my favorite probiotic, BG30, into a powder that mixes easily with water. It took me years of painstaking research to design this product and there is nothing else like it.

However, as all my patients know, I don't even sell my own products in my offices, choosing instead to point out alternative sources of polyphenols. Some of my favorite polyphenols in supplement form are grape seed extract, pine tree bark extract (sometimes marketed as pycnogenol), and resveratrol, the polyphenol in red wine. You can find supplements at Costco, Trader Joe's, Whole Foods, and online. My suggested doses are 100 mg of both grape seed extract and resveratrol, and 25 to 100 mg of pine tree bark extract a day. Other great additions are green tea extract, berberine, cocoa powder, cinnamon, mulberry, and pomegranate, all of which (and many more) are in Vital Reds, but can also be taken separately.

Green Plant Phytochemicals

Without a doubt, you cannot eat enough greens to satisfy your gut buddies, a fact that you will soon witness for yourself, when your cravings for greens will increase exponentially in the coming weeks on the Plant Paradox Program. An additional benefit of these greens is that they tend to suppress your appetite for the bad stuff that makes us fat. Studies have shown, for instance, that the phytochemicals in spinach dramatically reduce hunger for simple sugars and fats in humans,[5] which is one reason that it is a key ingredient in the Green Smoothie (page 315), which I usually have for breakfast. Spinach is an ingredient in a lot of the greens blend powders on the market, but a word of warning about these phytochemical powders. I have not been able to find a greens blend without wheatgrass, barley grass, or oat grass as an ingredient—and lectins in grains and grasses are the last things you need to swallow. Last year I finally designed my own green formula called GundryMD Primal Plants, combining spinach extract along with eleven other superfood greens, particularly DIM (diindolylmethane), a remarkable immune-stimulating compound found in only minute amounts in broccoli. My blend also includes modified citrus pectin and fructooligosaccharides (FOS) as hunger suppressants and gut buddy stimulators.

You can get the benefits without using this particular product. Spinach extract is available in 500 mg capsules, and I recommend you take two per day. DIM is available in capsule form, and the usual dose is 100 mg a day. Modified citrus pectin comes as a powder or in 500 mg capsules. Take two capsules or one scoop per day. My studies show that modified citrus pectin reduces elevated galectin 3 levels, a key marker of myocardial and kidney stress, by decreasing the types of bad bugs in your gut and improving the ratio of good guys.

Prebiotics

The nomenclature of what goes on in your intestinal tract is confusing at best. *Probiotics*, which you now know, refer to the bugs that live in and on you. But *prebiotics* are the compounds that the probiotics need to eat in order to survive and grow. I like to think of these compounds as the fertilizer for the grass seed (the probiotics). It turns out that many of the compounds that are used for the treatment of constipation, such as psyllium powder or husks, work not as a bowel stimulator laxative, but as a food for your gut buddies; this makes them grow and multiply, accounting for that bigger bowel movement. Even more interesting is the fact that the gang members in your gut can't eat psyllium husks and other fibers, so prebiotics feed the good guys and starve the bad guys.

One of the best prebiotics is inulin, an FOS that I have mentioned before. I like to call these fibrous sugars "friends of Steve"! And a mother's milk contains other important prebiotics known as galactooligosaccharides (GOS), which are designed to feed the gut bugs of a newborn. Yup, breast milk feeds the entire baby—not just the human part!

My good friend Dr. Terry Wahls believes that prebiotics primarily found in plants are so important that everyone should be eating nine cups of vegetables a day and, as a reminder, producing poops the size of coiled snakes twice a day. Now I applaud her efforts, but realistically, you are not going to eat that many vegetables every day, are you? However, because I completely agree with her, I designed a practical way around the need to get this stuff into you:

GundryMD PrebioThrive. It combines five prebiotics including FOS and GOS in a powder that you simply mix with water and drink daily. And believe me, you'll start seeing large "snakes" in the toilet bowl soon enough!

If you want to duplicate my recommendation yourself, try psyllium husks. Start with a teaspoon a day in water and work up to a tablespoon a day. Also consider ordering GOS, which is available online. Good brands include BiMuno and Probiota Immune. Take a packet or scoop each day. Then add a teaspoon of inulin powder a day. Also the sweetener Just Like Sugar is primarily inulin.

Lectin Blockers

Remember my saying, "Do what you can do, with what you've got, wherever you are"? Well, despite our best efforts, we all sometimes find ourselves in situations in which we must—or in which we accidentally—eat some foods that contain lectins. You saw such incidents in many of my patients' success stories. The good news is that there are a number of helpful lectin-absorbing compounds on the market. I designed a formula early in my career to help myself in such situations, and after many requests from my patients, I've recently released it as GundryMD Lectin Shield. It combines nine proven ingredients to absorb or block lectins from reaching your gut wall. Simply take two capsules before a suspect meal.

Alternatively, you could take glucosamine and MSM in tablet form, but they are not the same ingredients as those in my blend. That may explain why only 50 percent of people taking these supplements report lessening of arthritis pain. Products such as Osteo Bi-Flex or Move Free are available at Costco or other larger retailers. Also consider D-mannose, which is also in my Lectin Shield, in a dose of 500 mg twice a day, particularly if you are prone to urinary tract infections. D-mannose is the active ingredient in cranberries, although the juice provides ridiculously small amounts. And ignore no-sugar-added cranberry juice—that claim means there is so much sugar in there already that we didn't have to add any more!

Sugar Defense

Speaking of sugar, as you well know, we are awash in it—not only in its most familiar form, but also in high-fructose corn syrup and any simple carbohydrate that rapidly breaks down into sugar, including your favorite fruit. (That's why I want you to think of fruit as candy.) I have been impressed through the years that the addition of a few simple supplements has made a major difference in my compliant patients' glucose and HbA1C levels. Now in the past, this has meant acquiring and swallowing six different supplements, but after listening to the complaints of my patients, I finally formulated my own product, called GundryMD Glucose Defense. It combines chromium, zinc, selenium, cinnamon bark extract, berberine, turmeric extract, and black pepper extract. (The latter enhances absorbability. In fact, if you pick up a turmeric product without black pepper extract as an ingredient, return it.) You can take just two capsules, twice a day, to receive the whole spectrum of benefits. All these compounds change how your body and insulin handle the sugars you eat.

If you prefer, Costco sells a wonderful product called CinSulin, which combines chromium and cinnamon. Take two capsules a day. Combine this with 30 mg of zinc once a day, 150 mcg of selenium a day, 250 mg of berberine twice a day, and 200 mg of turmeric extract twice a day. Costco and online sources also offer Youtheory's Turmeric, which is an excellent product. Take three of those a day.

Because turmeric is so poorly absorbed, even when it includes a component of black pepper known as BioPerine, very little reaches your bloodstream. This is a shame because curcumin, the active ingredient in turmeric, is one of the few antioxidants to cross the blood-brain barrier into your brain. Because of this, I have developed BioMax Curcumin, my own formula of lipophilic curcumin, which is absorbed via a different mechanism, and thus reaches much higher blood levels, and which I currently take daily.

Long-Chain Omega-3s

I have been measuring RBC (red-blood-cell-bound) omega-3 levels in my patients for ten years, and what I see scares me. Most people are profoundly deficient in the omega-3 fatty acids EPA (eicosapentaenoic acid) and, more important, DHA (docosahexaenoic acid). In fact, the only people in my practice who have sufficient levels of these brain-boosting fats without taking supplements eat sardines or herring on a daily basis. Even my patients from Seattle and Vancouver who eat salmon daily do not achieve these results. Why should you worry? Well, your brain is approximately 60 percent fat. In other words, ladies, when you want to call your husband or boyfriend a "fathead," you unknowingly speak the truth! Half of the fat in your brain is DHA, and the other half arachidonic acid (AA)—a great source of which is egg yolks. Studies show that people with the highest levels of omega-3 fats in their blood have a better memory and a bigger brain than people with the lowest levels.[6] If that isn't persuasive enough, remember that fish oil helps repair your gut wall and keeps those nasty LPSs from getting across your gut border.

I recommend choosing a fish oil that is molecularly distilled and comes from small fish such as sardines and anchovies. I've been so impressed with the longevity data coming from the tiny fishing village of Acciaroli, in southern Italy, where the diet is heavily based on anchovies and rosemary, that I've formulated my own omega-3 supplement with DHA, EPA, and rosemary extract.

When taking fish oil, try to achieve 1000 mg of DHA per day. On the back of the bottle, you will find the serving size—either per capsule or per teaspoon if it is a liquid; then look under "ingredients" to find the DHA content per capsule or teaspoon. Calculate how many capsules or teaspoons will get you at or above 1000 mg of DHA per day.

There are several good national brands. Kirkland Signature Fish Oil, 1200 mg Enteric Coated, available at Costco and online, means no fishy burps. It has a blue (not yellow) label, and is the supplement I took for years before developing my own formula. OmegaVia DHA 600 is a nice small capsule that my female patients love. Carlson's Elite Gems can be swallowed or chewed. Carlson also makes an excellent lemon-flavored fish oil.

Other Supplements

IN MY PRACTICE, I have a two-page list of supplements that I recommend to people, many of which I have combined into a more convenient form available at www.GundryMD.com. Space does not permit my going into detail about all the fantastic things supplements can achieve for a host of issues. In fact, it would take an entire book to do the subject justice. But for those of you who are interested in my products to address brain health, longevity, mood support, circulation support, amino acid support, liver support, prostate support, specific polyphenols, estrogen blocking for men and women, acne, hair loss and thinning hair, and a complete line of unique polyphenol-based skin-care products that nurture your skin's microbiome, please visit my website. When I begin to see a common thread in patients' requests, or when I think I can design and provide a better or more convenient product than what is currently available in stores or online, I will make that product available on my website. Or you can always forward specific supplement questions to me at www.ThePlantParadox.com. To order any of my supplements, go to www.GundryMD.com.

Additional Supplements for the Keto Plant Paradox Intensive Care Program

IF YOU ARE adhering to the Keto Plant Paradox Intensive Care Program recommendations, you will rapidly, often within days, use up glycogen, the sugar stored in your liver and muscles. This form of sugar is stored with a water molecule attached, which accounts for the rapid weight loss in this program. But along with the water, two important minerals, potassium and magnesium, are washed out. Both of these elements are responsible for keeping muscle cells from cramping, so many people complain about leg cramps early in the program. While disturbing, I view them as a sign that you are being compliant and following the program. But the supplement potassium magnesium aspartate can stop the cramps. Several companies make this in a standard form, usually 99 mg of potassium and 299 or 300 mg of magnesium. I suggest taking one twice a day. Occasionally, the magnesium will cause loose stools, so back down to one in that event.

The Meaning of a Supplement

ONE FINAL THOUGHT on supplements: Many people still believe that there is a supplement magic bullet—in other words, that one or more supplements will somehow correct an ongoing reliance on the typical Western diet, as well as cause everything to magically reverse course and heal the body. I can assure you that this is nonsense, and I say that because I have witnessed this misconception in my patients' blood work far too many times over the last seventeen years. However, if you embark on the Plant Paradox Program, many of these supplements will and do provide measurable benefits. I have presented studies on such benefits at prestigious national and international meetings. Remember, true to their name, supplements enhance the results of the Plant Paradox Program— but they are not substitutes for the program.

—PART III—

Meal Plans
and
Recipes

Sample Meal Plans

Sample Meal Plans for Phase 1: The Three-Day Kick-Start Cleanse

RECIPES FOR ALL these meals appear on pages 315–324. An asterisk (*) indicates that the recipe contains chicken or salmon, and that there are vegan and/or vegetarian variations. Recipes set in bold can be found in the recipe section.

DAY 1

BREAKFAST	Green Smoothie
SNACK	Romaine Lettuce Boats Filled with Guacamole
LUNCH	Arugula Salad with Chicken and Lemon Vinaigrette*
SNACK	Romaine Lettuce Boats Filled with Guacamole
DINNER	Cabbage-Kale Sauté with Salmon and Avocado*

DAY 2

BREAKFAST	Green Smoothie
SNACK	Romaine Lettuce Boats Filled with Guacamole
LUNCH	Romaine Salad with Avocado and Cilantro-Pesto Chicken*
SNACK	Romaine Lettuce Boats Filled with Guacamole
DINNER	Lemony Brussels Sprouts, Kale, and Onions with Cabbage "Steak"

DAY 3

BREAKFAST	Green Smoothie
SNACK	Romaine Lettuce Boats Filled with Guacamole
LUNCH	Chicken-Arugula-Avocado Seaweed Wrap with Cilantro Dipping Sauce*

SNACK   **Romaine Lettuce Boats Filled with Guacamole**
DINNER   **Roasted Broccoli with Cauliflower "Rice" and Sautéed
               Onions**

Vegetarian modification: Replace animal protein with approved Quorn products (see page 308).
Vegan modification: Replace animal protein with grain-free tempeh, hemp
  tofu, or ¾-inch-thick cauliflower slice seared over high heat in avocado
  oil until golden brown on both sides.

Sample Meal Plans for Phase 2: Repair and Restore

THIS PHASE LASTS for a minimum of six weeks. You can alternate
these two weekly meal plans or create your own meal plan, following the guidelines in chapter 8.

Recipes appear on pages 315–363.

- Recipes marked with an asterisk (*) contain chicken, fish,
  shellfish, or eggs.
- Consume no more than 4 ounces of animal protein per meal.
- Vegetarians and vegans can refer to the vegetarian and vegan
  versions of recipes.
- For other dishes, vegans can substitute grain-free tempeh,
  hemp tofu, VeganEggs, pressure-cooked legumes, or cauliflower "steaks" for animal protein. Vegetarians can also substitute acceptable Quorn products (see page 308).

WEEK 1

DAY 1

BREAKFAST	**Green Smoothie**
SNACK	¼ cup raw nuts
LUNCH	Pastured chicken breast and cabbage slaw wrapped in lettuce leaves with sliced avocado*
SNACK	**Romaine Lettuce Boats Filled with Guacamole**
DINNER	**Spinach Pizza with a Cauliflower Crust**; mixed green salad with avocado vinaigrette dressing

DAY 2:

BREAKFAST	**Paradox Smoothie**
SNACK	¼ cup raw nuts
LUNCH	Small can of salmon mashed with ½ avocado and splash of balsamic vinegar, wrapped in lettuce leaves*
SNACK	**Romaine Lettuce Boats Filled with Guacamole**
DINNER	**Cassava Flour Waffles with a Collagen Kick***; grilled or stir-fried broccoli with perilla or avocado oil and 1 teaspoon sesame oil

DAY 3

BREAKFAST	**"Green" Egg-Sausage Muffin***
SNACK	¼ cup raw nuts
LUNCH	Two hard-boiled pastured eggs topped with **Basil Pesto*** (page 342); salad of your choice with vinaigrette
SNACK	**Romaine Lettuce Boats Filled with Guacamole**
DINNER	Grilled Alaska salmon*; **Roast Parmesan-Scented Cauliflower Mash**; asparagus salad topped with sesame seeds and dressed with sesame oil and vinegar

DAY 4

BREAKFAST	**Cinnamon-Flaxseed Muffin in a Mug***
SNACK	¼ cup raw nuts

LUNCH	**"Raw" Mushroom Soup**; salad of your choice with vinaigrette
SNACK	**Romaine Lettuce Boats Filled with Guacamole**
DINNER	**Sorghum Salad with Radicchio** topped with 3 or 4 grilled wild-caught shrimp or 4 oz. crabmeat*

DAY 5

BREAKFAST	**Green Smoothie**
SNACK	¼ cup raw nuts
LUNCH	Miracle Noodles or other konjac noodles tossed with olive oil, salt, and pepper; Boston lettuce salad with vinaigrette
SNACK	**Romaine Lettuce Boats Filled with Guacamole**
DINNER	**Baked Okra Lectin-Blocking Chips**; grilled pastured chicken breast*; spinach and red onion salad with vinaigrette dressing

DAY 6

BREAKFAST	**Perfect Plantain Pancakes***
SNACK	¼ cup raw nuts
LUNCH	**Tops and Bottoms Celery Soup**; salad of your choice with vinaigrette
SNACK	**Romaine Lettuce Boats Filled with Guacamole**
DINNER	**Grilled Portabella-Pesto Mini "Pizzas"**; salad of your choice with vinaigrette; steamed artichoke

DAY 7

BREAKFAST	Coconut-Almond Flour Muffin in a Mug*
SNACK	¼ cup raw nuts
LUNCH	**Chicken-Arugula-Avocado Seaweed Wrap with Cilantro Dipping Sauce***
SNACK	**Romaine Lettuce Boats Filled with Guacamole**
DINNER	**Veggie Curry with Sweet Potato "Noodles"; Cauliflower "Rice"**; salad of your choice with vinaigrette

WEEK 2

DAY 1

BREAKFAST	**Green Smoothie**
SNACK	¼ cup raw nuts
LUNCH	Grilled pastured chicken breast*; **Shaved Kohlrabi with Crispy Pear and Nuts**
SNACK	**Romaine Lettuce Boats Filled with Guacamole**
DINNER	Grilled Alaska salmon*; **Baked "Fried" Artichoke Hearts**; cabbage and carrot slaw with sesame oil and cider vinegar dressing

DAY 2

BREAKFAST	**Paradox Smoothie**
SNACK	¼ cup raw nuts
LUNCH	Canned sardines in olive oil mashed with ½ avocado and splash of balsamic vinegar, and wrapped in lettuce leaves*
SNACK	**Romaine Lettuce Boats Filled with Guacamole**
DINNER	**Nutty, Juicy Shroom Burgers, Protein Style**; grilled or stir-fried asparagus with perilla or avocado oil and 1 teaspoon sesame oil

DAY 3

BREAKFAST	**Cranberry-Orange Muffin***; 2 scrambled pastured eggs with sliced avocado
SNACK	¼ cup raw nuts
LUNCH	**3 Thoroughly Modern Millet Cakes***; salad of your choice with vinaigrette
SNACK	**Romaine Lettuce Boats Filled with Guacamole**
DINNER	Grilled Alaska salmon*; **Roast Parmesan–Scented Cauliflower Mash**; endive and arugula salad topped with sesame seeds and dressed with vinaigrette

DAY 4

BREAKFAST	**Cinnamon-Flaxseed Muffin in a Mug***
SNACK	¼ cup raw nuts
LUNCH	**Arugula Salad with Chicken and Lemon Vinaigrette***
SNACK	**Romaine Lettuce Boats Filled with Guacamole**
DINNER	**Sorghum Salad with Radicchio,** topped with Alaska salmon*

DAY 5

BREAKFAST	**Green Smoothie**
SNACK	¼ cup raw nuts
LUNCH	**Tops and Bottoms Celery Soup;** salad of your choice with vinaigrette
SNACK	**Romaine Lettuce Boats Filled with Guacamole**
DINNER	**Cabbage-Kale Sauté with Salmon and Avocado*; Cauliflower "Rice";** spinach and red onion salad with vinaigrette dressing

DAY 6

BREAKFAST	**Cassava Flour Waffles with a Collagen Kick***
SNACK	¼ cup raw nuts
LUNCH	**Romaine Salad with Avocado and Cilantro-Pesto Chicken***
SNACK	**Romaine Lettuce Boats Filled with Guacamole**
DINNER	**Marinated Grilled Cauliflower "Steaks";** watercress, jicama, and radish salad with vinaigrette; steamed artichoke with ghee

DAY 7

BREAKFAST	**Coconut-Almond Flour Muffin in a Mug**
SNACK	¼ cup raw nuts
LUNCH	Arugula salad topped with a small can of tuna* with perilla oil and vinegar dressing
SNACK	**Romaine Lettuce Boats Filled with Guacamole**
DINNER	**Veggie Curry with Sweet Potato "Noodles"; Baked Okra Lectin-Blocking Chips**

Sample Meal Plans for the Phase 3 Five-Day Modified Vegan Fast: Reap the Rewards

REAP THE REWARDS. For Phase 3, continue to follow the meal plans for Phase 2, but reduce your intake of animal protein to no more than 2 ounces per meal (a total of 4 ounces a day), modifying the recipes if necessary. Also review the Phase 3 program starting on page 229. If you wish, you can test your tolerance for foods that contain lectins by slowly—and one by one—adding small amounts back into your diet, including pressure-cooked legumes, as discussed on pages 233–235. If you choose to do so, you can follow the Five-Day Modified Vegan Fast, which is detailed below, once each month.

You can substitute a ¾-inch-thick cauliflower slice seared on high heat in avocado oil until golden brown on both sides for the hemp tofu or grain-free tempeh in any meal.

DAY 1

BREAKFAST	**Green Smoothie**
SNACK	**Romaine Lettuce Boats Filled with Guacamole**
LUNCH	Vegan version of **Arugula Salad with Chicken and Lemon Vinaigrette**, using hemp tofu
SNACK	**Romaine Lettuce Boats Filled with Guacamole**
DINNER	Vegan version of **Cabbage-Kale Sauté with Salmon and Avocado**, using grain-free tempeh

DAY 2

BREAKFAST	**Green Smoothie**
SNACK	**Romaine Lettuce Boats Filled with Guacamole**
LUNCH	Vegan version of **Romaine Salad with Avocado and Cilantro-Pesto Chicken**, using grain-free tempeh

SNACK	Romaine Lettuce Boats Filled with Guacamole
DINNER	Lemony Brussels Sprouts, Kale, and Onions with Cabbage "Steak"

DAY 3

BREAKFAST	Green Smoothie
SNACK	Romaine Lettuce Boats Filled with Guacamole
LUNCH	Vegan version of **Chicken-Arugula-Avocado Seaweed Wrap with Cilantro Dipping Sauce,** using hemp tofu
SNACK	Romaine Lettuce Boats Filled with Guacamole
DINNER	Roasted Broccoli with Cauliflower "Rice" and Sautéed Onions

DAY 4

BREAKFAST	Green Smoothie
SNACK	Romaine Lettuce Boats Filled with Guacamole
LUNCH	Vegan version of **Romaine Salad with Avocado and Cilantro-Pesto Chicken,** using hemp tofu for the chicken
SNACK	Romaine Lettuce Boats Filled with Guacamole
DINNER	Lemony Brussels Sprouts, Kale, and Onions with Cabbage "Steak"

DAY 5

BREAKFAST	Green Smoothie
SNACK	Romaine Lettuce Boats Filled with Guacamole
LUNCH	Vegan version of **Chicken-Arugula-Avocado Seaweed Wrap with Cilantro Dipping Sauce,** using grain-free tempeh
SNACK	Romaine Lettuce Boats Filled with Guacamole
DINNER	Roasted Broccoli with Cauliflower "Rice" and Sautéed Onion

Sample Meal Plans for the Keto Plant Paradox Intensive Care Program

REPEAT THESE MEAL plans every week, adding your own variations as long as you stay within the guidelines provided on pages 261–267. Modify the Phase 2 recipes to limit your intake of fish or other animal protein to a maximum of 4 ounces per day. Unless otherwise noted, dress all salads with "keto vinaigrette," which is a one-to-one mix of olive or perilla oil and MCT oil, plus the amount of vinegar you prefer.

Variations for vegetarians and vegans are provided in parentheses. Phase 2 recipes can be found on pages 315–363.

DAY 1

BREAKFAST	**Green Smoothie** with 1 tablespoon added MCT oil
SNACK	¼ cup macadamia nuts or **Romaine Lettuce Boats Filled with Guacamole**
LUNCH	Quorn Chik'n Cutlets and cabbage slaw wrapped in lettuce with 2 tablespoons avocado mayonnaise and sliced avocado. Drink 1 tablespoon MCT oil. (Vegan alternative to Chik'n: **Marinated Grilled Cauliflower "Steaks"**)
SNACK	1 packet single-serving coconut oil or 1 tablespoon MCT oil
DINNER	**Spinach Pizza with a Cauliflower Crust** smothered with olive oil and MCT oil. (Vegan alternative: **Marinated Grilled Cauliflower "Steaks"**); mixed green salad topped with avocado and "keto vinaigrette"

DAY 2

BREAKFAST   **Coconut-Almond Flour Muffin in a Mug** (vegan version), served in a bowl with 1/2 cup heavy cream (full-fat canned coconut cream or coconut milk) and eaten with a spoon

SNACK   1/4 cup macadamia nuts or **Romaine Lettuce Boats Filled with Guacamole**

LUNCH   Canned tuna or sardines in olive oil (hemp tofu, grain-free tempeh, or **Marinated Grilled Cauliflower "Steaks"**), mashed with 1/2 avocado and splash of balsamic vinegar, 1 tablespoon MCT oil, and wrapped in lettuce leaves

SNACK   1 packet single-serving coconut oil or 1 tablespoon MCT oil

DINNER   **Nutty, Juicy Shroom Burgers, Protein Style,** with grilled or stir-fried broccoli and perilla or avocado oil, 1 teaspoon sesame oil, and 1 tablespoon MCT oil

DAY 3

BREAKFAST   **"Green" Egg-Sausage Muffin** (vegan or vegetarian version), served in a bowl with 1 tablespoon MCT or coconut oil plus 1 tablespoon olive or perilla oil, and eaten with a spoon

SNACK   1/4 cup macadamia nuts or **Romaine Lettuce Boats Filled with Guacamole**

LUNCH   **3 Thoroughly Modern Millet Cakes** topped with sliced avocado; salad of your choice with "keto vinaigrette" plus 1 tablespoon MCT oil

SNACK   1 packet single-serving coconut oil or 1 tablespoon MCT oil

DINNER: Grilled Alaskan salmon (grilled grain-free tempeh or hemp tofu); **Roast Parmesan-Scented Cauliflower Mash** (omit Parmesan cheese); asparagus salad topped with sesame seeds and dressing of sesame oil and vinegar plus 1 tablespoon MCT oil

DAY 4

BREAKFAST   **Cinnamon-Flaxseed Muffin in a Mug,** served in a bowl with ½ cup heavy cream (coconut cream or canned coconut milk) and eaten with a spoon

SNACK   ¼ cup macadamia nuts or **Romaine Lettuce Boats Filled with Guacamole**

LUNCH   **"Raw" Mushroom Soup,** with 1 tablespoon MCT oil and 2 tablespoons olive or perilla oil added to recipe and more oil drizzled on top to serve; salad of your choice with "keto vinaigrette"

SNACK   1 packet single-serving coconut oil or 1 tablespoon MCT oil

DINNER   **Sorghum Salad with Radicchio** topped with 3 or 4 grilled wild shrimp or 4 oz. crabmeat, picked through, and 1 tablespoon MCT oil. (Replace shrimp with hemp seeds, hemp tofu, tempeh, or **Marinated Grilled Cauliflower "Steaks."**)

DAY 5

BREAKFAST   **Green Smoothie** with 1 tablespoon added MCT oil

SNACK   ¼ cup macadamia nuts or **Romaine Lettuce Boats Filled with Guacamole**

LUNCH   Miracle Noodles or other konjac noodles tossed with olive oil and MCT oil, or ½ cup sour cream or ¼ cup cream cheese (or ½ cup coconut cream or canned coconut milk), salt and pepper; Boston lettuce salad with "keto vinaigrette"

SNACK   1 packet single-serving coconut oil or 1 tablespoon MCT oil

DINNER   **Veggie Curry with Sweet Potato "Noodles";** Cauliflower "Rice," cooked in coconut cream or canned coconut milk; spinach and red onion salad with "keto vinaigrette"

DAY 6

BREAKFAST 2 avocado halves, each filled with 1 egg yolk and
1 tablespoon MCT oil, grilled under broiler until yolk
starts to thicken, and eaten with a spoon (fill avocado
with coconut cream.)

SNACK: ¼ cup macadamia nuts or **Romaine Lettuce Boats Filled
with Guacamole**

LUNCH: **Tops and Bottoms Celery Soup**, with ½ cup heavy cream
(or ½ cup coconut cream) added during cooking; salad of
your choice with "keto vinaigrette"

SNACK 1 packet single-serving coconut oil or 1 tablespoon MCT
oil

DINNER **Grilled Portabella-Pesto Mini "Pizzas"** (vegan
or vegetarian version); salad of choice with "keto
vinaigrette"; steamed artichoke with dipping sauce of
unlimited melted ghee with 1 tablespoon MCT oil (use
coconut oil or red palm oil as dipping sauce)

DAY 7

BREAKFAST 3-yolk omelet (toss the whites) plus 1 whole egg, filled
with mushrooms and spinach and cooked in coconut oil
and covered with perilla, avocado, or olive oil (vegan or
vegetarian version of **"Green" Egg-Sausage Muffin**)

SNACK ¼ cup macadamia nuts or **Romaine Lettuce Boats Filled
with Guacamole**

LUNCH Arugula salad topped with canned tuna, salmon, or
sardines (hemp tofu, grain-free tempeh, or **Marinated
Grilled Cauliflower "Steaks"**) and "keto vinaigrette"

SNACK 1 packet single-serving coconut oil or 1 tablespoon MCT
oil

DINNER Miracle Noodles or other konjac noodles tossed with
Kirkland Pesto Sauce (or vegan pesto), plus additional
1 tablespoon MCT oil

The Plant Paradox
Program Recipes

In this recipe section, I've provided thirty-six easy-to-prepare dishes. Irina Skoeries of Catalyst Cuisine developed the recipes for the Three-Day Kick-Start Cleanse, along with the meal plans for this initial phase, for which I owe her a debt of gratitude. The recipes for all three phases will guide you in selecting the kinds of foods that will help you achieve your goals, whether you want to lose or regain weight, or eliminate or alleviate one or more of a long list of health problems. All the recipes are also suitable for the Plant Paradox Intensive Care program, sometimes with small modifications. Please also regard the recipes as inspiration to devise your own meals suitable for the Plant Paradox Program. You can continue to use the Phase 1 recipes as you move through the program. The same applies to the Phase 2 recipes, which are also suitable for Phase 3 although you will want to reduce the amount of fish or other animal protein to 2 ounces per serving. Many of the recipes contain no animal protein. For those that do, I have provided vegetarian and vegan versions. One recipe contains pressure-cooked beans, making it suitable only for Phase 3. However, if you are a vegetarian or vegan, you can eat beans, as long as they are pressure cooked, in Phase 2, and I have provided suitable variations of this recipe for you.

I cannot stress enough the importance of eating a wide variety of vegetables, as well as those raised organically. Eat the vegetables and the few fruits on the Say "Yes Please" list in season. Feel free to substitute acceptable fresh ingredients depending upon what's available at your store or farmers' market, and don't hesitate to use organic frozen in place of fresh nonorganic ingredients.

How to Evolve Your Shopping Style

MOST OF THE ingredients in these recipes can be found in a well-stocked supermarket. However, some recipes may call for ingredients that may be new to you, such as cassava flour and millet—or you may not know where to find them. These products are usually found in a natural foods store. When such foods are not available locally, you can order them from Amazon, Vitacost, Thrive Market, and other online retailers. Some ingredients, such as natural (nonalkalized) cocoa powder or baking powder that does not contain aluminum, differ in important ways from those you may be currently using. Once you try some of these ingredients and realize how they increase your options and ability to follow the Plant Paradox Program, I think you will find them as essential as I do.

Valuable information on some of my favorites follows.

ALMOND BUTTER: Look for organic, unsweetened products made from raw and preferably non-GMO almonds. Avoid any products that contain partially hydrogenated oils (trans fats).

ALMOND FLOUR: Made of finely ground almonds, it is available in natural foods stores and online. Almond meal is less finely ground. Ideally, you want a product that uses non-GMO almonds.

ALMOND MILK: Use only unsweetened, organic unflavored products. Don't be fooled by terms like "lite" and "low-fat." Again, opt for a product that uses non-GMO almonds.

ARROWROOT FLOUR: Also called arrowroot starch, this flour made from the root of the arrowroot herb is free of gluten and other lectins and can be mixed with other "flours" in baked goods, waffles, and pancakes, as well as used for thickening sauces in lieu of cornstarch.

AVOCADO: My preference is for Hass avocados, which are dark green or black and have a pebbly skin. Several other acceptable varieties include the large, bright green Florida avocados with a smooth skin.

AVOCADO MAYONNAISE: Instead of traditional olive oil (or the various unacceptable oils usually used in prepared mayo), the basis of this condiment is avocado oil. Primal Kitchen makes a great avocado mayonnaise.

AVOCADO OIL: Full of monounsaturated fats, tasteless, and with one of the highest smoke points, avocado oil is an excellent all-purpose oil. Look for oil made from Hass avocados (see above). Costco and most supermarkets offer it.

BAKING POWDER, ALUMINUM-FREE: Conventional baking powder is basically a combination of sodium aluminum phosphate or sodium aluminum sulfate and baking soda. The acid and soda combine to create carbon dioxide gas, which makes baked goods rise. You do not want aluminum in your body! Bob's Red Mill and Rumford are two widely available aluminum-free brands.

BASMATI RICE: Acceptable in small amounts in Phase 3, white basmati rice from India (not Texas) has the lowest lectin content and most resistant starch of any rice.

BLACK PEPPER: Cracked black pepper has a more robust flavor than the more finely ground black pepper. You'll find it already cracked in the spice section of your supermarket; or you can simply crack whole peppercorns by mashing them with the side of a chef's knife. Jimmy Schmidt, a James Beard Award–winning chef, prefers Tellicherry peppercorns, which can be found at Costco, as well as many other stores.

CASSAVA FLOUR: Although they come from the same root (manioc or yuca), cassava flour is not the same thing as tapioca flour.

Cassava flour is the key to fluffy nongluten baking, and I have tried all the brands of it out there. Amazon sells Moon Rabbit, Otto's Naturals, and others if you cannot find it in your supermarket.

CAYENNE PEPPER: Like all bell and chili peppers, the peel and seeds of cayenne peppers contain lectins. However, the spice is ground only after both are removed, so its lectin content is limited. The same goes for *Capsicum annuum,* used to make paprika.

CHOCOLATE: You want to use an unsweetened product that is at least 72% cacao for making the occasional dessert. Trader Joe's, Lindt, Valrona, and many others make dark chocolate that is 85–90% cacao. Dagoba and Lily's make excellent chocolate chips and World Market offers a great 99% cacao baking chocolate that actually has a bit of sweet taste.

COCOA POWDER: Not to be confused with cocoa powder mix, which is sweetened. Use only natural (aka nonalkalized) products, which contain none of the potassium bromate or potassium carbonate used to neutralize the bitter polyphenols in the beans. Do not use Dutch process (alkalized) cocoa powder. Without the polyphenols, cocoa has little health benefit. My favorite brands are Dagoba and Scharffen Berger.

COCONUT CREAM: Don't confuse this with the beverage that comes in a cardboard package. Coconut cream is sometimes called coconut milk, but it is thicker than the beverage and comes in a can. Avoid any products with added sugar, such as Cocoloco, or that are labeled low fat, and ensure that the can is not lined with the deadly disruptor BPA. Trader Joe's makes a great thick coconut cream.

COCONUT FLOUR: You'll find this baking ingredient at most well-stocked supermarkets, natural foods stores, and online. It is much denser than grain flours, meaning it absorbs more liquid; therefore, it's best to follow a recipe closely until you become familiar with this flour's properties. Bob's Red Mill, Nutiva, and Let's Do all offer organic coconut flour.

COCONUT MILK: This nondairy beverage is increasingly available in both the refrigerated section of the supermarket and in a Tetra Pak that can be stored at room temperature until it is opened. It has the consistency more of whole milk than almond or hemp milk. Avoid any products with added sugar or flavors.

COCONUT OIL: Excellent for sautéing, coconut oil will be liquid in warm weather, and solid below about 70°F. To liquefy, place the jar in hot water for a few minutes or in a microwave oven for a few seconds. This oil is increasingly available in supermarkets, specialty markets, and of course online. Look for extra-virgin organic coconut oil from manufacturers such as Kirkland Viva Labs, Carrington Farms, and Nature's Way, among many others.

ERYTHRITOL: See Swerve.

FLAXSEED MEAL: Like flaxseed oil, this is a good source of omega-3 fats. But if you buy ground flaxseed, it should be cold-milled, meaning no heat was involved in the processing. (The reason is that heat can make the oils go rancid.) You can grind whole flaxseed yourself in a coffee mill or spice mill. In either case, once ground, keep it in the freezer or refrigerator to avoid rancidity.

GHEE: Clarified butter, or ghee, has been essential to Indian cuisine for centuries. Long before refrigeration became the norm, clarifying butter removed the milk solids (protein), making it shelf stable. This also means ghee contains no casein A-1, because it is 100 percent fat with no protein content. Nonetheless, do look for brands such as Pure or Pure Indian Foods, both from grass-fed cows, which have a better omega-3 profile than conventionally raised animals.

GOAT DAIRY PRODUCTS: Goat milk in liquid and powdered form (Meyenberg is one brand) is readily available at most supermarkets, as is soft goat cheese (also known as chèvre). Trader

Joe's and natural food markets offer goat yogurt, while goat butter is available at stores that carry more specialty products, such as Whole Foods.

HEMP MILK: Like coconut milk, hemp milk is an alternative to cow's milk and can be used in smoothies and baked goods. Pacific Natural and Living Harvest brands are both widely available. Hemp is a cousin of marijuana, but no, you will not get high from drinking it. Be sure to purchase the kind without sweeteners or added flavors.

HEMP PROTEIN POWDER: Great for smoothies, this powder contains all the essential amino acids, is high in heart-healthy omega-3s, and has all the benefits of whey protein powder without the downsides (many whey powders contain sugar or artificial sweeteners). Vegans who wish to avoid whey products can use hemp protein.

HEMP TOFU: Sometimes called hefu, this fermented product is made the same way that tofu is but with hemp seeds rather than soybeans. The result is somewhat denser and more textured than soy tofu. Living Harvest Tempt hemp tofu, which is non-GMO, is available at Whole Foods.

HONEY: In Phase 3 only, you can have a maximum of a teaspoon a day of local raw honey, or Manuka honey (from bees that feed on the nectar from the flowers of the manuka tree native to New Zealand and Australia). But remember, honey is not "natural sugar"—it is sugar. Period. Likewise, using ½ cup of honey or maple syrup in a dessert doesn't make it Paleo. It simply makes it full of sugar!

INULIN: See Just Like Sugar.

JUST LIKE SUGAR: This natural sweetener is made from chicory root or agave (not to be confused with agave, the sweetener), which contains the polysaccharide inulin that your gut bugs love but you cannot metabolize. It can be found in natural foods stores and online; it's also sold as Viv Agave Organic Blue Agave Inulin at Whole Foods.

MARINE COLLAGEN: Although made from fish, this collagen has no fishy taste or, in fact, any taste at all—repeat, it has no taste. Amazon sells the Vital Proteins version of this product.

MILLET: Millet has no hull, meaning—paradoxically—that it is a lectin-free grain. You can find it in most well-stocked supermarkets, from Bob's Red Mill and other manufacturers.

MIRACLE RICE: Made from the konjac root—the main ingredient is glucomannan—Miracle Rice is a good stand-in for rice. (The same manufacturer devised Miracle Noodles about a decade earlier.) You will find Miracle Rice in the refrigerated section near the tofu, but this product doesn't require refrigeration, unlike other konjac root products.

MOZZARELLA: Use only those products made from goat or water buffalo milk. It comes in baseball-sized balls packed in water. Buffalo mozzarella is easily found in most supermarkets or Italian grocery stores. You may have to order goat cheese mozzarella from Amazon or another online source.

NORI: The fish and rice in sushi are often wrapped in nori, seaweed that has been roasted, rolled, and flattened to the thickness of a piece of paper. Although it is a staple of Japanese cuisine, nori makes a great wrap (or cone) for my recipes, as well as for scrambled eggs or tuna salad and other sandwich fillings. You will find it in any supermarket, but to get an organic product, you may need to go to Whole Foods or shop online.

NUTRITIONAL YEAST: Not to be confused with the yeast that allows bread to rise, nutritional yeast is a great source of B vitamins and can lend a meat, egg, or cheese taste to vegan or vegetarian recipes. You'll find it in flake or powder form in natural foods stores and online.

OLIVE OIL: Use only extra-virgin olive oil (EVOO), preferably cold pressed (the same as first pressed) for cooking and dressing salads and other vegetables.

PAPRIKA: See cayenne pepper.

PARMIGIANO-REGGIANO: This aged, hard grating cheese is made from cow's milk collected only during the spring and fall grass-growing season. Use only a product imported from Italy, where the cows also do not have the casein A-1 mutation. Parmigiano-Reggiano is sometimes called the king of cheeses. Do not mistake generic Parmesan cheese for the real McCoy.

PECORINO-ROMANO: This readily available grating cheese from Tuscany is made from sheep's milk, making it acceptable on the Plant Paradox Program.

PERILLA OIL: Made from the seeds of the perilla plant, this is the most common oil used in most Asian countries, and it has the highest content of alpha linolenic acid, a form of omega-3 fat associated with protecting heart health, of any oil. Look for it in Asian markets, natural foods stores, and Whole Foods, as well as online.

QUORN PRODUCTS: These foods are made from a mushroom "root," which Quorn calls mycoprotein, and which has the texture and mild flavor of chicken or turkey. Use only approved versions on the Say "Yes Please" list. Offerings include patties, cutlets, and grounds. Certain products contain a small amount of egg white, making them unsuitable for vegans. Products in the vegan line contain a little potato and gluten, so they are unacceptable. Also avoid any breaded items. You'll find Quorn products in the vegetarian frozen foods section of any supermarket.

SEA SALT: Unlike standard table salt, which is mined and processed, sea salt is simply harvested from evaporated seawater. However, most table salt has added iodine, a nutrient essential for proper thyroid function. To get the best of both worlds, opt for iodized sea salt. Hain and Morton products are available in supermarkets, and you can find numerous offerings from different parts of the world in natural foods stores and online.

SORGHUM: One of only two grains without a hull, sorghum contains no lectins. It was the original staple grain in India until rice supplanted it. Bob's Red Mill sorghum can be found in any well-stocked supermarket. Sorghum can be used as a breakfast cereal, side dish, or salad, or it can be popped exactly like popcorn. You can find it online prepopped as Mini Pops.

STEVIA: Unlike artificial no-calorie sweeteners, stevia is a natural product. This herb, which is about three hundred times sweeter than sugar, comes in powdered form or as drops. Unlike other powdered brands, SweetLeaf contains no maltodextrin or other fillers, and the first ingredient in the powdered form is actually your gut buddies' friend inulin.

SWERVE: This natural sweetener is made from erythritol (which is also found in asparagus and certain other plant foods, as well as in fermented foods) and oligosaccharides (see inulin, above), which your gut buddies love. Erythritol is also less likely than other sugar alcohols to cause gastric upset. Unlike some sugar substitutes, Swerve is ideal for baking. Find it in bags and packets at Stop & Shop, Giant, Whole Foods, and natural foods stores.

TEMPEH: Tempeh is fermented soybeans formed into high-protein blocks. It's available refrigerated or frozen in natural foods stores and most supermarkets. Buy only tempeh made without grains.

VANILLA EXTRACT: Don't be fooled by little brown bottles filled with imitation vanilla extract, which are flavored with a concoction from a chemistry lab instead of vanilla beans. Look carefully at the label for the word "pure," because brands such as McCormick sell both the real deal and the imitation kind. Preferably you want the organic version.

VEGANEGG: Although this product mimics the taste and binding power of eggs for recipes, it's made from algal flour and algal protein, nutritional yeast, and other plant sources. It is lectin-free, dairy-free, non-GMO, and suitable for vegans. Still in limited distribution, it is available from Thrive Market, Amazon, and other online sources. For more information, visit www.follow yourheart.com.

WHEY PROTEIN POWDER: A by-product of cheese making, whey protein powder comes in plain or flavored versions. Read the labels carefully. Many whey powders are loaded with sugars or artificial sweeteners. Whey protein also elevates insulinlike growth factor (IGF), which explains why bodybuilders use it to build muscle. However, IGF stimulates cancer and ages you, so please be careful with your consumption.

YOGURT: Use only unsweetened, unflavored, organic yogurt made from goat or sheep milk. My preference, however, is "yogurt" made from fermented coconut milk or hemp milk.

Tools for Success

IF YOU HAVE some good pots and frying pans, sharp knives, and a vegetable peeler, you already have most of what you need in your kitchen to get cooking the healthy Plant Paradox way. A grill pan or grill, or a George Foreman–type indoor griller, is also invaluable. Other appliances, such as a blender, are essential, and there are other tools that can save you time and effort.

Here is the checklist of the tools you'll need.

BLENDER: A high-speed blender such as a Vitamix, Blendtec, or Ninja liquefies smoothie ingredients in seconds, enables you to make soups without needing to use the stove top, and simply speeds laborious tasks such as chopping and combining ingredients. A high-powered mini-blender such as a Magic Bullet or a Nutribullet can handle many of my recipes as well (see below). A standard blender will handle most jobs, but may take longer or require you to do the job in several steps (and it can't deliver warm soup).

FOOD PROCESSOR: Nothing beats a good food processor for chopping, slicing, combining ingredients for baked goods, making pesto, and dozens of other culinary tasks.

MAGIC BULLET: Inexpensive and easier to clean than a blender or a food processor, this powerful mini-blender can also handle most of the chopping chores a food processor does. If you use it mostly for single servings of smoothies, and don't do much cooking or cook for groups, this appliance may be the only blender or food processor you need.

MICROWAVE OVEN: Even a tiny countertop model will help you get Plant Paradox friendly breakfasts on the table in minutes.

MINI FOOD PROCESSOR: For a small investment, this small processor is ideal for chopping garlic, herbs, small portions of nuts, and the like.

PRESSURE COOKER: If you are able to reintroduce legumes, rice, and certain other grains in Phase 3, you should definitely consider purchasing a pressure cooker, which destroys their lectins. (See "Not Grandma's Pressure Cooker" on page 181.)

SALAD SPINNER: This is an indispensable tool for encouraging you to eat and enjoy more salad greens. Spinning removes as much residual moisture as possible from lettuce and other greens and allows the salad dressing to cling to the greens.

SPIRALIZER: When you say good-bye to pasta, this handy device turns carrots, daikon radishes, jicama, and root vegetables into "noodles." Don't bother buying a fancy and expensive electric spiralizer. Instead, a hand-operated spiralizer that costs about $15 will do the job.

List of Recipes

PHASE 1 RECIPES

Green Smoothie

Arugula Salad with Chicken and Lemon Vinaigrette

Romaine Salad with Avocado and Cilantro-Pesto Chicken

Chicken-Arugula-Avocado Seaweed Wrap with Cilantro Dipping Sauce

Romaine Lettuce Boats Filled with Guacamole

Lemony Brussels Sprouts, Kale, and Onions with Cabbage "Steak"

Cabbage-Kale Sauté with Salmon and Avocado

Roasted Broccoli with Cauliflower "Rice" and Sautéed Onions

PHASE 2 RECIPES

Breakfast

Coconut-Almond Flour Muffin in a Mug

Cranberry-Orange Muffins

Cinnamon-Flaxseed Muffin in a Mug

"Green" Egg-Sausage Muffins

Paradox Smoothie

Perfect Plantain Pancakes

Snacks and Beverages

Paradox Crackers

Dr. G.'s New and Improved World-Famous Nut Mix

Get Up and Go Cappuccino

Sparkling Balsamic Vinegar Spritzer

Main and Side Dishes

Tops and Bottoms Celery Soup

Sorghum Salad with Radicchio

"Raw" Mushroom Soup

Spinach Pizza with a Cauliflower Crust

Grilled Portabella-Pesto Mini "Pizzas"

Nutty, Juicy Shroom Burgers, Protein Style

Roast Parmesan-Scented Cauliflower Mash

Pressure-Cooked Lima Beans, Kale, and Turkey

Thoroughly Modern Millet Cakes

Shaved Kohlrabi with Crispy Pear and Nuts

Baked Okra Lectin-Blocking Chips

Veggie Curry with Sweet Potato "Noodles"

Baked "Fried" Artichoke Hearts

Cassava Flour Waffles with a Collagen Kick

Marinated Grilled Cauliflower "Steaks"

Desserts

Miracle Rice Pudding Two Ways

Mint Chocolate Chip–Avocado "Ice Cream"

Flourless Chocolate–Almond Butter Cake

PHASE 1: THREE-DAY KICK-START CLEANSE RECIPES

USE ORGANIC, LOCAL, sustainably grown ingredients whenever possible. When it comes to oil, turn to organic avocado oil and extra-virgin olive oil. All fish should be wild-caught and all chicken should be pastured. All recipes in this section make a single serving. If you are doing the cleanse with another person, be sure to double all the ingredients. Continue to enjoy these recipes in Phase 2 if you wish.

Make the Cleanse Easy

- You will have the same Green Smoothie for breakfast each day, so make three days' worth, divide in three portions, and refrigerate.
- The lunch suggestions are two salads and the seaweed wrap. Rolls travel more easily than salads, so you can have the wrap every day if you wish, perhaps swapping salmon for chicken on one day.
- If you start the cleanse on a Monday, you can make *all* the meals over the preceding weekend, warming each dinner in your microwave on the appropriate evening.
- You can make cauliflower "rice" ahead of time and reheat it before eating as a separate dish (see Roasted Broccoli with Cauliflower "Rice" and Sautéed Onions, page 323). If you are close to a Trader Joe's or Whole Foods, you'll find cauliflower rice in the refrigerated vegetable section.
- You'll use the same lemon vinaigrette on both lunch salads. Double the recipe and store the second portion in a glass jar overnight in the fridge if you wish.
- Costco sells single portions of guacamole (the brand is Wholly Guacamole), which are handy to have around when an avocado refuses to ripen on your schedule!

PHASE 1 RECIPES

Green Smoothie

Add a little more water if the smoothie is too thick. You can make a triple batch and refrigerate for up to three days in a covered glass container.

Phases 1–3
> *Serves 1*
> Total time: 5 minutes

  1 cup chopped romaine lettuce
  ½ cup baby spinach
  1 mint spring, with stem
  ½ avocado
  4 tablespoons freshly squeezed lemon juice
  3 to 6 drops stevia extract
  ¼ cup ice cubes
  1 cup tap or filtered water

Place all the ingredients in a high-powered blender and blend on high until smooth and fluffy, adding more ice cubes if desired.

Arugula Salad with Chicken and Lemon Vinaigrette

Note that the same dressing is used for Romaine Salad with Avocado and Cilantro-Pesto Chicken (page 317). You might therefore want to make two batches of dressing, storing the rest in a glass container to use the following day.

Phases 1–3
Serves 1
Total time: 15 minutes

CHICKEN
1 tablespoon avocado oil
4 ounces boneless, skinless pasture-raised chicken breast, cut into
    ½ -inch-thick strips
1 tablespoon freshly squeezed lemon juice
¼ teaspoon sea salt, preferably iodized
Zest of ½ lemon (optional)

DRESSING
2 tablespoons extra-virgin olive oil
1 tablespoon freshly squeezed lemon juice
Pinch sea salt, preferably iodized

SALAD
1½ cups arugula

MAKE THE CHICKEN. Heat the avocado oil in a small skillet over high heat. Place the chicken strips in the hot pan and sprinkle with the lemon juice and salt. Sauté the chicken strips for about 2 minutes; turn them and sauté for another 2 minutes, until cooked through. Remove from the pan and reserve.

MAKE THE DRESSING. Combine the ingredients in a mason jar with a tight-fitting lid. (Double the ingredients if making two batches.) Shake until well combined.

TO SERVE. Toss the arugula in the dressing and top with the chicken, adding the lemon zest, if desired.

VEGAN VERSION: Replace the chicken with grain-free tempeh, hemp tofu, or a cauliflower "steak," a ¾-inch-thick cauliflower slice seared over high heat in avocado oil until golden brown on both sides.

VEGETARIAN VERSION: Same as above or substitute acceptable Quorn products.

Romaine Salad with Avocado and Cilantro-Pesto Chicken

To save time, make the cilantro pesto in advance and store for up to three days in the refrigerator in a covered glass container. You can substitute basil or parsley for the cilantro.

This salad uses the same dressing as the preceding salad (page 316), so you may want to make two batches at once.

Phases 1–3
Serves 1
Total time: 15 minutes

CHICKEN
1 tablespoon avocado oil
4 ounces boneless, skinless pasture-raised chicken breast, cut into
    ½-inch-thick strips
1 tablespoon freshly squeezed lemon juice
¼ teaspoon sea salt, preferably iodized

PESTO
2 cups chopped cilantro
¼ cup extra-virgin olive oil
2 tablespoons freshly squeezed lemon juice
¼ teaspoon sea salt, preferably iodized

DRESSING
½ avocado, diced
2 tablespoons freshly squeezed lemon juice
2 tablespoons extra-virgin olive oil
Pinch sea salt, preferably iodized
Salad
1½ cups chopped romaine lettuce

MAKE THE CHICKEN. Heat the avocado oil in a small skillet over high heat. Place the chicken strips in the hot pan and sprinkle with the lemon juice and salt. Sauté the chicken strips for about 2 minutes; turn them and sauté for another 2 minutes, until cooked through. Remove from the pan and reserve.

MAKE THE PESTO. Place the ingredients in a high-powered blender. Process on high until very smooth.

MAKE THE DRESSING. Toss the avocado in 1 tablespoon of the lemon juice and set aside. Combine the remaining 1 tablespoon lemon juice, the olive oil, and salt in a mason jar with a tight-fitting lid. (Double the ingredients if making two batches.) Shake until well combined.

TO SERVE. Toss the romaine in the dressing. Arrange the avocado and chicken over the lettuce and spread the pesto on top.

> **VEGAN VERSION:** Replace the chicken with grain-free tempeh, hemp tofu, or a cauliflower "steak," a ¾-inch-thick cauliflower slice seared over high heat in avocado oil until golden brown on both sides.
>
> **VEGETARIAN VERSION:** Same as above or substitute acceptable Quorn products.

Chicken-Arugula-Avocado Seaweed Wrap with Cilantro Dipping Sauce

Nori is a form of seaweed that has been flattened into squares or strips. It makes a great stand-in for flatbread.

A bamboo mat, available in the Asian foods section of most supermarkets, can help you roll tight seaweed wraps.

Phases 1–3

Serves 1

Total time: 15 minutes

FILLING

1 tablespoon avocado oil

4 ounces boneless, skinless pasture-raised chicken breast, cut into ½-inch-thick strips

2 tablespoons freshly squeezed lemon juice

¼ teaspoon sea salt, preferably iodized, plus additional to taste

½ avocado, diced

1 cup arugula

1 sheet nori (sushi seaweed)

4 green olives, pitted and halved

CILANTRO DIPPING SAUCE

2 cups chopped cilantro

¼ cup extra-virgin olive oil

2 tablespoons freshly squeezed lemon juice

¼ teaspoon sea salt, preferably iodized

MAKE THE FILLING. Heat the avocado oil in a small skillet over high heat. Place the chicken strips in the hot pan and sprinkle with 1 tablespoon of the lemon juice and the salt. Sauté the chicken strips for about 2 minutes; turn them and sauté for another 2 minutes, until cooked through. Remove from the pan and reserve.

Toss the avocado in the remaining tablespoon lemon juice and season with salt.

MAKE THE DIPPING SAUCE. Place the ingredients in a high-powered blender. Process on high until very smooth.

TO SERVE. Arrange the arugula on the bottom half of the seaweed sheet. Top with the chicken, avocado, and olives. Sprinkle with salt. Carefully roll into a tight wrap, sealing the end with a little water. Cut in half and serve with the cilantro dipping sauce.

> **VEGAN VERSION:** Replace the chicken with grain-free tempeh, hemp tofu, or a cauliflower "steak," a ¾-inch-thick cauliflower slice seared over high heat in avocado oil until golden brown on both sides.
>
> **VEGETARIAN VERSION:** Same as above or substitute acceptable Quorn products.

Romaine Lettuce Boats Filled with Guacamole

I recommend you use Hass avocados for your guacamole (and other recipes). Hass have a black or dark green pebbly skin and contain more fat (the heart-healthy monounsaturated kind) than the larger, smooth-skinned Florida avocados, which tend to be more watery.

Phases 1–3
   Serves 1
   Total time: 5 minutes

   ½ avocado
   1 tablespoon finely chopped red onion
   1 teaspoon finely chopped cilantro
   1 tablespoon freshly squeezed lemon juice
   Pinch sea salt, preferably iodized
   4 romaine lettuce leaves, washed and patted dry

Place the avocado, onion, cilantro, lemon juice, and salt in a bowl. Mash with a fork until smooth.

To serve, scoop an equal amount of the guacamole into each lettuce leaf.

Lemony Brussels Sprouts, Kale, and Onions with Cabbage "Steak"

Use any of the many types of kale. Unless you're using baby kale, remove the stems before chopping. (There is no need to remove the stems or chop baby kale.)

Phases 1–3

Serves 1

Total time: 20 minutes

4 tablespoons avocado oil
One 1-inch-thick red cabbage slice
¼ teaspoon plus 1 pinch sea salt, preferably iodized
½ red onion, thinly sliced
1 cup Brussels sprouts, thinly sliced
1½ cups chopped kale
1 tablespoon freshly squeezed lemon juice
Extra-virgin olive oil (optional)

Heat a skillet over high heat. When it is hot, add 1 tablespoon of the avocado oil, reduce heat to medium, and sear the cabbage slice until it is golden brown on one side, about 3 minutes. Flip and brown it on the other side. Season with the pinch of salt, remove to a plate, and cover to keep warm. Wipe the skillet clean with a paper towel and return to the stove top.

Heat 2 tablespoons of the avocado oil in the skillet over medium heat. Add the onion and Brussels sprouts. Sauté until tender, about

3 minutes. Add the remaining 1 tablespoon avocado oil, the kale, and lemon juice, and sauté for another 3 minutes, until the kale is wilted. Season with the ¼ teaspoon salt.

To serve, top the cabbage "steak" with the sautéed vegetables. Add a drizzle of olive oil, if desired.

Cabbage-Kale Sauté with Salmon and Avocado

This recipe is very adaptable. Replace the salmon with another wild-caught fish or shellfish, or with pastured chicken. Or use bok choy or Napa cabbage instead of green cabbage.

Phases 1–3
Serves 1
Total time: 20 minutes

½ avocado, diced
3 tablespoons freshly squeezed lemon juice
4 pinches sea salt, preferably iodized
3 tablespoons avocado oil
1½ cups finely sliced green cabbage
½ red onion, thinly sliced
3 ounces wild-caught Alaska salmon

Toss the diced avocado in 1 tablespoon of the lemon juice and season with a pinch of salt. Set aside.

Heat a skillet over medium heat. When it is hot, add 2 tablespoons of the avocado oil and the cabbage and onion. Sauté until tender, about 10 minutes, stirring occasionally. Season with 2 more pinches of salt. Using a slotted spatula, remove from the skillet and set aside.

Add the remaining 1 tablespoon avocado oil to the skillet, raise the heat to high, and add the remaining 2 tablespoons lemon juice and the salmon. Sear the salmon, flipping after 3 minutes, until cooked through, about 6 minutes total. Season with the remaining pinch salt.

To serve, top the sautéed cabbage and onions with the salmon and avocado.

> **VEGAN VERSION:** Replace the salmon with grain-free tempeh, hemp tofu, or a cauliflower "steak," a ¾-inch-thick cauliflower slice seared over high heat in avocado oil until golden brown on both sides.
>
> **VEGETARIAN VERSION:** Same as above or substitute acceptable Quorn products.

Roasted Broccoli with Cauliflower "Rice" and Sautéed Onions

To make cauliflower "rice," grate the cauliflower with a cheese grater, using the largest holes, into rice-shaped pieces. You can also pulse it in a food processor, using the S-blade, cutting the cauliflower into chunks first and being careful not to overprocess it. You can also serve the cauliflower "rice" part of this recipe with other main course dishes.

Phases 1–3

Serves 1

Total time: 20 minutes

CAULIFLOWER "RICE"

½ head medium cauliflower, riced (see headnote)

1 tablespoon avocado oil

1 tablespoon freshly squeezed lemon juice

¼ teaspoon curry powder

1 pinch sea salt, preferably iodized

BROCCOLI
1½ cups cut-up broccoli florets
1½ tablespoons avocado oil
1 pinch sea salt, preferably iodized

CURRIED ONIONS
½ tablespoon avocado oil
½ red onion, thinly sliced
Pinch sea salt, preferably iodized

Heat the oven to 375°F.

Sauté the cauliflower in a medium skillet with 1 tablespoon of the avocado oil, the lemon juice, curry powder, and a pinch of salt until tender, 3 to 5 minutes. Do not let it get mushy by overcooking. Transfer the cauliflower "rice" to a plate and keep warm. Wipe the skillet clean with a paper towel.

Put the broccoli in a Pyrex dish with 1 tablespoon of the avocado oil. Roast in the oven for 15 minutes, stirring twice, until tender. Season with a pinch of salt.

Reheat the skillet over medium heat. When it is hot, add the remaining ½ tablespoon avocado oil and the sliced onion and sauté until tender, stirring frequently, for about 5 minutes. Season with a pinch of salt.

To serve, place the cauliflower "rice" on a plate and top with the broccoli and sautéed onions.

PHASE 2 RECIPES

Breakfast

Coconut-Almond Flour Muffin in a Mug

This tasty breakfast muffin takes just minutes to prepare. Double the recipe to make two muffins, and reheat the second muffin the following day to save even more time.

You can play with the basic recipe by adding 1 teaspoon cocoa powder, lemon or orange zest, mint leaves, or any other herb or berry to change the flavor and add polyphenols or flavonoids.

If you don't have a microwave, pour the batter in a frying pan and serve it up as a pancake.

Phases 2–3

Serves 1
Prep time: 3 minutes
Cook time: 1–2 minutes

1 tablespoon extra-virgin coconut oil, melted
1 tablespoon extra-virgin olive oil or macadamia nut oil
1 tablespoon coconut flour
1 tablespoon almond flour
½ teaspoon aluminum-free baking powder
Pinch sea salt, preferably iodized
1 packet stevia, or 2 teaspoons Just Like Sugar
1 tablespoon water
1 large pastured or omega-3 egg, lightly beaten

Place the ingredients in an 8- to 12-ounce microwave-safe mug, mixing well with a fork or spatula. Be sure to scrape the bottom and sides. Let it sit for a few seconds.

Microwave on high for 1 minute plus 25 to 30 seconds.

Using a pot holder, remove the mug from the microwave and invert, shaking out the muffin. Let cool for a couple of minutes before eating.

VEGAN VERSION: Replace the egg with a VeganEgg.

Cranberry-Orange Muffins

Both good sources of vitamin C, cranberries and oranges have a natural affinity. Most dried cranberries are sweetened with sugar or corn syrup, which you want to avoid at all costs. You can find freeze-dried unsweetened cranberries at Trader Joe's or Whole Foods, or online at Amazon.

To make orange zest, use a microplane or the finest side of a four-sided grater, being careful to avoid the bitter white pith beneath the skin.

Phases 2–3
  Serves 6
  Prep time: 10 minutes
  Cook time: 20 minutes

  ¼ cup coconut flour
  ¼ teaspoon sea salt, preferably iodized
  ¼ teaspoon baking soda
  ¼ cup extra-virgin coconut oil, melted
  ¼ cup Just Like Sugar or xylitol
  3 large pastured or omega-3 eggs
  1 tablespoon orange zest
  ½ cup dried, unsweetened cranberries

Heat the oven to 350°F. Line a standard 6-cup muffin tin with paper liners.

Place the coconut flour, salt, and baking soda in a food processor fitted with an S-blade. Add the coconut oil, Just Like Sugar, eggs, and orange zest. Pulse until blended. Remove the processor blade and stir in the cranberries by hand.

Scoop the batter into the muffin tins, filling to just beneath the rim. Bake for 20 minutes. Let cool on a rack for 15 minutes before serving.

VEGAN VERSION: Replace the eggs with 3 VeganEggs.

Cinnamon-Flaxseed Muffin in a Mug

Grind fresh flaxseeds in a coffee grinder or store ground flaxseed in the refrigerator.

Fresh flaxseeds have a nutty taste, but they are not the best-tasting ingredient in the world, which explains the generous amount of cinnamon in this recipe. If the taste is actually unpleasant, it means the flaxseed has turned rancid and should be discarded.

Phases 2–3
Serves 1
Prep time: 3 minutes
Cook time: 1 minute

¼ cup ground flaxseed
1 teaspoon cinnamon
1 large pastured or omega-3 egg
1 tablespoon extra-virgin coconut oil, melted
1 teaspoon aluminum-free baking powder
1 packet stevia

Place all the ingredients in an 8- to 12-ounce microwave-safe mug, and mix well with a fork or spatula. Be sure to scrape the bottom and sides. Let it sit for a few seconds.

Microwave on high for 1 minute. Check and cook for another 5 to 15 seconds if the muffin appears still wet in the center.

Using a pot holder, remove the mug from the microwave and invert, shaking out the muffin. Let cool for a couple of minutes before eating.

VEGAN VERSION: Replace the egg with a VeganEgg.

"Green" Egg-Sausage Muffins

I know how challenging breakfast can be when you begin the Plant Paradox Program, but this recipe is so easy, tasty, and portable that you just have to try it!

I like to put paper liners in the muffin pans, but they are not essential. Diestel Farms Turkey Italian Sausage or Turkey Chorizo, made from pastured turkey, is available at Whole Foods or other fine markets.

Keep leftovers in a covered glass casserole in the fridge or wrapped in wax paper in the freezer. You can reheat frozen muffins in the microwave, on high for 1 minute or until warm/hot to the touch. Or simply carry one to work and it will defrost by lunchtime. Peel off the liner and enjoy!

Phases 2–3
Makes 12 muffins
Prep time: 15 minutes
Cook time: 35 minutes

1 pound Diestel Farms Turkey Italian Sausage or Turkey Chorizo
One 10-ounce bag chopped organic frozen spinach (or chopped kale)
5 pastured or omega-3 eggs
2 tablespoons extra-virgin olive oil or perilla oil
2 cloves garlic, peeled, or 1 teaspoon garlic powder

2 tablespoons Italian seasoning
2 tablespoons dried minced onion
½ teaspoon sea salt, preferably iodized
½ teaspoon cracked black pepper

Heat the oven to 350°F. Line a standard-size 12-cup muffin tin with paper liners.

Crumble the sausage or chorizo and put in a non-Teflon frying pan. Cook over medium-high heat, stirring frequently, until browned, about 8 to 10 minutes. Set aside.

With a sharp knife, poke small holes in the bag of spinach, put in a microwavable bowl, and place in the microwave on high for 3 minutes.

Cut a tiny edge off the corner of the bag, and squeeze as much water out of the bag as possible.

Place the drained spinach, eggs, olive oil, garlic, Italian seasoning, onion, salt, and pepper in a high-speed blender and pulse/blend for about 1 minute, or until thoroughly mixed. Transfer to a large bowl and stir in the sausage until well mixed.

Fill the muffin tins to just beneath the rim. Bake for 30 to 35 minutes, until the tops start to brown. Remove from the oven and let cool before removing individual muffins from the liner.

VEGETARIAN VERSION: Substitute Quorn Grounds for the sausage. There is no need to fry them. Instead, briefly defrost and add to the spinach-egg mixture with 1 teaspoon fennel seeds.

VEGAN VERSION: Replace the eggs with 5 VeganEggs; substitute 1 block of tempeh, coarsely chopped, for the sausage, adding 1 teaspoon fennel seeds.

Paradox Smoothie

Margo Montelongo posted this recipe on my online discussion page, using several of my products, plus a green banana, which is a resistant starch. Thanks, Margo.

Phases 2–3
   Serves 1
   Total time: 2 minutes

   1 scoop GundryMD Vital Reds, or 1 tablespoon pomegranate powder
   1 scoop GundryMD PrebioThrive, or 2 tablespoons ground flaxseed
   1 scoop GundryMD Primal Plants (apple flavor), or 1 scoop modified
      citrus pectin
   ½ green banana, sliced
   1 tablespoon extra-virgin coconut oil
   1 teaspoon Just Like Sugar
   ½ cup sugar-free coconut milk
   1½ cups tap or filtered water
   3 or 4 ice cubes

Place the Vital Reds, PrebioThrive, and Primal Plants powders in a high-powered blender. Add the green banana, coconut oil, Just Like Sugar, coconut milk, water, and ice cubes, and blend on high until smooth and fluffy.

Perfect Plantain Pancakes

A close relative of the much sweeter banana, plantains are a good source of resistant starch, which your gut bugs thrive on.
   Vanilla enhances the flavors of the other ingredients. Read the la-

bel carefully on vanilla extract—some products use artificial flavoring, which you should avoid at all costs. I prefer to use organic vanilla extract, which is pricier than conventional products, but because you use very little in each recipe, it goes a long way.

Phases 2–3

Serves 4; makes about 8 pancakes
Prep time: 10 minutes
Cook time: 20 minutes

2 large green plantains, peeled and cut in pieces
4 large pastured or omega-3 eggs
2 teaspoons pure vanilla extract
4 to 5 tablespoons extra-virgin coconut oil, divided
¼ cup Just Like Sugar
⅛ teaspoon sea salt, preferably iodized
½ teaspoon baking soda

Place the plantain pieces in a blender or food processor and purée—you should have about 2 cups. Add the eggs and blend to form a smooth batter. Add the vanilla extract, 3 tablespoons of melted coconut oil, Just Like Sugar, the salt, and baking soda. Process on high for 2 to 3 minutes, until smooth.

Heat 1 tablespoon coconut oil in a pan or griddle over medium heat. When the oil shimmers, fill a ½ cup measure with batter and pour into the pan. Repeat for two to three more pancakes.

Cook 4 to 5 minutes, until the top looks fairly dry and has little bubbles. Flip and cook 1½ to 2 minutes more. Repeat with remaining batter, adding more oil as needed.

VEGAN VERSION: Replace the eggs with 4 VeganEggs.

Snacks

Paradox Crackers

When you need a little crunch in your life, these crispy wafers fit the bill. Use them as dippers with guacamole or as an accompaniment to scrambled eggs, soup, or a salad, or simply with a small piece of acceptable cheese. You can also experiment with different herbs, if you wish.

Phases 2–3

Serves 4; makes 16–20 crackers
Prep time: 15 minutes
Cook time: 20 minutes

2 large pastured or omega-3 eggs
1 teaspoon tap or filtered water
1 cup almond flour
½ cup coconut flour
½ teaspoon sea salt; preferably iodized
1 teaspoon Italian seasoning (optional)

Heat the oven to 350°F.

Whisk the eggs and water together in a small bowl.

In a medium bowl, mix the almond flour, coconut flour, and salt, adding the Italian seasoning, if desired. Add the egg mixture to the flour mixture and blend well with a spoon or spatula, eliminating any lumps.

Form into small balls about the size of a large marble, place on a cookie sheet, press flat with the back of a fork, and bake for about 20 minutes, until crisp.

Let cool on a baking rack before serving.

Dr. G.'s New and Improved World-Famous Nut Mix

Every patient who visits our office to give blood or see me is rewarded with ¼ cup of my nut mix to munch on. Based on copious data that nuts protect your heart, brain, and overall health, this mix has been a part of my program since its inception. We now know that the resistant starches in nuts are just what your gut buddies have been asking for! This is why they have the remarkable ability to make you feel full and satisfied for hours.

My recipe originally contained peanuts and pumpkin seeds, but after seeing the effects of their lectins in a number of my patients, we modified the original mix about ten years ago to make it Plant Paradox friendly.

Nuts are good for you, but only in moderation. Put them in snack bags in ¼ cup servings, or ladle them out with a ¼ cup measure.

Phases 2–3
   Makes 10 cups (40 servings)
   Prep time: 5 minutes

   1 pound raw shelled walnuts in halves and pieces
   1 pound raw shelled pistachios or salted and dry-roasted pistachios
   1 pound raw shelled macadamia nuts* or salted and dry-roasted
      macadamias

Put the nuts in a large bowl and stir with your hands or a spoon to mix well. Bag in individual servings and store in the refrigerator.

*If raw macadamia nuts are in halves, they are most likely rancid. Use roasted ones instead.

Beverages

Get Up and Go Cappuccino

Get your caffeine fix with this delicious treat.

Phases 2–3
  Serves 1
  Total time: 1 minute

  1 cup hot coffee
  1 tablespoon MCT oil
  1 tablespoon French or Italian butter, goat butter, or ghee
  1 packet stevia (optional)

Place the ingredients in a blender or Magic Bullet and blend for about 30 seconds. Pour into a mug and serve.

Sparkling Balsamic Vinegar Spritzer

Diet Coke, Diet Pepsi, Diet Dr. Pepper, Diet Root Beer, or diet whatever kills your gut buddies, but my surefire replacement is the color of your old cola and is similarly fizzy. The balsamic vinegar contains resveratrol, one of the most powerful polyphenol compounds, which does wonders for you—and the inner you.

Napa Valley Naturals Grand Reserve is my favorite balsamic vinegar, for its thick consistency and very smooth depth of flavor.

Once you've tried this spritzer, you'll never go back to cola! San Pellegrino is my sparking water of choice. Unlike most carbonated waters, it has a balanced pH. San Pellegrino also contains the highest sulfur content of any leading brand.

Phases 2–3

Serves 1

Total time: 1 minute

8 to 10 ounces San Pellegrino or other high-pH sparkling water,
  chilled
1 to 2 tablespoons balsamic vinegar de Modena

Combine the sparkling water and balsamic in a glass, stir, and enjoy this life-giving drink!

Main and Side Dishes

Tops and Bottoms Celery Soup

Celery root, aka celeriac, is a strong contender for the world's ugliest vegetable, but it makes up for its looks in taste. Plus tubers and roots of any kind make your gut buddies jump for joy. My challenge is to get you to eat these foods.

Everyone enjoys a hearty soup, but unfortunately, most creamy soups rely on cream, flour, and potatoes as thickening agents. Here's my take on Food & Wine's spotlight on chef Julianne Jones's recipe for Celeriac Soup. Note that it's suitable for vegans.

To prepare the celeriac, slice off the rough knobby portions with a knife or vegetable peeler.

Phases 2–3

Serves 4

Prep time: 25 minutes

Cook time: 35 minutes

3 tablespoons extra-virgin olive oil, or avocado or perilla oil, plus
  more for garnish (optional)
One 1-pound celery root, peeled and cut into 1-inch cubes
2 celery stalks with leaves, cut into 1-inch pieces
¼ cup minced dried onion, or ½ red onion, chopped
1 tablespoon chopped fresh rosemary leaves, or 1 teaspoon dried
  rosemary
¼ teaspoon sea salt, preferably iodized
½ teaspoon cracked black pepper
3 cups organic vegetable broth
½ lemon
3 tablespoons chopped flat-leaf parsley, for garnish

In a large Dutch oven or heavy saucepan, heat the 3 tablespoons of olive oil over medium heat. Add the chopped celery root, celery, onion, rosemary, salt, and pepper, and cook for about 5 minutes, until the celery root and celery start to soften and brown a bit.

Add the broth and lemon, and bring to a boil, Reduce the heat, cover, and simmer for 30 minutes. Stir occasionally and check to see when the celery root is tender. Once it is, remove from heat and discard the lemon half.

Transfer about half of the mixture to a high-speed blender and blend on the purée or soup setting until smooth and creamy. Repeat with the rest of the mixture and then reheat the whole batch in the Dutch oven for about 5 minutes.

To serve, pour into serving bowls and garnish with parsley. Drizzle 1 tablespoon olive oil over each bowl, if desired.

Sorghum Salad with Radicchio

Sorghum is used to make molasses, but the fact that it's a resistant starch is not well known. Unlike all other grains except millet, sorghum has no hull, meaning no lectins. What it does have is a cornucopia of polyphenols and anticancer properties. And it tastes great to boot!

Cook sorghum when you have an hour or so to spare, and freeze or refrigerate portions for later use. It never, ever goes mushy. Combine it with one of the greatest sources of inulin, radicchio (it is sometimes called Italian red lettuce, but it is really part of the chicory family), and some nuts, and you and your bugs will be ready for anything!

Perilla, macadamia, or avocado oil can be substituted for the olive oil.

Phases 2–3
　Serves 4
　Cook time: 2 hours for sorghum
　Prep time: 15 minutes for salad

BASIC SORGHUM
1 cup sorghum
3 cups vegetable broth or water, plus more if necessary
1 tablespoon extra-virgin olive oil
1 teaspoon sea salt, preferably iodized

DRESSING
3 tablespoons balsamic vinegar or other vinegar
4 tablespoons extra-virgin olive oil
3 tablespoons capers, rinsed
1 teaspoon coriander powder or seeds
1 clove garlic, peeled

SALAD
½ cup chopped walnuts or pecans
1 head radicchio, torn or chopped into bite-size pieces
½ cup chopped flat-leaf parsley

MAKE THE SORGHUM. Pick through the sorghum, rinse, and discard any debris.

Put the broth or water and oil in a medium saucepan, and bring to a boil. Stir in the sorghum and return to a boil. Reduce the heat to a simmer, cover, and cook for 1 to 2 hours, stirring every 15 minutes and adding broth or water as needed to keep it from drying out or sticking to the pan. To test for doneness, stir with a fork: the sorghum is done when it is light and fluffy.

You can make the recipe ahead of time up to this point. Refrigerate or freeze the cooked sorghum, and then thaw and let it come to room temperature when you want to use it. Alternatively, finish the dish immediately if you plan to serve while the sorghum is warm.

MAKE THE DRESSING. Using a Magic Bullet blender or a mini food processor fitted with an S-blade, combine the vinegar, olive oil, capers, coriander, and garlic and process until smooth.

TO SERVE. Mix the prepared sorghum, nuts, radicchio, and parsley in a large bowl. Add the dressing and toss to combine. Serve on dinner plates.

"Raw" Mushroom Soup

When my wife and I want comfort food, our thoughts turn to a hearty mushroom soup—but instead of waiting for several hours, we want it right away! We love raw food, but sometimes it just needs to be warmed up. After years of raw eating, we have come up with a medley of mushroom soups—this one is the easiest and our best yet. All you need is a food processor or a high-powered blender, and you'll have a warm or hot soup in minutes. Plus, it's vegan-friendly.

With a side salad, this soup makes a full meal. Choose your favorite mushroom—button, cremini, morels, chanterelles, shiitake, or portabella—or mix them up. Your gut buddies adore all mushrooms!

Truffle oil is optional, but I highly recommend it.

Phases 2–3

Serves 2

Prep time: 20 minutes

2 large handfuls of mushrooms with stems, approximately 2 ½ cups

1 cup water

½ cup raw walnuts (preferred), or ¼ cup almond butter or ¼ cup hemp seed hearts

1 tablespoon dried minced onion, or 3 tablespoons chopped red onion

½ teaspoon sea salt, preferably iodized, or Himalayan salt

¼ teaspoon cracked black pepper

2 sprigs fresh thyme leaves, or ½ teaspoon dried thyme

1 tablespoon truffle oil (optional)

Chop ½ cup of the mushrooms and set aside.

Place the remaining 2 cups mushrooms, the water, walnuts, onions, salt, pepper, and thyme in a food processor fitted with the S-blade or in a high-speed blender. Pulse for 30 seconds, and then blend for 2 minutes. Check for temperature—it should be warm but not hot. If you prefer, blend on high for another minute or longer, until it gets hotter.

Pour or spoon the soup into two bowls. It should be thick and gravylike. Top with the chopped mushrooms, drizzle with the truffle oil, if desired, and serve.

Spinach Pizza with a Cauliflower Crust

Riced cauliflower makes up the crust in this delicious pizza. To rice cauliflower, chop it evenly but do not completely pulverize it. You can grate the cauliflower with a cheese grater, using the largest holes, into rice-shaped pieces. Or pulse it in a food processor, using the S-blade and being careful not to overprocess it. If you use a food processor, cut the cauliflower into chunks first. You'll need to extract as much water from the cooked riced cauliflower as possible. (It may yield as much as 1 cup liquid.) Unless the cauliflower is completely dry, the pizza "dough" will be mushy.

Goat milk mozzarella is available from Amazon and other online sources.

Feel free to add some other lectin-free vegetables but don't overload the pizza crust with more veggies than it can support.

Phases 2–3
Serves 2
Prep time: 30 minutes
Cook time: 35 minutes

CRUST
Extra-virgin olive oil for greasing the pan
1 small head cauliflower, cut into small florets
1 pastured or omega-3 egg, lightly beaten
½ cup shredded buffalo or goat mozzarella
½ teaspoon sea salt, preferably iodized
½ teaspoon cracked black pepper
½ teaspoon dried oregano

TOPPING
¾ cup shredded buffalo or goat mozzarella
½ cup cooked and drained spinach

Chopped vegetables of your choice (optional)
¼ cup grated Pecorino-Romano cheese
Pinch sea salt, preferably iodized

Rice the cauliflower. You will have approximately 3 cups. Transfer to a microwave-safe dish and microwave on high for 8 minutes, until cooked. Allow to cool, stirring occasionally.

Place a rack in the middle of the oven. Heat the oven to 450°F. Grease a 10-inch ovenproof frying pan with olive oil.

Place the cooled riced cauliflower in a dishtowel, and twist and squeeze to remove all the moisture. Transfer to a mixing bowl. Add the egg, mozzarella, salt, pepper, and oregano. Mix well. Press the mixture evenly in the frying pan.

Over medium heat on the stove top, crisp the cauliflower crust for a few minutes. Transfer to the oven and bake for 15 minutes, until golden. Let cool for 5 minutes, and add the topping. Scatter the mozzarella evenly over the pizza base and spread the spinach over this. Add any additional vegetables. Sprinkle with the Pecorino-Romano cheese and add a pinch of salt. Bake for an additional 10 minutes, until the cheese has melted.

VEGAN VERSION: Replace the egg with 1 VeganEgg and use Kite Hill Ricotta "cheese" in lieu of the cheeses.

Grilled Portabella-Pesto Mini "Pizzas"

Probably the first thought that went through your head when you realized you were omitting wheat flour, tomatoes, and cow milk cheese was "I can't live without pizza!" In fact, you can live better without it, but I feel your pain. Here is a replacement that I cooked up over my wife Penny's initial objections, but it is now her favorite way to have pizza.

While you make your own pesto here, honestly, the one that comes closest to the true pesto of Liguria (a section of Italy where Penny and I have hiked extensively) is Kirkland's refrigerated pesto, sold at Costco, which uses only Ligurian basil. So feel free to substitute that.

Save or freeze the portabella mushroom stems for "Raw" Mushroom Soup (pages 338–339).

Phases 2–3
Serves 2
Prep time: 30 minutes (only 5 minutes if using store-bought pesto)
Cook time: 20 minutes

BASIL PESTO
1 cup packed fresh basil leaves
¼ cup extra-virgin olive oil
¼ cup pine nuts or walnuts
Two 1-inch cubes Parmigiano-Reggiano

MINI "PIZZAS"
2 large portabella mushroom, stems removed
Extra-virgin coconut or olive oil
2 slices Italian prosciutto
1 ball buffalo mozzarella, cut into ¼- to ½-inch-thick slices
Sea salt, preferably iodized, to taste
Cracked black pepper, to taste

MAKE THE PESTO. In a mini food processor, pulse the basil, olive oil, pine nuts, and cheese until well blended.

MAKE THE "PIZZAS." Set one burner of a gas grill to high or place a grill pan on the stove with burner set to medium-high heat with the exhaust fan on.

Rub the cap side of the mushrooms with oil, place on the grill or grill pan, cap side up, and grill for about 5 minutes, until the caps begin to brown slightly. Flip over and grill, gill side up, for another 5 minutes. Remove the mushrooms from the grill or burner. Leave the heat on.

Spoon 3 tablespoons of pesto onto the gill side of one mushroom, add 1 slice prosciutto, arranging it to fit neatly in the gill cup, and then top with half the mozzarella slices. Repeat with the other mushroom.

If cooking on a grill, return the mushrooms to the grill, close the hood, and grill until the cheese begins to melt, about 5 minutes. If cooking indoors, return the grill pan to the stove top for about 5 minutes; alternatively, cover the grill pan with a glass casserole cover to "steam" for 5 minutes.

TO SERVE. Season to taste with salt and pepper.

VEGETARIAN VERSION: Omit the prosciutto.

VEGAN VERSION: In making the pesto, substitute 1 tablespoon nutritional yeast for the Parmigiano-Reggiano. In making the "pizzas," replace the mozzarella with Kite Hill Ricotta "cheese." Top the grilled mushrooms with this pesto, then spoon scoops of the ricotta over pesto and follow final grilling directions above.

Nutty, Juicy Shroom Burgers, Protein Style

You have probably heard about the new veggie burger that bleeds "blood." Sounds good until you read the list of ingredients, which read like a who's who of lectins.

My wife and I make raw taco "meat" with walnuts and mushrooms, so I decided to do a "bloody burger" using my taco recipe and adding red beets for the crimson hue. Pick a beet about the size of a baseball. Use any kind of mushroom, but portabella or cremini have a meatier texture. Lettuce leaves stand in for "buns" (here in California, we call a burger served this way "protein style"). Then enjoy your meaty, red-tinged burger minus the meat.

For you die-hard carnivores, I've added a real meat version.

Phases 2–3

Serves 4
Prep time: 25 minutes
Cook time: 10 minutes

2 cups walnuts, halves and pieces
2 cups chopped mushrooms
1 cup chopped red beet
2 cloves garlic, peeled, or ¼ teaspoon garlic powder
½ cup chopped red onion, or 2 tablespoons dried minced onions
1 teaspoon paprika, preferably Hungarian
1 tablespoon dried parsley
Sea salt, preferably iodized
Cracked black pepper
½ cup finely chopped fresh basil or sage
2 tablespoons cassava or tapioca flour
3 tablespoons extra-virgin olive oil or avocado oil for frying, plus
    additional to shape the patties

8 romaine leaves or butter lettuce leaves
Avocado mayonnaise (optional)
1 Hass avocado, peeled, pit removed, and sliced

Put the walnuts, mushrooms, beet, garlic, ¼ cup of the onion, paprika, dried parsley, ¼ teaspoon salt, and ¼ teaspoon pepper in a food processor fitted with the S-blade. Pulse and blend until blended but still chunky.

Transfer this mixture to a mixing bowl and stir in the basil, the remaining ¼ cup onion, and the flour. Grease your hands with olive oil and knead the mixture to fully combine ingredients. On a sheet of wax paper, form into four patties, each about 4 inches in diameter and 1 inch thick. Use a coffee mug or lowball glass to shape the patties, if you wish.

Heat a large skillet over medium-high heat. Pour in 3 tablespoons of olive or avocado oil. Add the patties, cooking 4 to 5 minutes per side, until nicely browned.

To serve, place each patty on a lettuce leaf, add a dollop of avocado mayo, if desired, add salt and pepper to taste, top with slices of avocado, and cover with a second lettuce leaf.

MEAT VERSION: Add ½ pound of grass-fed ground beef or pastured chicken or turkey to the mixing bowl before forming into patties.

Roast Parmesan-Scented Cauliflower Mash

My best friend Jimmy Schmidt, the James Beard Award—winning chef at Morgan's in the Desert at the La Quinta Resort and Club, invented this recipe, which I have modified ever so slightly for the Plant Paradox Program.

This dish is a great accompaniment to salmon or another fish.

Phases 2–3

Serves 4
Prep Time: 10 minutes
Cook Time: 60 minutes

1 large head cauliflower, cored and cut into florets
¼ cup extra-virgin olive oil
Sea salt, preferably iodized
Cracked black pepper
2 tablespoons unsalted French or Italian butter, goat butter, or ghee
    (optional)
1 cup finely grated Parmigiano-Reggiano cheese

Heat the oven to 400°F.

Place the cauliflower florets in a large bowl, add the olive oil, and toss to coat well, seasoning generously with sea salt and black pepper.

Lay a large sheet of aluminum foil, shiny side up, on the countertop. Fold in half and then reopen the foil. Transfer the cauliflower to the center of one half of the foil. Fold over the other half and crimp the edges to seal the packet. Place on a cookie sheet and position on the middle rack of the oven.

Cook until very tender and slightly browned, about 1 hour. Remove from the oven, open the pouch carefully—do not let any juices flow out—and cool for about 10 minutes.

Transfer the cauliflower and its liquid to a food processor. Add the butter, if desired, and the Parmesan. Purée until smooth and thickened. Season with salt and pepper to taste. Serve immediately.

Pressure-Cooked Lima Beans, Kale, and Turkey

I am a frequent visitor to the tiny villages of Tuscany. In every town, beans cooked in deep glass flasks are a popular side dish, and one I cannot resist. I usually paid dearly later in the day when the "attack of the lectins" began, as did my wife, trapped in the car with me moaning. However, with the arrival of my pressure cooker, I can now have my beans and eat them, too—plus my gut buddies get the benefits of beans.

I modified this terrific recipe from one by the queen of pressure cooking, Lorna Sass, to make it even easier.

Vegans and vegetarians can try the variations given below in Phase 2, but omnivores should hold off until Phase 3.

Phase 3*
Serves 4–6
Prep time: 30 minutes
Cook time: 25 minutes

1 bunch Tuscan, black, or other kale
1 medium red or yellow onion, chopped
2 cloves garlic, minced, or ½ teaspoon garlic powder
2 tablespoons extra-virgin olive oil or avocado oil
4 cups vegetable stock
3 cups water
1 pound dried large lima beans, rinsed and picked through
2 teaspoons Italian seasoning
1 small pastured bone-in turkey thigh, about ¾ pound

2 tablespoons grainy mustard
2 teaspoons powdered sage
Sea salt, preferably iodized
Cracked black pepper
4 to 6 tablespoons extra-virgin olive oil or truffle oil, for drizzling

Slice the leaves off the stems of the kale. Chop the stems and chop the leaves into larger pieces. Set aside.

If your pressure cooker has a sauté feature, sauté the onions and the garlic in the oil for about 5 minutes. Alternatively, sauté them in a non-Teflon frying pan or wok over medium heat.

Transfer the garlic and onions to the pressure cooker. Add the vegetable stock and water. Add the beans, Italian seasoning, and turkey thigh. Cook at high pressure for 14 minutes, then allow the pressure to come down naturally. Remove the turkey, and stir in the kale leaves, mustard, sage, and salt and pepper to taste.

Shred the turkey and return to the pot. Stir until well blended, and ladle into serving bowls. Drizzle each serving with a tablespoon of olive oil or truffle oil.

VEGETARIAN VERSION: Replace the turkey with ½ package thawed Quorn Grounds.
VEGAN VERSION: Replace the turkey with 1 block grain-free tempeh, crumbled.

*Vegans and vegetarians can consume pressure-cooked legumes in Phase 2.

Thoroughly Modern Millet Cakes

I am one of the world's experts on the dietary treatment of the ApoE4 gene, which 30 percent of all people carry. It is unfortunately named the Alzheimer's gene, because of its strong association with that disease. Nigerians have the highest proportion of this gene in their population, but they have a very low incidence of dementia, a fact often attributed to their mostly plant-based diet. Their grain of choice is millet, sometimes called birdseed, which is free of lectins.

I have spent the last fifteen years formulating user-friendly vegaquarian recipes for the large population with the ApoE4 gene, and I wanted to share some of that with you—so here is a great way to consume millet without having to raid your bird feeder!

With a salad, three patties make a complete meal.

Phases 2–3

> *Serves 4*
> Prep time: 45 minutes
> Cook time: 10 minutes

½ cup millet
2 cups vegetable stock or water
¾ teaspoon sea salt, preferably iodized
¼ cup chopped red onion
¼ cup chopped carrots
¼ cup chopped basil
1 cup chopped mushrooms
1 clove garlic, chopped
½ teaspoon Italian seasoning
2 tablespoons extra-virgin olive oil or perilla oil
1 pastured or omega-3 egg, beaten
1 tablespoon coconut flour

In a large dry saucepan, toast the millet over medium heat for about 5 minutes, stirring or shaking frequently, until golden brown and fragrant. Do not burn. Slowly add the vegetable stock and salt, being careful not to get burned from the rising steam. Stir and bring to boil. Lower the heat to simmer, cover the pan, and cook for about 15 minutes, until all the water is absorbed. Remove from the heat and let stand covered for 10 minutes, then fluff with a fork.

Meanwhile, place the onion, carrots, basil, mushrooms, garlic, and Italian seasoning in a food processor fitted with the S-blade and pulse into fine pieces.

Place 1 tablespoon of the oil in a large skillet over medium heat, add the vegetable mixture, and sauté for 3 to 4 minutes, until tender. Transfer to a large bowl. Wipe the skillet clean with a paper towel. Add the millet, beaten egg, and coconut flour to the mixing bowl. Stir to combine and thicken.

With greased hands, form the mixture into 2-inch balls, and then press down with the palm of your hand to form into 12 patties.

Add the remaining 1 tablespoon oil to the skillet. Add the patties and sauté over medium heat for 5 minutes per side. Drain on a paper-towel-covered plate before serving.

VEGAN VERSION: Replace the egg with 1 VeganEgg.

Shaved Kohlrabi with Crispy Pear and Nuts

Kohlrabi is a member of the cruciferous vegetable family that no one seems to know what to do with. Fear not—one taste of this easy-to-make salad and you'll be hooked!

To grate the kohlrabi and pear, use the side of a box grater with the largest holes or the grating blade of a food processor.

Phases 2–3
Serves 4
Prep time: 30 minutes

½ cup blanched hazelnuts, walnuts, macadamia nuts, or pistachios
2 medium kohlrabi, peeled and grated
1 crisp pear (Comice, Bosc, or Anjou), cored and grated
½ teaspoon finely grated lemon zest
1 tablespoon fresh lemon juice
1 tablespoon white balsamic vinegar
Kosher salt
½ cup torn fresh mint leaves, plus additional for serving
1 tablespoon extra-virgin olive oil
2 ounces Pecorino de Fossa or Parmigiano-Reggiano cheese, shaved

Heat the oven to 350°F.

On a baking sheet, toast the nuts for 10 to 12 minutes, tossing occasionally, until golden brown. Cool and coarsely chop.

Meanwhile, toss the kohlrabi, pear, lemon zest, lemon juice, and vinegar in a bowl. Season with kosher salt. Add the ½ cup mint leaves and toss to combine.

Put the toasted nuts in a small bowl and toss with the olive oil to coat. Season with more salt, if desired.

To serve, divide the salad among four plates and top with seasoned nuts, cheese, and more mint.

Baked Okra Lectin-Blocking Chips

Most people know okra as that slimy vegetable that's found in gumbo or stewed with tomatoes. But you probably don't know that the slimy stuff is actually one of the most effective trappers of lectins ever discovered. It is so powerful that it is a major ingredient in my GundryMD Lectin Shield, part of my supplement line.

This recipe is another great way to get the benefits of okra without the slime. I modified it from a wonderful one at www.eatingbird food.com.

If you are using frozen okra, defrost it first. These chips are absolutely addictive, so you may want to double the recipe! Although I often prepare this as a side dish, it almost never makes it to the table.

Phases 2–3
Serves 4
Prep time: 15 minutes
Cook time: 25–30 minutes

1 pound fresh or whole frozen okra, rinsed and patted dry
1 to 2 tablespoons extra-virgin olive oil
2 teaspoons fresh thyme, or ½ teaspoon dried thyme leaves
½ teaspoon dried crushed or ground rosemary
¼ teaspoon garlic powder
¼ teaspoon sea salt, preferably iodized
Cracked black pepper
Pinch cayenne pepper (optional)

Heat the oven to 450°F.

Cut off the stem ends of the okra and then cut in half lengthwise. Place in a large bowl. Add the olive oil, thyme, rosemary, garlic powder, and salt. Add black pepper and optional cayenne pepper powder to taste and stir to coat the okra.

Place the okra on a baking sheet in a single layer. Roast in the oven for 15 minutes, then shake the pan or, using a spatula, stir the okra. Roast another 10 to 15 minutes, until the okra is lightly browned and tender. Serve hot.

Veggie Curry with Sweet Potato "Noodles"

I'm a huge fan of curry as a way to consume turmeric, but since most curries are served over rice, that's a nonstarter—at least until you are in Phase 3. Spiralized sweet potatoes to the rescue! Spiralizers can transform firm tubers, roots, or even broccoli stems into noodles. Don't have a spiralizer? Just use a vegetable peeler to make "noodles."

This is my variation on a recipe from www.foodfaithfitness.com, Taylor Kiser's site. I've eliminated the nasty nightshades and kicked up the curry, making it Plant Paradox–friendly and vegan-friendly.

Phases 2–3
Serves 2
Prep time: 10 minutes
Cook time: 25 minutes

CURRY
½ tablespoon extra-virgin coconut oil
1 large carrot, spiralized or julienned
1 cup broccoli, cut into bite-size pieces
⅓ cup chopped onion, or 2 tablespoons dried minced onion
1 teaspoon minced fresh ginger, or ½ teaspoon dried ginger
1 tablespoon yellow curry powder
One 13.5-ounce BPA-free can full-fat coconut milk or coconut cream
Pinch sea salt, preferably iodized

SWEET POTATO "NOODLES"
½ tablespoon coconut oil
1 large sweet potato, peeled and spiralized with the 3-mm blade
Pinch salt
4 tablespoons chopped cilantro or flat-leaf parsley, for garnish

MAKE THE CURRY. Heat the coconut oil on medium-high heat. Add the carrot and cook about 3 minutes, until it just begins to soften. Turn the heat down to medium, add the broccoli, onion, and ginger, and cook until they begin to soften and brown, about 5 minutes. Add the yellow curry powder and cook 1 minute. Then add the coconut milk and salt, stirring to mix well.

Raise the heat to medium-high again and bring to a boil. Turn the heat down to medium-low and simmer for 15 minutes, stirring occasionally, until the sauce begins to thicken.

MAKE THE NOODLES. While the sauce is cooking, heat the coconut oil in a skillet over medium heat. Add the spiralized sweet potato noodles, and cook, stirring often, until they just begin to wilt, about 10 minutes. Season with salt.

TO SERVE. Divide the noodles between two plates and top with the curry. Or combine before serving. Sprinkle with the cilantro and serve.

Baked "Fried" Artichoke Hearts

Artichokes are an amazing source of inulin to feed your gut buddies, but steaming and then tediously pulling off each leaf to scrape out a meager amount of meat with your teeth is a pain in the neck. Inspired by Jimmy Schmidt, of Morgan's in the Desert at the La Quinta Resort and Club, I've simplified his dish and omitted the deep-frying for a baked version.

Phases 2–3
Serves 2
Prep time: 20 minutes
Cook time: 25 minutes

4 tablespoons extra-virgin olive oil (or perilla oil)
Juice of ½ lemon, or 2 tablespoons bottled lemon juice

⅛ teaspoon cayenne pepper powder

10 frozen artichoke hearts, defrosted and patted dry with paper
   towels

¼ cup almond, coconut, or cassava flour

¼ teaspoon sea salt, preferably iodized, plus additional for serving

¼ teaspoon cracked black pepper

Lemon wedges

Heat the oven to 400°F.

Place 3 tablespoons of the olive oil, the lemon juice, and cayenne pepper in a mixing bowl and whisk until blended. Add the artichoke hearts to the bowl and stir until well coated.

Coat a rimmed baking sheet with the remaining 1 tablespoon olive oil. Place the flour, the ¼ teaspoon salt, and the pepper in a 1 quart resealable plastic bag. Using tongs or your hands, add the artichokes to the bag and shake to lightly cover. (Alternatively, mix the flour, the ¼ teaspoon salt, and the pepper in a glass casserole with a tight-fitting lid. Add the artichokes and, holding the top firmly, shake to cover.)

Place the artichoke hearts on the baking sheet and bake for 20 to 25 minutes, turning the artichokes or shaking the pan two or three times, until the artichokes are golden brown and crispy.

Remove to a serving dish, sprinkle with more salt, if desired, and serve with lemon wedges.

Cassava Flour Waffles with a Collagen Kick

If you want to eat like a Kitavan Islander, you've got to use cassava flour. You may equate it with tapioca flour, because they come from the same root, but cassava flour is the key to fluffy, nongluten baking. (Trust me, I've tried them all.)

I've modified this great recipe by blogger Heather Resler, after meeting with my good friends at Vital Proteins to get some help for vegaquarians like me (and hopefully you). Have it for breakfast, lunch, or dinner.

The folks at Vital Proteins have come up with marine collagen from wild salmon that just blows me away! It has no fishy taste or any taste— repeat, none. Have it for breakfast, lunch, or dinner. The marine collagen adds fish protein.

If necessary, melt the coconut oil in the microwave on high for 30 seconds or set into a bowl of hot water until melted.

Phases 2–3

Serves 4; makes 4 to 8 waffles, depending on the size and shape of the waffle iron
Prep time: 5 minutes
Cook time: 15 minutes

4 pastured or omega-3 eggs
¼ cup Vital Proteins marine collagen (optional)
½ cup cassava flour
¼ cup extra-virgin coconut oil
1 tablespoon local honey or Manuka honey, or 3 tablespoons Just
    Like Sugar
½ teaspoon baking soda
¼ teaspoon salt
Just Like Sugar, for dusting waffles (optional)
One 12-oz. package Trader Joe's frozen wild blueberries (optional)

Heat a waffle iron.

Place the eggs, marine collagen, if desired, cassava flour, coconut oil, honey, baking soda, and salt in a high-powered blender or regular blender and mix on high for 45 seconds or until well blended and slightly foamy. If you don't have a blender, whisk the eggs, coconut oil, marine collagen, and honey until well blended, and then whisk or stir in the cassava flour, baking soda, and salt.

Using a ¼ cup measure, ladle batter into the waffle iron and cook, following the manufacturer's instructions. Check periodically, since they cook quickly.

If serving as a dessert (phase 3 only), you may want to sprinkle a light coating of Just like Sugar and add ¼ cup wild blueberries on top of each waffle. But always remember, it is best to retreat from sweet!

VEGAN VERSION: Replace the eggs with 4 VeganEggs and omit the collagen.

VEGETARIAN VERSION: Omit the collagen.

Marinated Grilled Cauliflower "Steaks"

A few years ago, my wife and I sat down for lunch at Da Silvano's in Manhattan, one of our favorite Italian restaurants. My friend Silvano Marchetto is the owner, and that afternoon he walked over to our table with a glint in his eye, placing a plate, two forks, and a bottle of his own Tuscan olive oil in front of us. "Try this," he said. The rest is history. Cauliflower "steak" is now a permanent fixture on the Da Silvano's menu—and in our house. I've adapted his brilliant idea for you here.

Substitute avocado, perilla oil, or macadamia nut oil for the olive oil, if you wish.

Phases 2–3

Serves 4
Prep time: 15 minutes
Cook time: 10–15 minutes

½ cup extra-virgin olive oil, plus additional for serving
2 teaspoons minced onion
½ teaspoon garlic powder
2 teaspoons Italian seasoning
¼ teaspoon cayenne pepper
Sea salt, preferably iodized
Cracked black pepper
Juice of 1 lemon
2 heads cauliflower

Place the ½ cup olive oil, the onion, garlic powder, Italian seasoning, and cayenne pepper in a medium bowl. Add salt and black pepper to taste and the lemon juice. Whisk to combine. Transfer to a shallow pan.

Using a large chef's knife, cut off the cauliflower stems flush with the head. Place the stem ends down on a cutting board. Slice each cauliflower in half. Then cut into slices ½ to 1 inch thick (steaks).

Turn on the exhaust fan if cooking indoors. Heat the grill to medium, or place a grill pan over medium-high heat on the stove top.

Using tongs, dip the cauliflower steaks in the marinade. Place on the grill or grill pan and cook 5 to 8 minutes per side, until browned on the outside and tender inside. Transfer to a serving platter. Adjust the seasonings and serve with more olive oil.

Desserts

Miracle Rice Pudding Two Ways

Saying good-bye to the sugars and lectins in grains is never easy on your taste buds, particularly if your mother made a great rice pudding. But your gut and the rest of your body will thank you for changing. The folks at Miracle Noodles, whose products I featured in my first book as "foodles," have developed Miracle Rice, which makes a good stand-in for rice and is widely available. Miracle Rice is made from the konjac root, whose main ingredient is glucomannan, an amazing resistant starch that your gut buddies adore. On the few occasions when you decide to have dessert, how about having something that feeds the good guys, and not the gang members? You even get to pick between the chocolate and vanilla versions.

Phases 2–3

Serves 4
Prep time: 30 minutes
Cook time: 20 minutes

2 bags of Miracle Rice
4 to 5 tablespoons arrowroot powder
3½ cups canned unsweetened, full-fat coconut milk or coconut cream
1 teaspoon ghee or French or Italian butter, plus additional for oiling the pan
1 cup Just Like Sugar, or ½ cup Swerve
1 tablespoon pure vanilla extract
¼ cup (nonalkalized) cocoa powder
1 pastured or omega-3 egg, whisked

Heat the oven to 350°F.

Drain the Miracle Rice in a colander and rinse under running water for about a minute. Set aside to drain further.

Put 4 tablespoons of the arrowroot powder and ½ cup of the coconut milk or cream in a small bowl, and stir to dissolve. Add more arrowroot if necessary.

In a medium saucepan, place the ghee or butter and the remaining 3 cups coconut milk. Cook over medium heat, stirring frequently. As the milk heats, slowly and one at a time, stirring to break up any lumps (particularly in the cocoa powder), add the Just Like Sugar, vanilla extract, cocoa powder, egg, and finally the drained Miracle Rice.

Add about 1 tablespoon of the dissolved arrowroot mixture to the "rice," stirring to incorporate. Repeat 1 tablespoon at a time until you achieve the desired thickness. Add a bit more coconut milk if it seems too thick.

Lightly grease an 8-by-8-inch Pyrex baking dish or 8-inch bowl with butter or ghee. Pour the pudding into the dish and bake for 15 to 20 minutes, until the top is golden brown. Remove from the oven and cool a bit before serving, or refrigerate and serve cold.

VARIATION: VANILLA RICE PUDDING: Omit the cocoa powder and add 1 teaspoon cinnamon and ½ teaspoon nutmeg.

VEGAN VERSION: Replace the ghee or butter with 1 teaspoon coconut oil. Omit the egg or substitute 1 VeganEgg.

Mint Chocolate Chip–Avocado "Ice Cream"

Okay, I admit it. I love ice cream and there's not a lot out there that passes the Plant Paradox Program test, except the So Delicious brand's Coconut Milk blue label. Let's bring the plants to ice cream and sweeten it with the best gut buddy food there is, inulin. What a paradox!

Here's my fabulous version of a recipe on www.allldayIdreamabout food.com, a blog by "Carolyn." I made some adaptations to get even more plant goodness into you. This delectable dessert will satisfy your cravings for ice cream and chocolate without derailing your new way of eating.

Be sure that the coconut milk can is not lined with the deadly disruptor BPA. Trader Joe's makes a great thick coconut cream.

Phases 2–3

Serves 6
Prep time: 20 minutes
Chill time: 2 hours

One 15-ounce can coconut milk or coconut cream
¾ cup Just Like Sugar, or ⅓ cup Swerve
1 teaspoon instant coffee powder or finely ground espresso beans
2 tablespoons (nonalkalized) unsweetened cocoa powder
3 ounces (about one bar) 85% to 90% sugar-free dark chocolate, chopped
1 teaspoon pure vanilla extract
2 Hass avocados, peeled and pits removed.
3 tablespoons chopped fresh mint, or 10 drops SweetLeaf Mint Stevia drops, or to taste
½ cup 72% or more sugar-free extra-dark chocolate chips, or ½ cup chopped 100% percent cocoa baking chocolate

Put the coconut milk, sweetener, coffee powder, and cocoa powder in a medium saucepan. Whisk over medium heat, until the sweetener has dissolved and the mixture is blended.

Turn off the heat. Add the chopped chocolate and stir until melted.

Place the chocolate mixture in a food processor fitted with the S-blade or a blender. Add the vanilla extract, avocados, and mint, and blend until smooth. Pour into a bowl, cover, and refrigerate for 2 hours, until cool.

Stir in the chocolate chips until well dispersed. Spoon or pour into an ice cream maker (see Note) and churn until thick and set. It will be the consistency of soft-serve ice cream.

Serve immediately. You can also freeze to a firmer consistency and serve later: transfer to a metal or glass container and cover with wax paper secured with a rubber band.

VEGAN VERSION: Omit the egg and substitute one VeganEgg.

NOTE: If you don't have an ice cream maker, put the ice cream mixture into a metal loaf pan or a glass or ceramic casserole pan and place in the freezer. Stir every ½ hour to break up ice crystals and keep stirring until desired consistency is reached.

Flourless Chocolate–Almond Butter Cake

Make your own personal mini cake that boasts a symphony of flavors when you need a special treat. Because cream is 100 percent fat, the breed of cow does not matter as it does with milk (it is the protein portion of the milk that is impacted by the casein A-1 mutation in most cows).

Phases 2–3
Serves 1
Prep time: 10 minutes
Cook time: 1 minute

2 tablespoons (nonalkalized) unsweetened cocoa powder
2 tablespoons Just Like Sugar, Swerve, or xylitol
¼ teaspoon aluminum-free baking powder
1 large pastured or omega-3 egg
1 tablespoon heavy cow cream
½ teaspoon pure vanilla extract
1 teaspoon salted French or Italian butter, goat butter, or ghee
1 tablespoon organic smooth or crunchy almond butter

Put the cocoa powder, sweetener, and baking powder in a small mixing bowl. Using a fork, whisk to combine and mash up any clumps of baking powder.

Put the egg, heavy cream, and vanilla extract in another small bowl, and whisk to combine.

Pour the wet ingredients into the dry ingredients and mix until all ingredients are well incorporated.

Grease the bottom and sides of a 4½-inch-diameter ramekin with the butter. Pour in the batter.

Microwave on high for 1 minute 20 seconds and remove. Soften the almond butter in the microwave oven, drizzle over the top of the cake, and serve.

VEGAN VERSION: Replace the cow cream with 1 tablespoon coconut milk or coconut cream. Replace the butter with 1 teaspoon coconut oil. Replace the egg with 1 VeganEgg.

Acknowledgments

Without a doubt, my encounter with the patient who changed my life's arc, "Big Ed," started me on the path that led from my first book, *Dr. Gundry's Diet Evolution,* to the one you now hold in your hands. Thank you again, Ed. Since the publication of my earlier book, tens of thousands of patients have come to Palm Springs or Santa Barbara to see me at the International Heart and Lung Institute, and within it, the Center for Restorative Medicine. Hundreds of thousands of other people have written to tell me about the success they have experienced by following *Diet Evolution* and the subsequent program, "Matrix," on which this book is based. Without my patients' tireless search for health and their willingness to let me examine their blood test results every three months for years on end, *The Plant Paradox* would never have come to fruition. As my dedication says, everything I know, or learned, is because of you.

Once again, my wonderful wife and soul mate, Penny, has not only endured many days and nights without the presence of my brain and attention while I was writing this book, but also the many days and nights without my physical presence while I traveled to present the results of my research to a worldwide audience. She has also been my best critic of my early versions of the manuscript and "crazy" ideas for supplements. Thank you again for your patience and love. I have banked that love and promise to repay it with interest!

As with my first book, this one would not have been possible without the tireless efforts of my collaborator, Olivia Bell Buehl, who takes my wordy manuscripts and employs her word-smithing magic to transform them into readable and usable books. This one has been more of a challenge on many levels than our first, but I'm so glad we both persevered to deliver to you this wonderful guide for your health.

My office is under the direction of Susan Lokken, my right-hand woman aka administrative assistant and office manager, who somehow gets me where I need to be, gets patients what they need, and keeps order in an environment that is constantly besieged by requests from people worldwide to somehow get them past the seven-month waiting list and in to see me "tomorrow" to address a life-threatening health issue. Without Susan, nothing in this book would have happened.

Another huge thank-you to Adda Harris, who reversed her own personal health issues by following the Plant Paradox, and now somehow juggles patient care and training while always showing a welcoming concern for any issue a patient might have. As we say, "You go, girl!"

I cannot say enough about my former nurse practitioner, Jean Epstein, who collaborated on many of my research papers, and brought joy and comfort to so many of our mutual patients. Not a day goes by that we don't all miss you.

I cannot resist mentioning my younger daughter, Melissa Perko, who manages my wife's store Zense on El Paseo Drive in Palm Desert, but who also dives into my office for four months every summer to bring order to chaos. I know how much it means to you to have a chance to boss your father around! And how much it means to me to have you nearby!

The kickoff for the Plant Paradox Program couldn't have happened without my dear friend and supporter, the great chef Irina Skoeries—and I thank her for her enthusiasm and tireless commitment to making vibrant health a reality for everyone. Having witnessed her skill in salvaging several of my toughest patients with nourishing and delectable food, I knew she had to develop the Three-Day Kick-Start Cleanse for Phase 1! Thank you, Irina!

Another heartfelt thanks to Celia Hamilton of Palm Springs, who has guided so many of my patients back from the brink of despair and toward thriving health with her loving care in teaching and living my principles.

Any of you who have visited my office have encountered my fantastic team of "Blood Suckers," who have convinced you to relinquish up to a dozen vials of blood every few months without pain! Believe me, nothing I have learned and written here would have been possible without Laurie Acuna and her team. Thank you all.

I owe a huge debt to my agent, Shannon Marven, president of Dupree-Miller, and her great associate, Dabney Rice, who connected me with Harper Wave and who then consistently and calmly kept everything on track.

Thank you to my editors, Julie Will and Sarah Murphy, as well as publisher Karen Rinaldi at Harper Wave. You took my all-encompassing ideas and gently, but firmly, brought forth this guide to achieving great health! And thank you to the great support team at Harper Wave, Hannah Robinson and Elizabeth Preske, my copy editor Trent Duffy and production editor Nikki Baldauf, Brian Perrin in marketing, and my publicists, Victoria Comella and Nick Davies.

You may have never heard of me, or my work, without the amazing team at GoldenHippoMedia, who collectively made www.GundryMD.com the premier health information portal it has become. They are also responsible for producing and marketing my formulas for supplements and skin-care products for GundryMD. To all 450 team members—and you know who you are—thank you, each and every one! I wanted to name you all, but, well, that would take a whole other book!

Notes

Introduction

1. Gundry, S.R. 2015. Abstract 309: Twelve year followup for managing coronary artery diease using a nutrigenomics based diet and supplement program with quarterly assessment of biomarkers. *Arteriosclerosis, Thrombosis, and Vascular Biology* 35: A309.

   Gundry, S.R., and Epstein, J. 2013. Abstract 137: Reversal of endothelial dysfunction using polyphenol rich foods and supplements coupled with avoidance of major dietary lectins. *Arteriosclerosis, Thrombosis, and Vascular Biology* 33: A137.

Chapter 1: The War Between Plants and Animals

1. Childs et al. 1990. Effects of shellfish consumption on lipoproteins in normolipidemic men. *The American Journal of Clinical Nutrition* 51(6): 1020–1027.
2. Wellman et al. 2003. Fragments of the earliest land plants. *Nature* 425(6955): 282–285.
3. Monahan, P. 2016. Plants defend themselves with armor made of sand. http://www.sciencemag.org/news/2016/03/plants-defend-themselves-armor-made-sand. Accessed 12/10/2016.
4. Nelson, H.E. 2016. Why can't many carnivores and herbivores see color? https://www.quora.com/Why-cant-many-carnivores-and-herbivores-see-color. Accessed 11/26/2016.

   Schaefer et al. 2007. Are fruit colors adapted to consumer vision and birds equally efficient in detecting colorful signals? *The American Naturalist* 169(Suppl. 1): S159-S69.
5. Bennett, C. 2014. Chewing vibrations prompt plant to react with chemical releases. http://www.agweb.com/article/plants-can-hear-pests-attack/. Accessed 11/26/2016.
6. Gagliano et al. 2014. Experience teaches plants to learn faster and forget slower in environments where it matters. *Oecologia* 175(1): 63–72.
7. Meireles-Filho, A.C.A., and Kyriacou, C.P. 2013. Circadian rhythms in insect disease vectors. *Memórias do Instituto Oswaldo Cruz* 108(Suppl. I): 48–58.
8. Boevé et al. 2013. Invertebrate and avian predators as drivers of chemical defensive strategies in tenthredinid sawflies. *BMC Evolutionary Biology* 13: 198.
9. Chatterjee et al. 2007. A BELL1-like gene of potato is light activated and wound inducible. *Plant Physiology* 145(4): 1435–1443.
10. Pierini, C. 2009. Lectin lock: Natural defense against a hidden cause of digestive

concerns and weight gain. http://www.vrp.co.za/Public/ViewArticle.aspx?Article
ID=102. Accessed 11/26/2016.

11. The Beef Site. 2009. Ground limestone in beef cattle diets. http://www.thebeefsite
.com/articles/1936/ground-limestone-in-beef-cattle-diets/. Accessed 12/10/2016.

12. Barański et al. 2014. Higher antioxidant and lower cadmium concentrations and
lower incidence of pesticide residues in organically grown crops: A systematic literature review and meta-analyses. *British Journal of Nutrition* 112(5): 794–811.

    Faller, A.L.K., and Fialho, E. 2010. Polyphenol content and antioxidant capac-
ity in organic and conventional plant foods. *Journal of Food Composition and Analysis*
23(6): 561–568.

13. Leiber et al. 2005. A study on the causes for the elevated n-3 fatty acids in cows' milk
of alpine origin. *Lipids* 40(2): 191–202.

14. Goodman, R. 2012. Ask a farmer: Does feeding corn harm cattle? https://agricul
tureproud.com/2012/09/27/ask-a-farmer-does-feeding-corn-harm-cattle/. Accessed
11/26/2016.

15. Sanz, Y. 2010. Effects of a gluten-free diet on gut microbiota and immune function
in healthy adult humans. *Gut Microbes* 1(3): 135–137.

16. Children's Hospital of Pittsburgh of UPMC. 2016. About the small and large intestines. http://www.chp.edu/our-services/transplant/intestine/education/about
-small-large-intestines. Accessed 11/27/2016.

    Diep, F. 2014. Human gut has the surface area of a studio apartment. Revising
an old biology analogy. http://www.popsci.com/article/science/human-gut-has
-surface-area-studio-apartment. Accessed 11/27/2016.

    Magsanide, S. 2016. Digestive 6. https://quizlet.com/11845442/digestive-6-flash
-cards/. Accessed 11/27/2016.

17. Patel et al. 2002. Potato glycoalkaloids adversely affect intestinal permeability and
aggravate inflammatory bowel disease. *Inflammatory Bowel Diseases* 8(5): 340–346.

18. Mogensen, T.H. 2009. Pathogen recognition and inflammatory signaling in innate
immune defenses. *Clinical Microbiology Reviews* 22(2): 240–273.

19. Fälth-Magnusson, K., and Magnusson, K.E. 1995. Elevated levels of serum antibodies to the lectin wheat germ agglutinin in celiac children lend support to the
gluten-lectin theory of celiac disease. *Pediatric Allergy and Immunology* 6(2): 98–102.

    Hollander et al. 1986. Increased intestinal permeability in patients with
Crohn's disease and their relatives. A possible etiologic factor. *Annals of Internal
Medicine* 105(6): 883–885.

    Livingston, J.N., and Purvis, B.J. 1980. Effects of wheat germ agglutinin on in-
sulin binding and insulin sensitivity of fat cells. *The American Journal of Physiology*
238(3): E267-E275.

Chapter 2: Lectins on the Loose

1. Azvolinsky, A. 2016. Primates, gut microbes evolved together. Symbiotic gut bacteria evolved and diverged along with ape and human lineages, researchers find.

http://mobile.the-scientist.com/article/46603/primates-gut-microbes-evolved
-together. Accessed 11/27/2016.

2. Elsevier. 2016. Uterine microbiota play a key role in implantation and pregnancy
    success in in vitro fertilization. https://www.sciencedaily.com/releases/2016/12
    /161206124717.htm. Accessed 12/10/2016.

3. Eades, M.R. 2007. Obesity in ancient Egypt. https://proteinpower.com/drmike
    /2007/07/01/obesity-in-ancient-egypt/#more-782. Accessed 11/27/2016.

4. Mellanby, M., and Pattison, C.L. 1932. Remarks on the influence of a cereal-free
    diet rich in vitamin D and calcium on dental caries in children. *The British Medical
    Journal* 1(3715): 507–510.

5. Pal et al. 2015. Milk intolerance, beta-casein and lactose. *Nutrients* 7(9): 7285–7297.

6. Woodford, K. 2009. *Devil in the Milk: Illness, Health and the Politics of A1 and A2 Milk.*
    White River Junction, VT: Chelsea Green Publishing.

7. Gross et al. 2004. Increased consumption of refined carbohydrates and the epi-
    demic of type 2 diabetes in the United States: an ecologic assessment. *The American
    Journal of Clinical Nutrition* 79(5): 774–779.

8. United States Department of Agriculture Economic Research Service. 2016.
    Food—away—from—home. https://www.ers.usda.gov/topics/food-choices-health
    /food-consumption-demand/food-away-from-home.aspx. Accessed 11/28/2016.

9. Scientific American. 2016. Dirt poor: Have fruits and vegetables become less nutri-
    tious? https://www.scientificamerican.com/article/soil-depletion-and-nutrition
    -loss/. Accessed 11/28/2016.

10. Gundry, S.R. 2016. Curing/remission of multiple autoimmune diseases is possible
    by manipulation of the human gut microbiome: The effect of a lectin limited, poly-
    phenol enriched, prebiotic/probiotic regimen in 78 patients. *Journal of International
    Society of Microbiota* 3(1).

11. Müller et al. 2001. Fasting followed by vegetarian diet in patients with rheumatoid
    arthritis: A systematic review. *Scandinavian Journal of Rheumatology* 30(1): 1–10.

12. Lanzini et al. 2009. Complete recovery of intestinal mucosa occurs very rarely in
    adult coeliac patients despite adherence to gluten-free diet. *Alimentary Pharmacol-
    ogy & Therapeutics* 29(12): 1299–1308.

13. Sanz, Y. 2010. Effects of a gluten-free diet on gut microbiota and immune function
    in healthy adult humans. *Gut Microbes* 1(3): 135–137.

14. Centers for Disease Control and Prevention. 2016. Obesity and overweight. http://
    www.cdc.gov/nchs/fastats/obesity-overweight.htm. Accessed 11/28/2016.

15. Engel et al. 1997. Lectin staining of renal tubules in normal kidney. *Acta Patholog-
    ica, Microbiologica et Immunologica Scandinavica* 105(1): 31–34.

16. Campbell, T.C., and Campbell, T.M. 2006. *The China Study: The Most Comprehensive
    Study of Nutrition Ever Conducted and the Startling Implications for Diet, Weight Loss and
    Long-Term Health.* Dallas, TX: BenBella Books.

17. Bebee, B. 2008. *The Hundred-Year DIET: Guidelines and Recipes for a Long and Vigorous
    Life.* Bloomington, IN: iUniverse.

18. Blum, D. 2010. Early puberty in girls. https://truthjunkie.wordpress.com/2010
/06/06/early-puberty-in-girls/. Accessed 12/10/2016.

Hood, E. 2005. Are EDCs blurring issues of gender? *Environmental Health Perspectives* 113(10): A670-A677.

Chapter 3: Your Gut Under Attack

1. Goldman, B. 2016. Low-fiber diet may cause irreversible depletion of gut bacteria over generations. https://med.stanford.edu/news/all-news/2016/01/low-fiber-diet-may-cause-irreversible-depletion-of-gut-bacteria.html. Accessed 11/28/2016.
2. Sampson et al. 2016. Gut microbiota regulate motor deficits and neuroinflammation in a model of Parkinson's disease. *Cell* 167(6): 1469–1480.
3. Matsui et al. 2011. The pathophysiology of non-steroidal anti-inflammatory drug (NSAID)-induced mucosal injuries in stomach and small intestine. *Journal of Clinical Biochemistry and Nutrition* 48(2): 107–111.
4. Tillisch, K. 2014. The effects of gut microbiota on CNS function in humans. *Gut Microbes* 5(3): 404–410.
5. Zheng et al. 2016. Dietary plant lectins appear to be transported from the gut to gain access to and alter dopaminergic neurons of Caenorhabditis elegans, a potential etiology of Parkinson's disease. *Frontiers in Nutrition* 3: 7.
6. Sonnenburg, J., and Sonnenburg, E. 2015. *The Good Gut: Taking Control of Your Weight, Your Mood, and Your Long-Term Health.* New York, NY: Penguin Books.

Chapter 4: Know Thy Enemy

1. Whiteman, H. 2014. CDC: Life expectancy in the US reaches record high. http://www.medicalnewstoday.com/articles/283625.php. Accessed 11/28/2016.
2. Centers for Disease Control and Prevention. 2016. Infant mortality. http://www.cdc.gov/reproductivehealth/MaternalInfantHealth/InfantMortality.htm. Accessed 11/28/2016.
3. Kaplan, K. 2014. Premature births a big factor in high U.S. infant mortality rate. http://www.latimes.com/science/sciencenow/la-sci-sn-infant-mortality-us-ranks-26th-20140924-story.html. Accessed 11/28/2016.
4. Duke Health. 2016. Physical declines begin earlier than expected among U.S. adults. https://www.sciencedaily.com/releases/2016/07/160721144805.htm. Accessed 11/28/2016.
5. Kane, J. 2012. Health costs: How the U.S. compares with other countries. http://www.pbs.org/newshour/rundown/health-costs-how-the-us-compares-with-other-countries/. Accessed 11/28/2016.
6. Blaser, M.J. 2014. *Missing Microbes: How the Overuse of Antibiotics Is Fueling Our Modern Plagues.* New York, NY: Henry Holt and Company.
7. Gonzalez, R. 2012. Maryland politicians chicken out on arsenic ban. http://www.treehugger.com/health/maryland-politicians-chicken-out-on-arsenic-ban.html. Accessed 12/10/2016.

8. Ly, L. 2013. FDA finally bans most arsenic in chicken feed—oh, by the way, there's arsenic in your chicken. https://www.kcet.org/food/fda-finally-bans-most-arse nic-in-chicken-feed-oh-by-the-way-theres-arsenic-in-your-chicken. Accessed 12/10/2016.

9. Reyes-Herrera, I., and Donoghue, D.J. 2008. Antibiotic residues distribute uniformly in broiler chicken breast muscle tissue. 71(1): 223–225.

10. Tajima, A. 2014. Non-steroidal anti-inflammatory drug (NSAID)-induced small intestinal injury. *Pharmaceutica Analytica Acta* 5(1): 282.

11. Gomm et al. 2016. Association of proton pump inhibitors with risk of dementia: A pharmacoepidemiological claims data analysis. *JAMA Neurology* 73(4): 410–416.

12. Morrison et al. 2011. Risk factors associated with complications and mortality in patients with clostridium difficile infection. *Clinical Infectious Diseases* 53(12): 1173–1178.

13. Laheij et al. 2004. Risk of community-acquired pneumonia and use of gastric acid-suppressive drugs. *JAMA* 292(16): 1955–1960.

14. Abou-Donia et al. 2008. Splenda alters gut microflora and increases intestinal p-glycoprotein and cytochrome p-450 in male rats. *Journal of Toxicology and Environmental Health* 71(21): 1415–1429.

15. Axe, J. 2016. How endocrine disruptors destroy your body + the dirty dozen to avoid. https://draxe.com/endocrine-disruptors-how-to-avoid-excess-estrogen/?utm _source=promotional&utm_medium=email&utm_campaign=20161102_newsletter _curated_bbp+healingprotein. Accessed 11/28/2016.

16. Gore et al. 2015. EDC-2: The Endocrine Society's second scientific statement on endocrine-disrupting chemicals. *Endocrine Reviews* 36(6): E1-E150.

17. American Chemical Society. 2016. Baby teethers soothe, but many contain low levels of BPA. https://www.sciencedaily.com/releases/2016/12/161207092920.htm. Accessed 12/10/2016.

18. News-Medical.Net. 2016. Food additive tBHQ may be linked to increase in food allergies. http://www.news-medical.net/news/20160711/Food-additive-tBHQ-may -be-linked-to-increase-in-food-allergies.aspx. Accessed 11/28/2016.

19. Kapil et al. 2013. Physiological role for nitrate-reducing oral bacteria in blood pressure control. *Free Radical Biology & Medicine* 55: 93–100.

20. Hanley, D.A., and Davison, K.S. 2005. Vitamin D insufficiency in North America. *The Journal of Nutrition* 135(2): 332–337.

21. Janesick, A., and Blumberg, B. 2011. Endocrine disrupting chemicals and the developmental programming of adipogenesis and obesity. *Birth Defects Research Part C: Embryo Today: Reviews* 93(1): 34–50.

22. Union of Concerned Scientists. 2015. Bad chemistry: How the chemical industry's trade association undermines the policies that protect us. http://www.ucsusa.org /center-science-and-democracy/fighting-misinformation/american-chemistry -council-report#.WD3f9MkabES. Accessed 11/29/2016.

23. Foster et al. 2000. Effects of di-n-butyl phthalate (DBP) on male reproductive de-

velopment in the rat: implications for human risk assessment. *Food and Chemical Toxicology* 38(1 Suppl.): S97–S99.

24. Duty et al. 2003. The relationship between environmental exposures to phthalates and DNA damage in human sperm using the neutral comet assay. *Environmental Health Perspectives* 111(9): 1164–1169.

25. Colón et al. 2000. Identification of phthalate esters in the serum of young Puerto Rican girls with premature breast development. *Environmental Health Perspectives* 108(9): 895–900.

26. Latini et al. 2003. In utero exposure to di-(2-ethylhexyl) phthalate and duration of human pregnancy. *Environmental Health Perspectives* 111(14): 1783–1785.

27. Schecter et al. 2013. Phthalate concentrations and dietary exposure from food purchased in New York State. *Environmental Health Perspectives* 121(4): 473–479.

28. Greger, M. 2011. Chicken consumption & the feminization of male genitalia. http://nutritionfacts.org/video/chicken-consumption-and-the-feminization-of-male-genitalia/. Accessed 11/29/2016.

29. Swan et al. 2010. Prenatal phthalate exposure and reduced masculine play in boys. *International Journal of Andrology* 33(2): 259–269.

30. Maranghi et al. 2009. Effects of the food contaminant semicarbazide following oral administration in juvenile Sprague-Dawley rats. *Food and Chemical Toxicology* 47(2): 472–479.

Maranghi et al. 2010. The food contaminant semicarbazide acts as an endocrine disrupter: Evidence from an integrated in vivo/in vitro approach. *Chemico-Biological Interactions* 183(1): 40–48.

31. European Food Safety Authority. 2005. EFSA publishes further evaluation on semicarbazide in food. https://www.efsa.europa.eu/en/press/news/afc050701. Accessed 11/29/2016.

32. Landau, E. 2004. Subway to remove 'dough conditioner' chemical from bread. http://www.cnn.com/2014/02/06/health/subway-bread-chemical/. Accessed 1/15/2017.

33. Kim et al. 2004. Occupational asthma due to azodicarbonamide. *Yonsei Medical Journal* 45(2): 325–329.

Cary et al. 1999. Azodicarbonamide. http://apps.who.int/iris/bitstream/10665/42200/1/9241530162.pdf. Accessed 11/29/2016.

34. Tassignon et al. 2001. Azodicarbonamide as a new T cell immunosuppressant: Synergy with cyclosporin A. *Clinical Immunology* 100(1): 24–30.

35. Chen et al. 2016. Exposure to the BPA-Substitute Bisphenol S causes unique alterations of germline function. *PLoS Genetics* 12(7): e1006223.

36. Gammon, C. 2009. Weed-whacking herbicide proves deadly to human cells. https://www.scientificamerican.com/article/weed-whacking-herbicide-p/. Accessed 11/29/2016.

37. Food Democracy Now. 2016. Glysophosphate: Unsafe on any plate. Food testing results and scientific reasons for concern. https://s3.amazonaws.com/media.food democracynow.org/images/FDN_Glyphosate_FoodTesting_Report_p2016.pdf. Accessed 11/29/2016.

38. Samsel, A., and Seneff, S. 2013. Glyphosate, pathways to modern diseases II: Celiac sprue and gluten intolerance. *Interdisciplinary Toxicology* 6(4): 159–184.

39. Cantorna et al. 2014. Vitamin D, immune regulation, the microbiota, and inflammatory bowel disease. *Experimental Biology & Medicine* 239(11): 1524–1530.

40. Van Hoesen, S. 2015. World Health Organization labels glyphosate probable carcinogen. http://www.ewg.org/release/world-health-organization-labels-glyphosate-probable-carcinogen. Accessed 11/29/2016.

41. Gillam, C. 2016. FDA to start testing for glyphosate in food. http://civileats.com/2016/02/17/fda-to-start-testing-for-glyphosate-in-food. Accessed 2/15/17.

42. University of California San Francisco. 2016. UCSF presentation reveals glyphosate contamination in people across America. https://www.organicconsumers.org/news/ucsf-presentation-reveals-glyphosate-contamination-people-across-america. Accessed 11/29/2016.

43. Gale, R., and Null, G. 2015. Monsanto's sealed documents reveal the truth behind roundup's toxicological dangers. https://www.organicconsumers.org/news/monsantos-sealed-documents-reveal-truth-behind-roundups-toxicological-dangers. Accessed 11/29/2016.

44. Organic Consumers Association. 2015. World's first public testing for Monsanto's glyphosate begins today. https://www.organicconsumers.org/press/world%E2%80%99s-first-public-testing-monsanto%E2%80%99s-glyphosate-begins-today. Accessed 11/29/2016.

45. Hakim, D. 2016. Doubts about the promised bounty of genetically modified crops. http://www.nytimes.com/2016/10/30/business/gmo-promise-falls-short.html?_r=1. Accessed 11/29/2016.

46. Reid et al. 2014. Timing and intensity of light correlate with body weight in adults, *PLoS One* 9(4): e92251.

Chapter 5: How the Modern Diet Makes You Fat (and Sick)

1. National Institute of Diabetes and Digestive and Kidney Diseases. 2012. Overweight and obesity statistics. https://www.niddk.nih.gov/health-information/health-statistics/Pages/overweight-obesity-statistics.aspx. Accessed 11/29/2016.

2. Wing, R.R., and Phelan, S. 2005. Long-term weight loss maintenance. *The American Journal of Clinical Nutrition* 82(1 Suppl.): 222S-225S.

3. Zheng et al. 2016. Dietary plant lectins appear to be transported from the gut to gain access to and alter dopaminergic neurons of Caenorhabditis Elegans, a potential etiology of Parkinson's disease. *Frontiers in Nutrition* 3: 7.

4. Svensson et al. 2015. Vagotomy and subsequent risk of Parkinson's disease. *Annals of Neurology* 78(4): 522–529.

5. Aslanabadi et al. 2014. Epicardial and pericardial fat volume correlate with the severity of coronary artery stenosis. *Journal of Cardiovascular and Thoracic Research* 6(4): 235–239.

6. Aune et al. 2016. Nut consumption and risk of cardiovascular disease, total can-

cer, all-cause and cause-specific mortality: a systematic review and dose-response meta-analysis of prospective studies. *BMC Medicine* 14(1): 207.

7. Lindeberg, Staffan. *Food and Western Disease*. John Wiley and Sons, 2010.

8. Martinez et al. 2010. Resistant starches types 2 and 4 have differential effects on the composition of the fecal microbiota in human subjects. *PLoS One* 5: e15046.

9. University of Michigan Health System. 2016. High-fiber diet keeps gut microbes from eating the colon's lining, protects against infection, animal study shows. https://www.sciencedaily.com/releases/2016/11/161117134626.htm. Accessed 11/20/2016.

10. Aust et al. 2001. Estimation of available energy of dietary fibres by indirect calorimetry in rats. *European Journal of Nutrition* 40(1): 23–29.

    Anderson et al. 2010. Relation between estimates of cornstarch digestibility by the Englyst in vitro method and glycemic response, subjective appetite, and short-term food intake in young men. *The American Journal of Clinical Nutrition* 91(4): 932–939.

11. Bodinham et al. 2010. Acute ingestion of resistant starch reduces food intake in healthy adults. *British Journal of Nutrition* 103(6): 917–922.

    Willis et al. 2009. Greater satiety response with resistant starch and corn bran in human subjects. *Nutrition Research* 29(2): 100–105.

    Nilsson et al. 2008. Including indigestible carbohydrates in the evening meal of healthy subjects improves glucose tolerance, lowers inflammatory markers, and increases satiety after a subsequent standardized breakfast. *Journal of Nutrition* 138(4): 732–739.

12. Higgins et al. 2004. Resistant starch consumption promotes lipid oxidation. *Nutrition & Metabolism* 1(1): 8.

    Robertson et al. 2012. Insulin-sensitizing effects on muscle and adipose tissue after dietary fiber intake in men and women with metabolic syndrome. *The Journal of Clinical Endocrinology & Metabolism* 97(9): 3326–3332.

13. Gittner, L.S. 2009. *From farm to fat kids: The intersection of agricultural and health policy* (Doctoral dissertation). Retrieved from https://etd.ohiolink.edu/ap/10?0::NO:10:P10_ACCESSION_NUM:akron1254251814#abstract-files. Accessed 11/30/2016.

Chapter 6: Revamp Your Habits

1. Cheng et al. 2014. Prolonged fasting reduces IGF-1/PKA to promote hematopoietic-stem-cell-based regeneration and reverse immunosuppression. *Cell Stem Cell* 14(6): 810–823.

2. Gersch et al. 2007. Fructose, but not dextrose, accelerates the progression of chronic kidney disease. *American Journal of Physiology. Renal Physiology* 293(4): F1256–1261.

3. Jahren, A.H., and Kraft, R.A. 2008. Carbon and nitrogen stable isotopes in fast food: signatures of corn and confinement. *Proceedings of the National Academy of Sciences of the United States of America* 105(46): 17855–17860.

    Biello, D. 2008. That burger you're eating is mostly corn. http://www.scientificamerican.com/article/that-burger-youre-eating-is-mostly-corn/. Accessed 09/01/2016.

4. Bellows, S. 2008. The hair detective. http://uvamagazine.org/articles/the_hair_detective. Accessed 09/01/2016.

5. Gupta, S. 2007. If we are what we eat, Americans are corn and soy. http://www.cnn .com/2007/HEALTH/diet.fitness/09/22/kd.gupta.column/. Accessed 09/01/2016.

6. Brickett et al. 2007. The impact of nutrient density, feed form, and photoperiod on the walking ability and skeletal quality of broiler chickens. *Poultry Science* 86(10): 2117–2125.

7. Jakobsen et al. 2012. Is Escherichia coli urinary tract infection a zoonosis? Proof of direct link with production animals and meat. *European Journal of Clinical Microbiology & Infectious Diseases* 31(6): 1121–1129.

8. Gutleb et al. 2015. Detection of multiple mycotoxin occurrences in soy animal feed by traditional mycological identification combined with molecular species identification. *Toxicology Reports* 2: 275–279.

9. Piotrowska et al. 2013. Mycotoxins in cereal and soybean-based food and feed. In H.A. El-Shemy (Ed.), *Soybean-Pest Resistance*. Rijeka, Croatia: InTech.

10. Viggiano et al. 2016. Effects of an high-fat diet enriched in lard or in fish oil on the hypothalamic amp-activated protein kinase and inflammatory mediators. *Frontiers in Cellular Neuroscience* 10: 150.

11. Aune et al. 2016. Nut consumption and risk of cardiovascular disease, total cancer, all-cause and cause-specific mortality: a systematic review and dose-response meta-analysis of prospective studies. *BMC Medicine* 14(1): 207.

12. Fontana et al. 2008. Long-term effects of calorie or protein restriction on serum IGF-1 and IGFBP-3 concentration in humans. *Aging Cell* 7(5): 681–687.

    Conn, C.S., and Qian, S.B. 2011. mTOR signaling in protein homeostasis: Less is more? *Cell Cycle* 10(12): 1940–1947.

13. Ananieva, E. 2015. Targeting amino acid metabolism in cancer growth and anti-tumor immune response. *World Journal of Biological Chemistry* 6(4): 281–289.

14. The Low Histamine Chef. 2015. Interview: Fasting mimicking diets for mast cell activation & allergies. http://thelowhistaminechef.com/interview-fasting-mimicking -diets-for-mast-cell-activation-allergies/. Accessed 09/01/2016.

Chapter 7: Phase 1

1. Thompson, L. 2016. What does a three-day dietary cleanse do to your gut microbiome? http://americangut.org/what-does-a-three-day-dietary-cleanse-do-to-your -gut-microbiome/. Accessed 09/03/2016.

2. Angelakis et al. 2015. A Metagenomic investigation of the duodenal microbiota reveals links with obesity. *PLos One* 10(9): e0137784.

    Collins, F. 2013. New take on how gastric bypass cures diabetes. https://directors blog.nih.gov/2013/07/30/new-take-on-how-gastric-bypass-cures-diabetes/. Accessed 09/03/2016.

Chapter 8: Phase 2

1. University of California–Berkeley. 2016. Biologists home in on paleo gut for clues to our evolutionary history: Evolution of gut bacteria in humans and hominids parallels ape evolution. www.sciencedaily.com/releases/2016/07/160721151457.htm. Accessed 09/03/2016.
2. Walderhaug, M. 2012. *Bad bug book, foodborne pathogenic microorganisms and natural toxins.* Second Edition. K.A. Lampel (Ed.). Silver Spring, MD: U.S. Food and Drug Administration.
3. Centers for Disease Control and Prevention. 2012. Pathogens causing US foodborne illnesses, hospitalizations, and deaths, 2000–2008. http://www.cdc.gov/foodborne burden/pdfs/pathogens-complete-list-04–12.pdf. Accessed 09/04/2016.
4. Bae, S., and Hong, Y.C. 2015. Exposure to bisphenol A from drinking canned beverages increases blood pressure: randomized crossover trial. *Hypertension* 65(2): 313–319.
5. Lebowitz, N. 2015. Nightshades & toxicity: Are "healthy" vegetables poisoning you? http://www.drnoahlebowitz.com/2015/01/02/nightshades/. Accessed 09/04/2016.
6. Parker et al. 1992. A new enzyme-linked lectin/mucin antibody sandwich assay (CAM 17.1/WGA) assessed in combination with CA 19–9 and peanut lectin binding assay for the diagnosis of pancreatic cancer. *Cancer* 70(5): 1062–1068.

   Patel et al. 2002. Potato glycoalkaloids adversely affect intestinal permeability and aggravate inflammatory bowel disease. *Inflammatory Bowel Diseases* 8(5): 340–346.
7. Cordain, L. 2013. Are chia seeds permitted on the paleo diet? http://thepaleodiet.com/paleo-diet-special-report-chia-seeds/. Accessed 1/15/17.
8. Kannan et al. 2003. Expression of peanut agglutinin-binding mucin-type glycoprotein in human esophageal squamous cell carcinoma as a marker. *Molecular Cancer* 2: 38.
9. Wang et al. 1998. Identification of intact peanut lectin in peripheral venous blood. *Lancet* 352(9143): 1831–1832.
10. Singh et al. 2006. Peanut lectin stimulates proliferation of colon cancer cells by interaction with glycosylated CD44v6 isoforms and consequential activation of c-Met and MAPK: functional implications for disease-associated glycosylation changes. *Glycobiology* 16(7): 594–601.

    Gabius, H-J., and Gabius, S. (Eds.) 1996. *Glycosciences: Status & perspectives.* Weinheim, Germany: Wiley-VCH.
11. Centers for Disease Control and Prevention. 1983. Dermatitis associated with cashew nut consumption—Pennsylvania. http://www.cdc.gov/mmwr/preview/mmwrhtml/00001269.htm. Accessed 09/04/2016.
12. Goodman, R. 2012. Ask a farmer: Does feeding corn harm cattle? https://agricultureproud.com/2012/09/27/ask-a-farmer-does-feeding-corn-harm-cattle/. Accessed 09/04/2016.
13. Rizzello et al. 2007. Highly efficient gluten degradation by lactobacilli and fungal

proteases during food processing: New perspectives for celiac disease. *Applied and Environmental Microbiology* 73(14): 4499–4507.

14. Cuadrado et al. 2002. Effect of natural fermentation on the lectin of lentils measured by immunological methods. *Food and Agricultural Immunology* 14(1): 41–44.

15. Fontes, M. 2010. Are sprouted legumes paleo? http://thepaleodiet.com/paleo-diet-q-a-sprouted-legumes/#.VmNKHF876nM. Accessed 09/04/2016.

16. Buchmann et al. 2007. Dihydroxy-7-methoxy-1,4-benzoxazin-3-one (DIMBOA) and 2,4-dihydroxy-1,4-benzoxazin-3-one (DIBOA), two naturally occurring benzoxazinones contained in sprouts of Gramineae are potent aneugens in human-derived liver cells (HepG2). *Cancer Letters* 246(1–2): 290–299.

17. You, W., and Henneberg, M. 2016. Meat consumption providing a surplus energy in modern diet contributes to obesity prevalence: an ecological analysis. *BMC Nutrition* 2: 22.

     You, W., and Henneberg, M. 2016. Meat in modern diet, just as bad as sugar, correlates with worldwide obesity: an ecological analysis. *Journal of Nutrition & Food Sciences* 6: 517.

18. Fonteles et al. 2016. Rosemarinic acid prevents against memory deficits in ischemic mice. *Behavioural Brain Research* 297: 91–103.

19. Kim et al. 2016. Effects of linolenic acid supplementation in perilla oil on collagen-epinephrine closure time, activated partial thromboplastin time and Lp-PLA2 activity in non-diabetic and hypercholesterolaemic subjects. *Journal of Functional Foods* 23: 95–104.

20. de Lorgeril, M., and Salen, P. 2005. Dietary prevention of coronary heart disease: The Lyon diet heart study and after. *World Review of Nutrition and Dietetics* 95: 103–114.

21. Fahs et al. 2010. The effect of acute fish-oil supplementation on endothelial function and arterial stiffness following a high-fat meal. *Applied Physiology, Nutrition, and Metabolism* 35(3): 294–302.

22. Joelving, F. 2009. Lard lesson: Why fat lubricates your appetite. https://www.scientificamerican.com/article/lard-lesson-why-fat-lubri/#. Accessed 12/11/2016.

     University of Michigan Health System. 2016. High-fiber diet keeps gut microbes from eating the colon's lining, protects against infection, animal study shows. https://www.sciencedaily.com/releases/2016/11/161117134626.htm. Accessed 12/11/2016.

23. Viggiano et al. 2016. Effects of an high-fat diet enriched in lard or in fish oil on the hypothalamic amp-activated protein kinase and inflammatory mediators. *Frontiers in Cellular Neuroscience* 10: 150.

24. Bao et al. 2013. Association of nut consumption with total and cause-specific mortality. *The New England Journal of Medicine* 369: 2001–2011.

     Aune et al. 2016. Nut consumption and risk of cardiovascular disease, total cancer, all-cause and cause-specific mortality: a systematic review and dose-response meta-analysis of prospective studies. *BMC Medicine* 14(1): 207.

25. Chen et al. 2016. Resveratrol attenuates trimethylamine-N-oxide (TMAO)-induced atherosclerosis by regulating TMAO synthesis and bile acid metabolism via remodeling of the gut microbiota. *mBio* 7(2): e02210-e02215.

26. Pottala et al. 2014. Higher RBC EPA + DHA corresponds with larger total brain and hippocampal volumes: WHIMS-MRI study. *Neurology* 82(5): 435–442.

27. Hanley, D.A., and Davison, K.S. 2005. Vitamin D insufficiency in North America. *The Journal of Nutrition* 135(2): 332–337. 26.

    Cantorna et al. 2014. Vitamin D, immune regulation, the microbiota, and inflammatory bowel disease. *Experimental Biology & Medicine* 239(11): 1524–1530. 27.

Chapter 9: Phase 3

1. Nichols, H. 2016. Worldwide obesity: Meat protein has as much effect as sugar. http://www.medicalnewstoday.com/articles/312080.php. Accessed 09/06/2016.

    You, W., and Henneberg, M. 2016. Meat consumption providing a surplus energy in modern diet contributes to obesity prevalence: an ecological analysis. *BMC Nutrition* 2: 22.

    You, W., and Henneberg, M. 2016. Meat in modern diet, just as bad as sugar, correlates with worldwide obesity: an ecological analysis. *Journal of Nutrition & Food Sciences* 6: 517.

    Vernaud et al. 2010. Meat consumption and prospective weight change in participants of the EPIC-PANACEA study. *The American Journal of Clinical Nutrition* 92(2): 398-407.

2. Pan et al. 2012. Red meat consumption and mortality: Results from 2 prospective cohort studies. *Archives of Internal Medicine* 172(7): 555–563.

3. Zamora-Ros et. al. "Mediterranean Diet and Non Enzymatic Antioxidant Capacity in the PREDIMED Study." *National Center for Biotechnology Information*. U.S. National Library of Medicine, 2013. Web. 16 Feb. 2017.

4. Martínez-González et al. 2011. "Mediterranean diet and the incidence of cardiovascular disease: a Spanish cohort." *Nutrition, Metabolism, and Cardiovascular Diseases* 21(4): 237–244.

    Martínez-González et al. 2011. "Low consumption of fruit and vegetables and risk of chronic disease." *Public Health Nutrition* 14(12A): 2309-15.

5. Schünke et al. 1985. Lectin-binding in normal and fibrillated articular cartilage of human patellae. *Virchows Archiv A Pathological Anatomy and Histopathology* 407(2): 221–31.

6. National Institute on Aging. 2012. NIH study finds calorie restriction does not affect survival. https://www.nia.nih.gov/newsroom/2012/08/nih-study-finds-calorie-restriction-does-not-affect-survival. Accessed 09/06/2016.

7. Colman et al. 2014. Caloric restriction reduces age-related and all-cause mortality in rhesus monkeys. *Nature Communications* 5: 3557.

8. Fontana et al. 2008. Long-term effects of calorie or protein restriction on serum IGF-1 and IGFBP-3 concentration in humans. *Aging Cell* 7(5): 681–687.
9. Vitale et al. 2012. Low circulating IGF-I bioactivity is associated with human longevity: findings in centenarians' offspring. *Aging* 4(9): 580–589.
10. Conn, C.S., and Qian, S.B. 2011. mTOR signaling in protein homeostasis: less is more? *Cell Cycle* 10(12): 1940–1947.
11. Orlich et al. 2013. Vegetarian dietary patterns and mortality in Adventist health study 2. *JAMA International Medicine* 173(13): 1230–1238.
12. Grant, W.B. 2016. Using multicountry ecological and observational studies to determine dietary risk factors for Alzheimer's disease. *Journal of the American College of Nutrition* 35(5): 476–489.
13. Drenick et al. 1972. Resistance to symptomatic insulin reactions after fasting. *The Journal of Clinical Investigation* 51(10): 2757–2762.
14. Owen, O.E. 2005. Ketone bodies as fuel for the brain during starvation. *Biochemistry and Molecular Biology Education* 33(4): 246–251.

    Cahill, G.F., Jr. 2006. Fuel metabolism in starvation. *Annual Review of Nutrition* 26: 1–22.
15. McClure et al. 2007. Abstract 3642: Fasting, a novel indicator of religiosity, may reduce the risk of coronary artery disease. *Circulation* 116: II_826–II_827.
16. Choi et al. A diet mimicking fasting promotes regeneration and reduces autoimmunity and Multiple Sclerosis symptoms. *Cell Reports* 5(10): 2136–2146.
17. Bhammar et al. 2012. Effects of fractionized and continuous exercise on 24-h ambulatory blood pressure. *Medicine and Science in Sports and Exercise* 44(12): 2270–2276.
18. Obesity Society. 2016. Eating dinner early, or skipping it, may be effective in fighting body fat. https://www.sciencedaily.com/releases/2016/11/161103091229.htm. Accessed 12/01/2016.

Chapter 10: The Keto Plant Paradox Intensive Care Program

1. Nichols, H. 2016. Worldwide obesity: Meat protein has as much effect as sugar. http://www.medicalnewstoday.com/articles/312080.php. Accessed 09/06/2016.

    You, W., and Henneberg, M. 2016. Meat consumption providing a surplus energy in modern diet contributes to obesity prevalence: an ecological analysis. *BMC Nutrition* 2: 22.

    You, W., and Henneberg, M. 2016. Meat in modern diet, just as bad as sugar, correlates with worldwide obesity: an ecological analysis. *Journal of Nutrition & Food Sciences* 6: 517.
2. Vander Heiden et al. 2009. Understanding the Warburg effect: the metabolic requirements of cell proliferation. *Science* 324(5930): 1029–1033.
3. Fox, M. 2010. Cancer cells slurp up fructose, US study finds. http://mobile.reuters.com/article/idAFN0210830520100802?irpc=932. Accessed 09/06/2016.
4. Maalouf et al. 2009. The neuroprotective properties of calorie restriction, the ketogenic diet, and ketone bodies. *Brain Research Reviews* 59(2): 293–315.

5. Drenick et al. 1972. Resistance to symptomatic insulin reactions after fasting. *Journal of Clinical Investigation* 51(10): 2757–2762.

6. Gersch et al. 2007. Fructose, but not dextrose, accelerates the progression of chronic kidney disease. *American Journal of Physiology. Renal Physiology* 293(4): F1256-F1261.

7. Johnson et al. 2010. The effect of fructose on renal biology and disease. *Journal of the American Society of Nephrology* 21(12): 2036–2039.

8. Ananieva, E. 2015. Targeting amino acid metabolism in cancer growth and anti-tumor response. *World Journal of Biological Chemistry* 6(4): 281-289.

9. Mercola, J. 2014. Seven benefits of walnuts. http://articles.mercola.com/sites/arti cles/archive/2014/05/19/7-walnuts-benefits.aspx. Accessed 1/15/2017.

Chapter 11: Plant Paradox Supplement Recommendations

1. American Heart Association. 2013. A diet low in grains, beans and certain vegetables—combined with "anti-aging" supplements—improved blood vessel function, in a new study. https://www.sciencedaily.com/releases/2013/05/13050 1193127.htm. Accessed 09/08/2016.

2. United States Government. 1936. Senate document #264. http://www.betterhealth thruresearch.com/document264.htm. Accessed 09/08/2016.

3. Thomas, D. 2003. A study on the mineral depletion of the foods available to us as a nation over the period 1940 to 1991. *Nutrition and Health* 17(2): 85–115.

4. Cantorna et al. 2014. Vitamin D, immune regulation, the microbiota, and inflammatory bowel disease. *Experimental Biology & Medicine* 239(11): 1524–1530.

5. Stenblom et al. 2015. Consumption of thylakoid-rich spinach extract reduces hunger, increases satiety and reduces cravings for palatable food in overweight women. *Appetite* 91: 209–219.

6. Pottala et al. 2014. Higher RBC EPA + DHA corresponds with larger total brain and hippocampal volumes: WHIMS-MRI study. *Neurology* 82(5): 435–442.

Index

About the Author

Steven R. Gundry, MD, is a cum laude graduate of Yale University, with special honors in human biological and social evolution. After graduating Alpha Omega Alpha from the Medical College of Georgia, Dr. Gundry completed residencies in general surgery and cardiothoracic surgery at the University of Michigan and served as a clinical associate at the National Institutes of Health. He invented devices that reverse the cell death seen in heart attacks; variations of these devices became the Medtronic Gundry Retrograde Cardioplegia Cannula, the most widely used device of its kind worldwide to protect the heart during open-heart surgery. After completing a fellowship in congenital heart surgery at the Hospital for Sick Children, Great Ormond Street, in London, and two years as a professor at the University of Maryland School of Medicine, Dr. Gundry was recruited as professor and chairman of cardiothoracic surgery at Loma Linda University School of Medicine.

During his tenure at Loma Linda, Dr. Gundry pioneered the field of xenotransplantation, the study of how the immune system and blood vessel proteins of one species react to the transplanted heart of a foreign species. He was one of the original twenty investigators of the first FDA-approved implantable left ventricular assist device. Dr. Gundry is the inventor of the Gundry Ministernotomy, the most widely used minimally invasive surgical technique to operate on the aortic valve; the Gundry Lateral Tunnel, a living tissue that can rebuild parts of the heart in children with severe congenital heart malformations; and the Skoosh

Venous Cannula, the most widely used cannula in minimally invasive heart operations.

As a consultant to Computer Motion (now Intuitive Surgical), Dr. Gundry was one of the fathers of robotic heart surgery. He received early FDA approval for robotic-assisted minimally invasive surgery for coronary artery bypass and mitral valve operations. He holds patents on connecting blood vessels and coronary artery bypasses without the need for sutures, as well as on repairing the mitral valve without the need for sutures and the heart-lung machine.

Dr. Gundry has served on the Board of Directors of the American Society of Artificial Internal Organs and was a founding board member and treasurer of the International Society of Minimally Invasive Cardiothoracic Surgery. He also served two successive terms as president of the Board of Directors of the American Heart Association, Desert Division. Dr. Gundry has been elected a Fellow of the American College of Surgeons, the American College of Cardiology, the American Surgical Association, the American Academy of Pediatrics, and the College of Chest Physicians. He has served numerous times as an abstract reviewer for the American Heart Association annual meetings. The author of more than three hundred articles, chapters, and abstracts in peer-reviewed journals on surgical, immunologic, genetic, nutritional, and lipid investigations, he has also operated in more than thirty countries, including on multiple charitable missions.

In 2000, inspired by the stunning reversal of coronary artery disease in an "inoperable" patient by using a combination of dietary changes and nutriceutical supplements, Dr. Gundry changed the arc of his career. An obese chronic diet failure himself, he adapted his Yale University thesis to design a diet based on evolutionary coding and the interaction of our ancestral microbiome, genes, and environment. Following this program enabled him to reverse his own numerous medical problems. In the process, he effortlessly lost seventy pounds and has kept them off for seventeen years. These discoveries led him to establish the International Heart and Lung Institute—and, as part of it, the Center for Restorative Medicine—in Palm Springs and Santa Barbara,